Pharmacological Screening Methods and Toxicology

Pharmacological Screening Methods and Toxicology

Dr. Avanapu Srinivasa Rao
M.Pharm., Ph.D., F.I.C.
Professor of Pharmacology
Principal, Bhaskar Pharmacy College, Hyderabad.

Namburi Bhagya Lakshmi
M. Pharm.
Assistant Professor, Bhaskar Pharmacy College, Hyderabad.

PharmaMed Press
An imprint of Pharma Book Syndicate
A unit of BSP Books Pvt. Ltd.
4-4-309/316, Giriraj Lane,
Sultan Bazar, Hyderabad - 500 095.

Published by

PharmaMed Press

An imprint of Pharma Book Syndicate

A unit of BSP Books Pvt. Ltd.

4-4-309/316, Giriraj Lane, Sultan Bazar, Hyderabad - 500 095.

Phone: 040-23445605, 23445688; Fax: 91+40-23445611

E-mail: info@pharmamedpress.com

ISBN: 978-93-85433-81-8 (HB)

Dedication

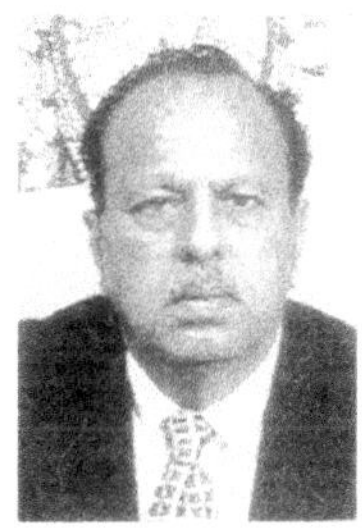

We feel extremely proud to dedicate this book to Sri. Joginpally Bhaskar Rao, B.Com, LLB, Chairman, J.B. Group of Educational Institutions, Hyderabad. His vision and dedication towards the improvement of professional and higher educational in Andhra Pradesh has always matured our thoughts and supported our career and motivated us in professional development. His confidence in us has been the best encouragement in finishing this task of writing the book on Pharmacological Screening Methods and Toxicology.

Man has so many questions
It may be frustration
It may be anguish
It may be sadness, sometimes it may be meaninglessness
The problems may be many but the answer is "Medication".

Preface

The purpose of this present book is to provide fundamental knowledge of practical aspects of subject ranging from screening methods of different drugs by using several laboratory animals and for practical implications of various important recent advances. In new drug development process to perform preclinical evaluation (animal screening methods) is very essential to estimate pharmacokinetic and pharmacodynamic parameters.

Topics covered in this book have been carefully selected based on most of useful aspects which are placed main role in preclinical evaluation of newly discovered drugs and the topics are not covered in any other text books. We are hopeful for all the postgraduates related to pharmacology, trainees and research workers during their day to day activities including allied health disciplines and scientists in industrial drug discovery set-up.

Several simple and newer experimental models have been incorporated which will help the students to engage in drug discovery in future, especially in preclinical studies. In new drug discovery process, preclinical studies are very important step while a drug is invented. Prior to administration to human being it should be administered to any animal which has similar type of organ systems as like humans with respect to pharmacokinetics (absorption, distribution, metabolism, excretion) and pharmacodynamics (therapeutic effects and adverse drug reactions) and for dose estimation.

Experience with students of various streams of Pharmacy, Medical and other health sciences strengthened our opinion that too little attention is paid to the details that are necessary for screening of various new drug molecules. Hence, we decided that there is a genuine need for a different kind of text book which would highlight certain key areas. In writing this book our intention is to help the candidate by providing basic and accurate knowledge of *Pharmacological Screening Methods and Toxicology*, so that the understanding of the subject gets stronger.

-Authors

Contents

Preface .... (vii)
Abbrevations .... (xv)

CHAPTER 1

DRUG DISCOVERY

1.1 Introduction 1
1.2 Drug Discovery Process 2
1.2.1 Steps in Drug Discoveries 3
1.2.2 Lead 5
1.2.3 Synthesis of Lead Compound 8
1.2.4 Preclinical Development 9
1.2.5 FDA Requirements for Preclinical Studies 10
1.2.6 Protocol Design 13
1.2.7 Clinical Development 14
1.2.8 Ethics in Preclinical Research 15
1.3 High Throughput Screening 16
1.3.1 *In vitro* Matrix-Ligand Interactions Studies 18
1.3.2 HTS Binding Assay 19
1.4 Pharmacogenomics, Proteomics and Array Technology 20
1.4.1 Pharmacogenomics 20
1.4.2 Proteomics 28
1.4.3 Array Technology 32

CHAPTER 2

LABORATORY ANIMALS

2.1 Laboratory Animals Care 33
2.2 Experimental Animals 36
2.3 Collection of Blood from Laboratory Animals 42

2.4 Laboratory Animals 57
2.4.1 Breeding Techniques..........57
2.4.2 GLP (Good Laboratory Practices) 61
2.5 Transgenic Animals 62
2.6 Knockout Animals 67

CHAPTER 3

ALTERNATIVE TO ANIMALS

3.1 Introduction..........73
3.1.1 *In vitro* Methods..........75
3.1.2 *In silico* Methods..........75
3.1.3 Cell Line Techniques 75
3.1.4 Patch Clamp Technique 75
3.1.5 Computer Aid Drug Designing 76
3.2 Cell Line Techniques 77
3.2.1 Types of Cells used in Cell Line 77
3.2.2 Characteristics of Cell Culture 77
3.2.3 Requirements 78
3.2.4 Equipments Required..........78
3.2.5 Culture Vessels 78
3.2.6 Materials used for Culture Vessels 78
3.2.7 Types of Culture Vessels 78
3.2.8 Culture Media used in Cell Line Technique 78
3.2.9 Physicochemical Properties of Culture Media..........80
3.2.10 Types of Cell Culture..........80
3.2.11 Source of Explants Tissue..........83
3.2.12 Sub Culturing..........85
3.2.13 Applications of Cell Line Techniques..........85
3.2.14 List of some Vaccines Prepared by Cell Culture are 85
3.3 Patch Clamp Technique 86
3.3.1 Variations in Patch Clamp Techniques 87
3.3.2 Patch–Clamp Technique in Kidney Cells 88
3.3.3 Applications of Patch Clamp Technique..........89

3.4 *In vitro* Models.....90
3.4.1 Advantages of *In vitro* Studies.....90
3.4.2 Disadvantages of *In vitro* Studies.....90
3.4.3 *In vitro* Models are 3 Types that include.....91
3.4.4 Some of the Alternatives to Animal Tests are as Follows.....93
3.5 Molecular Biology Techniques.....95

CHAPTER 4

BIOASSAY

4.1 Introduction.....101
4.1.1 Bioassay of Vasopressin.....106
4.1.2 Bioassay of Oxytocin.....109
4.1.3 Bioassay of Insulin.....112
4.1.4 Bioassay of D-Tubocurarine.....115
4.1.5 Bioassay of Acetylcholine.....117
4.1.6 Bioassay of Adrenaline.....120
4.1.7 Bioassay of Autacoids.....123
4.1.8 Bioassay of Corticotrophin.....124
4.1.9 Bioassay of Pertussis Vaccine.....126
4.1.10 Bioassay of Plague Vaccine.....127
4.1.11 Bioassay of Rabies Vaccine.....128
4.1.12 Bioassay of Hyaluronidase.....130
4.1.13 Bioassay of Tetanus Antitoxin.....132
4.1.14 Bioassay of Diphtheria Vaccine (ADSORBED).....133
4.1.15 Bioassay of Digitalis.....135
4.1.16 Bioassay of HCG.....137

CHAPTER 5

SCREENING METHODS

5.1 Introduction.....139
5.2 Screening Methods for Drugs Acting on CNS.....143
5.2.1 Screening Methods for Sedatives.....143

5.2.2 Screening Methods for Hypnotics....................................146
5.2.3 Screening Methods for Anti Epileptic Activity..................148
5.2.4 Screening Methods for Anxiolytic Activity........................156
5.2.5 Screening Methods for Neuroleptics and Anti Psychotic Activity..160
5.2.6 Screening Methods for Anti Depressants...........................164
5.2.7 Screening Methods for Anti Parkinsonism Activity 168
5.2.8 Screening Methods for Drugs Influencing Learning and Memory (NOOTROPICS)............................172
5.2.9 Screening Methods for CNS Stimulants 176

5.3 Screening Methods of Drugs Acting on Autonomic Nervous System 181
5.3.1 Screening Methods for Sympathomimetics 181
5.3.2 Screening Methods for Parasympathomimetics..................186
5.3.3 Screening Methods of Local Anaesthetic Activity 189
5.3.4 Screening Methods for Muscle Relaxants...........................193

5.4 Screening of Drugs Acting on Cardiovascular System....................196
5.4.1 Screening Methods for Anti Hypertensive Agents 196
5.4.2 Screening Methods of Anti Arrhythmic Activity................201
5.4.3 Screening Methods for Cardiac Stimulants.........................207
5.4.4 Screening Methods for Atherosclerosis 213

5.5 Screening for Drug Acting on Respiratory System..........................218
5.5.1 Screening Methods for Anti Asthmatics and Bronchodilators 218
5.5.2 Screening Methods for Antitussives and Expectorants..223

5.6 Screening Methods for Analgesics, Atipyretics and Anti Inflammatory Agents 225
5.6.1 Screening Methods for Analgesics and Antipyretics 225
5.6.2 Screening Methods for Inflammatory Drugs 229

5.7 Screening Methods for Drugs Acting on Urinary System 234
5.7.1 Diuretic Activity 234
5.7.2 Anti Urolithiatic Activity 237
5.8 Screening Methods of Drugs Acting on Gastro Intestinal System 239
5.8.1 Screening Methods for Antiulcer Agents 239
5.9 Screening Methods for Drugs Acting on Liver 244
5.10 Screening Methods for Diabetic Drugs 246
5.11 Screening Methods for Antifertility Drugs 250
5.12 Screening Methods of Drugs for Malaria 256
5.13 Screening Methods of Drugs Acting on Eye 258
5.14 Screening Methods of Anti Stressor and Anti Oxidant Activity 262

CHAPTER 6

TOXICOLOGY

6.1 Principles of Toxicology 265
6.2 Mutagenesis 269
6.3 Multistage Carcinogenesis 270
6.4 Teratogenicity 273
6.4.1 Predictable Toxic Drug Actions in the Fetus 273
6.4.2 Teratogenic Drug Actions 273
6.4.3 Defining a Teratogen 273
6.4.4 Teratogenic Mechanisms 275
6.4.5 Counseling of Women about Teratogenic Risk 275
6.5 Acute, Sub Acute, Chronic Toxicity Studies 277
6.5.1 Acute Toxicology Testing 277
6.5.2 Sub-Acute/Sub-Chronic Studies 280
6.5.3 Chronic Toxicity Tests 283

CHAPTER 7

POISONS

7.1 Classification of Poisonous Substances 287

7.2 Common Poisoning Agents 290

7.3 Principles of Management of Acute Poisoning,
Treatment of Poisoning 296

7.4 General Treatment of Poisoning 300

7.5 Special Treatment of Poisoning 304

Index 311

Abbreviations

1K1C	-	One Kidney One Clip Method
2-DE	-	2 Dimensional Proteins Electrophoresis
2D-PAGE	-	Two Dimensional Polyacrylamide Gel Electrophoresis
2K2C	-	Two Kidney Two Clip Method
A.A	-	Arachidonic Acid
AA	-	Amino Acid
ACE inhibitors	-	Angiotensine Converting Enzyme Inhibitors
ACH	-	Acetyl Choline
ACLAM	-	American College of Laboratory Animal Medicine
ACP	-	Acid phosphate
ADME	-	Absorption, Distribution, Metabolism, Excretion
ALB	-	Albumin
ALP	-	Alkaline Phosphatase
Anorexia	-	Loss of Appetite
ANOVA	-	Analysis of Variance
AV Node	-	Atrio Ventricular Node
AWRs	-	Animal Welfare and Regulations
BAC	-	British Anti – Lewisite (Dimercaprol)
BBB	-	Blood Brain Barrier
Be	-	Beryllium
BHR	-	Borderline Hypertensive Rats
BSA	-	Bovine Serum Albumin
BSS	-	Balanced Salt Solution
CAAT	-	Center for Alternatives to Animal Testing
Cachexia	-	Loss of body Weight
CAD	-	Coronary Artery Diseases
Cd	-	Cadmium
CBZ	-	Carbomarzepien
CCK_2	-	Cholecystokinin receptor
CCl_4	-	Carbon Tetra Chloride
CDER	-	Center for Drug Evaluation and Research

CHF	-	Congestive Heart Failure
CK	-	Creatinine Kinase
CMC	-	Carboxy Methyl Cellulose
CNS	-	Central Nervous System
CO	-	Carbon Monoxide
COX	-	Cyclo Oxygenase
CPCSEA	-	Committee for the Purpose of Control and Supervision for Experiments on Animals
CS	-	Calf Serum
CTs	-	Computed Tomography Scan
CVS	-	Cardiovascular System
CyP_{450}	-	Cytochrome P_{450}
d NTPs	-	Deoxy Nucleotide Triphosphate
DCC	-	Dextran Coated Charcoal
DEM	-	Dulbecco's Enriched Modification
DHHS	-	Department of Health and Human Services
DHR	-	Drug Hypersensitivity Reactions
DIGE	-	Difference Gel Electrophoresis
DKO	-	Double Knock Out
DM and PK	-	Drug Metabolism and Pharmacokinetics
DMSO	-	Dimethyl Sulphoxide
DNA	-	Deoxyribo Neucleic Acid
DOCA	-	Deoxy Corticosterone Acetate
DPPH	-	2, 2-diphenyl-1-picryl Hydroxyl Radical
DSBs	-	Double Standard Breaks
DTNB	-	5,5-Dithiobis-(2-Nitrobenzoic Acid)
ECG	-	Electro Cardio Graph
ED_{50}	-	Effective Dose
EDTA	-	Ethylene Diamine Tetra Acetic acid
EEG	-	Electro Encephalo Graph
ELISA	-	Enzyme Linked Immunosorbent assay
EMEM	-	Egle's Minimal Essential Medium
EMF	-	Electro Magnetic Fields
ES Cells	-	Embryonic Stem Cells
EST	-	Embryonic Stem cell Test

FA	-	Fluorescence Anisotropy
FB	-	Fetal Bovine
FDA	-	Food and Drug Administration
FEV	-	Forced Expirators Volume
FIA	-	Fluorescence Intensity Assay
FMLP	-	Peptide N-formyl-methionyl-leucyl-phenylalanine
FSH	-	Follicule Stimulating Hormone
GCC	-	Ganglion Cells Complex
GIT	-	Gastro Intestinal System
GLP	-	Good Laboratory Practice
GMEM	-	Glargow's Modification of Eagle's Medium
GMO	-	Genetically Modified Organism
GRF	-	Glomerular Filtration Rate
GSH	-	Glutathione
HCG	-	Human Chorionic Gonadotropin
HETP	-	Hexaethyl Tetraphosphate
HMG-CoA	-	Hydroxy Methyl Glutaryl Coenzyme A
HR	-	Homologous Recombination
HTS	-	High Throughput Screening
IAEC	-	Institutional Animal Ethics Committee
IC_{50}	-	Inhibition Concentration
ICAT	-	Isotope Coded Affinity Tag
IDDM	-	Insulin Dependent Diabetes Mellitus
IgG	-	Immuno globulin G
IL	-	Inter Lenkines
INDA	-	Investigational New Drug Application
IOP	-	Intra Ocular Pressure
IPG	-	Immobilized pH Gradient
ISO	-	International Organization for Standardization
IUPAC	-	International Union for Pure and Applied Chemistry
L.A	-	Local Anesthetics
LAL test	-	Limulus Amebocyte Lysate Test
LD_{50}	-	Lethal Dose
LDL	-	Low Density Lipoprotein

LH	-	Luteinizing Hormone
LLNA	-	Local Lymphnode Assay
LPS	-	Lipo polysaccharide
LVEDP	-	Left Ventricular End Diastolic Pressure
M.I	-	Miocardial Infraction
MAO	-	Mono Amino Oxidase
MAT test	-	Monocyte Activation Test
mCPP	-	Metabolite (1-(3-Chlorphenyl) piperazine)
MIC	-	Minimum Inhibitory Concentration
MP	-	Multiplexed Proteomics
MRI	-	Magnetic Resonance Imaging
MS	-	Mass Spectrometer
MTT	-	3-(4,5-Dimethylthiazol-2-yl)-2,5-Di phenyl tetrazolium Bromide
NDA	-	New Drug Application
NDD	-	New Drug Discovery
NIDDM	-	Non Insulin Dependent Diabetes Mellitus
NIH	-	National Institutes of Health
NK Cells	-	Natural Killer Cells
NMR	-	Nuclear Magnatic Resonance
NNK	-	Nicotine Derived Nitrosaminoketone
NNN	-	N-Nitrosonoricotine
NRU	-	Neutral Red Uptake
O_3	-	Ozone
OECD	-	Organization of Economic Cooperation and Development
OHT	-	Ocular Hypertension
OLAW	-	Office of Laboratory Animal Welfare
OMPA	-	Octamethyl Pyrophosphoramide
PAM	-	Pyridine Aldoxime Methyl Chloride
PAS	-	Para Amino Salicylic acid
PCBs	-	Poly Chlorinated Biphenyls
PCR	-	Polymerase Chain Reaction
PDGF	-	Platelet Derived Growth Factor
PG	-	Prostaglandines

P_{gp}	-	P-glycoprotein
PHS Policy	-	Public Health Service Policy
PK and PD	-	Pharmacokinetics, Pharmacodynamics
PMNs	-	Poly Morpho Nuclear Cells
PRA	-	Plasma Renin Activity
QKO	-	Quadrapole Knock Out
QSAR	-	Quantitative Structure Activity Relationship
RAAS	-	Renin Angiotensin Aldosteron System
RBC	-	Red Blood Cells
RGCs	-	Retinal Ganglion Cells
RIA	-	Radio Immune Assay
RPMI	-	Roswell Park Memorial Institute
RSA	-	Radical Scavenging Activity
SA Node	-	Sino Atrial node or Sino Auricular Node
SD-OCT	-	Spectral Domain Optical Coherence Tomography
SDS	-	Second Dimension Seperation
SDS-PAGE	-	Second Dimension Seperation- Polyacrylamide Gel Electrophoresis
SEM	-	Scanning Electron Microscopy
SGOT	-	Serum Glutamate Oxaloacetate Transaminase
SGPT	-	Serum Glutamate Pyruvate Transaminase
SHE assay	-	Syrian Hamster Embryo
SHR	-	Spontaneous Hypertensive Rats
SNC	-	Substantia Nigra Compacta (A_9)
SNP	-	Single Nucleotide Polymorphism
SO_2	-	Sulphur Dioxide
SOPs	-	Standard Operating Procedures
SPA	-	Scintillation Proximity Assay
STZ	-	Streptozotocin
$t_{1/2}$	-	Half Life
TBARs	-	Thiobarbituric Acid Reactive substance
TCDD	-	2,3,7,8-Tetra Chlorodibenzo Digoxin and Phenobarbital
TDDR	-	Traditional Drug Discovery Research
TEPP	-	Tetra Ethyl Pyrophosphate
TGF	-	Tissue Growth Factor

TKO	-	Triple Knock Out
TMPD	-	N, N, N_1 N_1 Tetramethyl-P-Phenylenediamine Dichloride
TNF	-	α Tumour Necrosis Factor
TOF-Ms	-	Time of Flight Mass Spectrophotometer
TP	-	Total Proteins
TPA	-	Tetradecanoyl Phorbol Acetate
TPMT	-	Thiopurine Methyl Transferase
uHTS	-	Ultra High Throughput Screening
UV light	-	Ultra Violet Light
VKOR	-	Vitamin K Epoxide Reductase
VTA	-	Ventral Tegmental Area (A_{10})
WBC	-	White Blood Cells
WFR	-	Wistar Fatty Rats
WHO	-	World Health Organisation
WST Assay	-	Writing Skill Test

CHAPTER 1

DRUG DISCOVERY

1.1 INTRODUCTION

The drug discovery is very important process. At the time of invention of new molecule there is necessity of related fields like medicine, biotechnology, chemistry, pharmacology.

In previous histories of drug discovery, more drugs were discovered by serendipity or in process of identification of active constant in traditional plants or medicinal plants. Later according to classical pharmacology, substance which has desirable therapeutic effect is identified. Chemical libraries of synthesis small molecules, natural products and extracts were screened.

Later in reverse pharmacology, sequencing of human genomes which allowed rapid cloning and synthesis of large quantities of purified proteins are identified. High throughput screening is very useful method for this process to screening of large amount of compounds. These methods are very useful against isolated biological targets which are hypothesized to disease modifying process. In recent identifications also so many newer inventions are able to known about biological molecules at the atomic level.

Modern drug discovery involves the identification of screening hits, optimization techniques to increase affinity, bioavailability and also to increase half life of drugs to decreasing of dose at the same techniques for reduction of side effects.

Prior to clinical trails only the compound should fulfill all requirements, and then only it will begin the process of drugs developments.

Computer aid drug design is a very important process. It is a very useful thing in new drug discovery. After understanding of all these biological systems and advances in technologies only then it is possible to a new drug discovery. But this new drug discovery is still a lengthy, expensive and also inefficient process.

1.2 DRUG DISCOVERY PROCESS

Drug design also sometimes referred to as rational drugs design, is the inventive process of finding new medications based on the knowledge of biological target. In the most basic sense drug design involves design of small molecules that are complementary in shape and charge to the bimolecular target to which they interact and therefore will bind to it.

Basic considerations in drug design: The drug is most commonly an organic small molecule which activates or inhibits the function of a bimolecular such as a protein which in turn results in therapeutic benefit to the patient.

Table 1.1 Time involved in drug discovery.

Target discovery (2.5 years)

↓

Lead generation & lead optimization (3 years)

↓

Preclinical development (1 year)

↓

Phase I, II & III clinical trials (6 years)

↓

FDA review and approval (1 year)

↓

Drug to the market (14 years)

During the last 50 years the philosophy of valuable drugs discovery has evolved from one that was mostly around chemistry to one that has more biological approach to treat a disease. These changes were not only driven by strategic imperative but were enabled also by the significant changes in technology that has occurred during the past half century.

1.2.1 Steps in Drug Discoveries

The advent of molecular biology, coupled with advances in screening and synthetic chemistry technologies has allowed a combination of both knowledge around the receptor and random screening to be used for drug discovery.

Target identification

Once a thematic area has been identified, the next stage is to identify a suitable drug target. Example: Receptor, Enzyme or Nucleic acid.

Many early drugs such as the morphine just happen to interact with a molecule target in the human body. As this involves coincidence more than design, the detection of drug targets was very much a hit and miss affair.

By using **Genomics and Proteomics** many proteins were found to be drug targets and still research is going on them to find further new targets.

Target specificity and selectivity between species

- The more selective a drug is for its target, the less chance there is that it will interact with different targets and have undesirable side effects.

  Example: Penicillin targets an enzyme involved in bacterial cell wall biosynthesis.
- Target specificity & selectivity within the body: Enzyme inhibitors should inhibit only the target enzyme and not some other enzyme.
- Receptor agonists and antagonists should only show selectivity for a particular receptor (Example: An adrenergic receptor) or even a particular receptor subtype. (Example : β_2 adrenergic receptors)
- Targeting drugs to specific organs and tissues.

  Example: The adrenergic receptors in heart are predominantly β_1, where as those in the lung are β_2.
- Multi target drug:

  Example: Olanzapine binds to more receptors like Serotonin, Dopamine, Muscarine, Noradrenalin's and Histamine.
- This kind of profile would normally be unacceptable in schizophrenia, probably because it blocks both Serotonin and Dopamine receptors. Drugs which interact with a range of targets are called promiscuous ligand or dirty drugs.

Table 1.2 Steps in drug development.

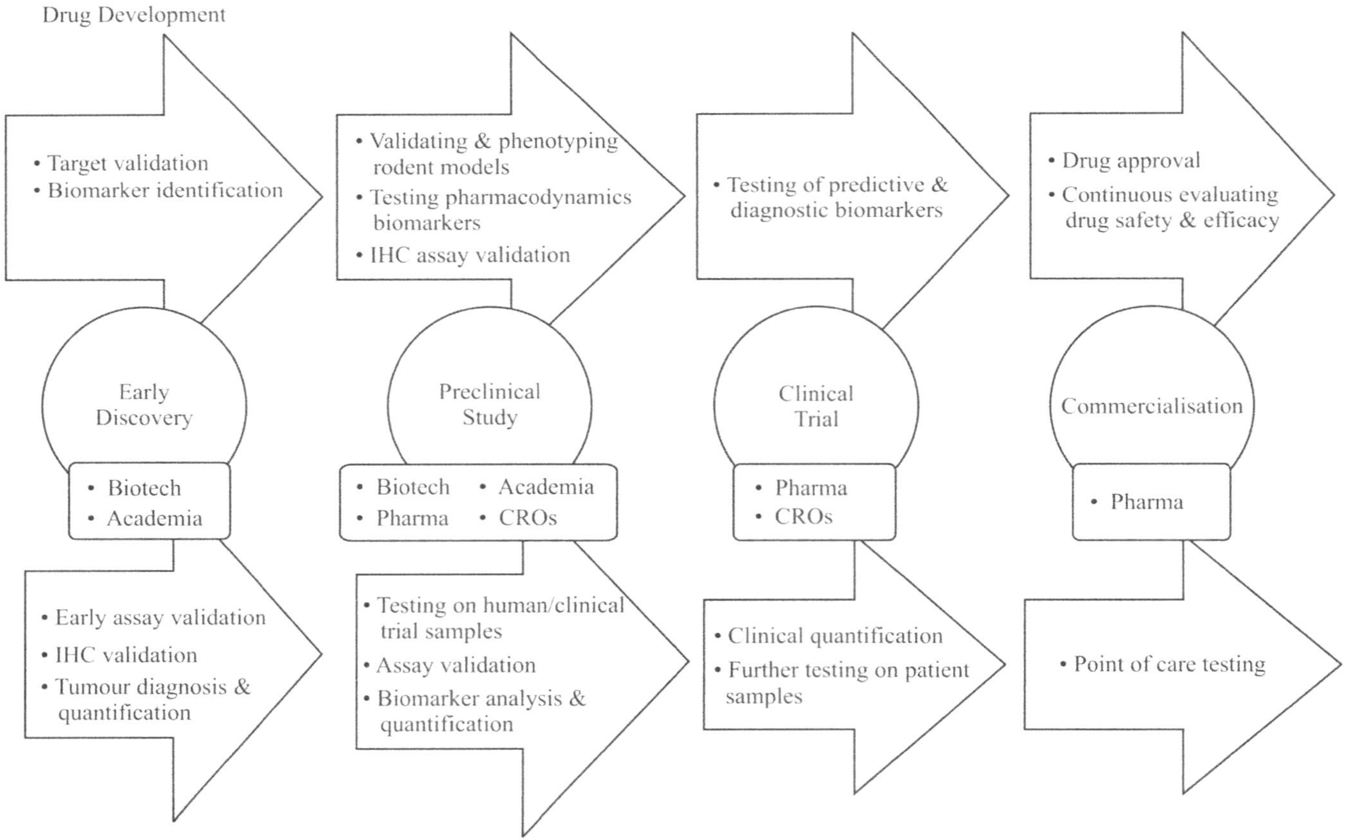

Structural properties of drug molecules: Also involves in target specificity.

Physical properties of drug molecules may be categorized

- Physicochemical properties
- Shape (Geometric, Steric, Conformation, Topological)
- Stereo chemical properties
- Electronic properties

Physico-chemical properties of drug molecules are

- Role and structure of water on drug structure
- Solubility properties of drug molecules
- Partition coefficient of drug molecule
- Surface activity effects of drug molecule.
- The clinical molecular interface: Bio availability and drug hydration etc.

1.2.2 Lead

A lead is a compound from a series of related compounds, which has some of a desired biological activity. This molecule can be characterized and modified to produce another molecule with a better profile.

The lead seeking methods: (used to selection of lead molecules)

- Lead compound identification by serendipity.
- Lead compound identification from existing drugs.
- Lead compound identification by endogenous sources.
- Lead compound identification by exogenous sources.
- Lead compound identification by rational drug design.
- Lead compound identification by combinatorial chemistry with high throughput screening.
- Lead compound identification through genomics and proteomics.
- Pharmacogenomics and the future of lead compound discovery.

(a) ***Lead compound identification by serendipity:*** Serendipity actual meaning is unexpected discovery by accident. If the scientist is working for any known action, sometimes may chances of invention of other things, for example Alexander Fleming is working for examination of systemic fluids, while doing that experiment accidentally he observed the *Penicillin notatum*. This is one of famous example of serendipity reaction. This serendipity has important role in psychotic disorders, hallocinogenation. So examples of drugs discovered by serendipity are aniline purple, penicillin, lysergic acid, diethylamide, meprobamate, chlorpramazine

(b) ***Lead compound identification from existing drugs:*** Many companies use established drugs from their competitor as lead compounds in order to design a drug disparaged, they can after implement, forms as better drug than original drug.

Example: Modern penicillin is more selective, more potent and more capable than original penicillin's.

(c) ***Lead compound identification from endogenous sources:***

- Endogenous source means natural ligand for receptors. Example: Histamine was used as original lead compound in the development of H_2 Histamine Antagonist, (Cimetidine).
- Natural substrates for enzymes. Example: Enkephalins have been used as lead comp for the design of Enkephalinase inhibitors.
- Enzyme products as lead compounds. Example: Design of carboxypeptidase inhibitor.
- Natural compounds as lead compounds, allosteric site of GABA.

(d) ***Lead compound identification from exogenous sources:***

- **Plant kingdom:** Plants have always been a rich source of lead compound. Example: Morphine, Cocaine, Digitalis, Quinine, Tubocurairne, Nicotine, Muscarine. Many of these lead compounds are useful drugs in themselves.
- Others have been the basis for synthetic drugs. Example: Local anaesthetics developed from cocaine.
- Clinically useful drugs which have recently been isolated from plants include anticancer agent paclitaxol from few trees Taxol, and the antimalarial agent Artemisinin from Chinese plant.

(e) ***Lead compound identification from Micro organism source:***

Example: Cephalosporin, Tetracycline, Amino glycosides, Rifampcin, Chloramphenicol & Vancomycin etc.

(f) ***Lead compound identification from Marine sources:*** Antitumor agents derived from marine sources include Discodermolide, Bryostatin, Dolaostatins and Cephalostatins etc.

(g) ***Lead compound identification from Animal sources:*** Antibiotics polypeptides known as the magainins were extracted from skin of the African clawed frog *Xenopus laevis* etc.

(h) ***Lead compound identification from Venoms and toxins:*** Teprotide, a peptide isolated from the venom of the Brazilian viper was a lead compound for the development of the Antihypertensive agent's Cilazapril and Captopril etc.

(i) ***Lead compound identification by combinatorial chemistry:*** Lead compound identification by combinatorial chemistry with high through put screening. A key to success in drug discovery by screening is the availability of a large and structurally diverse library of compound. .

(j) ***HTS Assays:*** HTS (High Throughput Screening) have been developed and perfected over the past 10-20 years it includes

- *Micro plate activity assay:* Assay is in solution in a well, the result of the assay, such as enzyme inhibitors is linked to some observable, such as colour change to enable identification of bio availability.
- *Gel diffusion assay:* Biological target is mixed in soft agar and spread on the surface of the film, after allowing the compound to diffusion, an appropriate developing agent is sprayed on the agar surface and areas in which bioactivity has occurred will show up as distinct zones.
- *Affinity selection assays:* Compound library is applied to a protein target receptor, all compounds that do not bind are removed, and compounds that do bind are then identified. Of these micro plate assays are probably the most widely used. Screening of combinatorial libraries in 96 or even 384 well micro plates is time & cost efficient.
- Using modern robotic techniques, it is possible to perform more than 1,00,000 bio assays per wheel in a micro plate system.

(k) ***Lead compound identification through genomics and proteomics:***

- Taking **Genomics** one step further for the purpose of drug discovery will require linking specific proteins to those specific genes which helps in treating specific diseases and in development of new drug.
- *Proteomics and lead compound discovery:* Proteomics is the molecular biology discipline that seeks to elucidate the structure and function profiles of all proteins encoded with in a specific genome.
- DNA microarray technology is a powerful technique with which to monitor the relative abundance of a specific mRNA in an individual cell and to correlate this with a specific protein.

(I) ***Bioinformatics and cheminformatics in lead compound discovery:***

- Bioinformatics and cheminformatics will apply knowledge discovery and pattern recognition algorithms to the genome wide and proteome wide experimental data, there by facilitating drug design.
- Pharmacogenomics represents a new conceptual approach to target identification and drug development. Pharmacogenomics and the future of lead compound discovery. Conventional drug design attempts to discovery drugs to treat particular diseases, Pharmacogenomics attempts to design individualized drugs to treat particular people with particular diseases. Single Nucleotide Polymorphism (SNP) is crucial to the task of individualized drug design.

1.2.3 Synthesis of Lead Compound

- Organic synthesis is preparation of complicated organic molecules from other, simplex, organic compounds. Because of the ability of carbon atoms to form chains, multiple bonds and rings an almost unimaginably large number of organic compounds can be conceived and created.
- In planning a synthetic route for the preparation of desired molecule the organic chemist devices a synthetic tree an outline of multiple available routes to get to the target molecule from a available starting materials. An organic synthesis may be either linear or convergent. A linear synthesis constructs the target molecule from a single starting material and progresses in a sequential step by step fashion.

Some lead optimization methods

- Variation of substituent.
- Extension of the structure.
- Chain extension or contraction.
- Ring expansion or contraction.
- Ring variations.
- Ring fusions.
- Isosteres and Bioisosteres.
- Simplification of structure.
- Conformational blockers.
- Drug design by NMR.
- Structure based drug design and molecular modelling.
- The elements of lack and inspiration.

1.2.4 Preclinical Development

- Pre-clinical development is a stage that explains before clinical trials (testing in humans) during which important safety and pharmacology data are collected. Most regulatory decisions on whether a new drug can be approved for marketing. Most regulatory toxicity studies request in a rodent (Example: Rats) and non rodents (Example: Dogs).
- Choice of animal species based on the similarities of its metabolism to humans or the applicability of desired pharmacological properties to humans. It is not possible or ethical to use animals in large numbers, to compensate for the same it is assumed that increasing the dose and prolonging the duration of exposure will improve both sensitivity and productivity of the tests.
- Main goals of preclinical studies are to determine a drugs Pharmacodynamics, Pharmacokinetics & toxicity through animals testing. This data allow researchers to estimate a safe starting dose of the drug for clinical trials in humans.

Types of preclinical studies

- *In vitro* studies
- *In vivo* studies
- *Ex vivo* studies

In vitro studies: *In vitro* studies are done for testing of a drug or chemicals effect on a specific isolated tissue or organ maintaining its body functions in laboratories, also called test tube experiments.

Examples: Langendroff's Heart Preparation, Ileum Preparation, Rectus Abdominal Muscle Preparation.

In vivo studies: In Latin meaning is "in the living" it indicates the use of a whole organism or animals (for an experiment) purpose of model is chosen because it is believed to be appropriate to the condition being investigated and is thought likely to respond in the same way as human to the proposed treatment for the character being investigated.

These studies used to measure

- Therapeutic potential
- Toxicity potential
- Pharmaceutical properties & metabolic pathway
- Mechanism and specification.

***In vivo* are preferable than *In vitro* because**

- Greater similarity to human studies when compared to *in vitro*.
- Drug effects modified by physiological mechanism can be calculated.

- Absorption, Distribution, Metabolism and Excretion also calculated.
- Most animal systems are similar to human systems.
- Effects of drug are studies on complete system rather than tissues and organs.
- Drugs acting on Central Nervous System, Cardio Vascular System, Gastro Intestinal System and other systems are studied.
- Results easier to interpret and extrapolate.

Some of **examples of *in vivo*** studies is

- Non invasive methods – rat tail cuff method.
- Invasive methods – BP recording in anaesthetized dog or cat.

Ex vivo studies: Experiment is performed *in vivo* and then analyzed *in vitro*.

General requirements for conducting preclinical studies

- Toxicity studies should comply with Good Laboratory Practice (GLP).
- Standard Operating Procedures (SOPs) should be followed.
- All documents belonging to each study including its approved protocol, raw data, draft report and histology slides and paraffin tissue blocks should be preserved for a minimum of 5 years after marketing of drug.
- ***Animal toxicity studies:*** Toxicity studies also preformed to assess systemic exposure achieved in animals and its relationship to dose level and the time course of toxicity studies. Some toxicity studies like
    - Systemic toxicity studies
    - Male fertility studies
    - Female reproductive & development toxicity studies
    - Teratogenicity studies
    - Prenatal studies
    - Local toxicity
    - Genotoxicity and carcinogenicity

1.2.5 FDA Requirements for Preclinical Studies

It is essential to ensure the quality and reliability of safety studies and this can be achieved by adhering to Good Laboratory Practices (GLP). The purpose of GLP is to obtain data on properties and safety of these substances with respect to human health and environment, to promote development of quality test data, such comparable data from the basis of mutual acceptance across organizations or countries, confidence in and reliability of data from different countries will prevent duplication tests, save time, energy and resources.

- For every 5000 drug compounds that enter preclinical tests in the United States, only about 5 will eventually be considered acceptable to test in humans.
- Of those final 5 drugs only how many out of 5 drugs may actually receive approval for use in patient care.
- Under FDA requirements, a sponsor must first submit data showing that the drug is reasonably safe for use in initial, small scale clinical studies.
- Depending on whether the compound has been studies or marketed previously, the sponsor may have several options for fulfilling these requirements.
- Compiling existing non clinical data from past *in vitro* laboratory or animal studies on the compound.
- Compiling data from previous clinical testing or markets of the drug in the United States or another country whose population is relevant to the US population.
- Undertaking new preclinical studies designed to provide the evidence necessary to support the safety of administering the compound to humans.
- At the pre-clinical stage, the FDA will generally ask, at a minimum that sponsors.
- Develop a pharmacological profile of the drug.
- Determine the acute toxicity of the drug at least 2 species of animals.
- Conduct short term toxicity studies ranging from 2 weeks to 3 months depending of the proposed duration of use of the substance in the proposed clinical studies.
- Organization of Economic Cooperation & Development (OECD) framed guidelines known as Good Laboratory Practices (GLP).
- GLP gives guidelines for animal test facilities, housing the animals, responsibilities & duties of personnel conducting the animal studies, equipment, quality control etc.
- In India, the Committee for the Purpose of Control and Supervision for Experiments on Animals (CPCSEA) ensures that the animal facilities are well maintained and experiments are conducted as per internationally accepted norms.
- An Institutional Animal Ethical Committee (IAEC) must be established by an institution (or group of organization) which has an approved code of ethical conduct.
- Final report shall be prepared for each non clinical/pre clinical laboratory study and shall include:

- Names and address of facility performing the study and the dates on which the study was initiated & completed.
- Objectives and procedures stated in approved protocol, including any changes in original protocol.
- Statistical methods employed for analyzing the data.
- The test and control articles identified by name, chemical abstracts no. or code number, strength, purity and composition or other appropriate characteristics. Stability of test and control articles under the conditions of administration.
- A description of the methods used.
- A description of the test system used where applicable the final report shall include the no. of animals used, sex, body weight range, source of supplies, species, strain and sub strain, age and procedure used of identification.
- A description of the dosage, dosage regimen, rate of administration and duration.
- The description of all circumstances that may have affected the quality or integrity of the data.
- The name of study director, the name of the other scientists or other professionals and the names of all supervisory personnel involved in the study.
- A description of transformation calculations or operations performed on the data, a summary and analysis of data, statement of conclusions drawn from analysis.
- The signed and data reports of each of the individual's scientists or other professional involved in the study.
- The location where all specimens, raw data and the final report are to be stored.
- A statement prepared and signed by quality assurance unit & the final report signed and dated by study director.

Drug discovery and drug development is being revolutionized due to changes in technology. Technologies like genomics, proteomics high throughput screening and structure based design have enabled the process of discover to evolve into a system where new lead molecules can be rapidly found against novel and difficult targets. FDA's role in the development of a new drug begins when the drug's sponsor (usually the manufacturer or potential markers) having screened the new molecules for pharmacological activity and acute toxicity potential in animals, wants to test its diagnostically or therapeutic potential in humans. At that point the molecule changes in legal study under the federal food, drug and cosmetic act. Before the sponsor proceeds to study a new drug in human, approval has to be obtained by IND.

Applications

- IND application (Investigational New Drug application) is to provide the data showing that it is reasonable to begin tests of a new drug on humans.
- IND application is result of successful preclinical development programme and it is also the vehicle through which a sponsor advances to next stage of drug development known as clinical trials.
- IND application categories: Commercial Research.

There are 3 types of IND application.

- Investigator IND application.
- Emergency use IND application.
- Treatment IND application.

The IND application must contain information in 3 bridge areas.

- Animal pharmacology and toxicology studies.
- Manufacturing information.
- Clinical protocol & investigator information.

Sponsor files the IND application in form 1571 to the FDA for review once successful series of preclinical studies are completed.

Along with IND application the sponsor submits the statement of the investigator in form 1572. Once the IND application is submitted, the sponsor must wait 30 calendar days before initiating any clinical trials. If the sponsor hears nothing from CDER (Center for Drug Evaluation & Research) then on day 31 after submission of IND application, the study may proceed as submitted. The CDER is a division of FDA that reviews "New Drug Applications" to ensure that drug are safe and effective. After medical review, chemical reviewers, pharmacological toxicology review, statistical analysis, safety review only they promoted to clinical investigation.

1.2.6 Protocol Design

The following topics should be considered in the preparation and review of animals care and protocols:

- Rationale and purpose of the proposed use of animals.
- Justification of the spices and number of animals requested. Whenever possible, the number of animals requested should be justified spastically.

- Availability or appropriateness of the use of less-invasive procedures, the other spices, isolated organ preparation, cell or tissue culture, or computer simulation (see appendix A alternatives).
- Adequacy of training and experience of personnel in procedures used.
- Usual housing and husbandry requirements.
- Appropriate sedation, analgesia, and anaesthesia (scales of pain or invasiveness might aid in the preparation and review of protocols; see appendix A, "anaesthesia, pain and surgery").
- Unnecessary duplication of experiments.
- Conduct of multiple major operative procedures.
- Criteria and process for timely intervention, removal of animals from a study, or euthanasia if painful or stressful outcomes are anticipated.
- Post procedure Care.
- Method of euthanasia or disposition of animal.
- Safety of working environment for personal.

Occasionally, protocols include procedure that have not been previous study or that have potential to cause pain or distress that cannot be reliably controlled such procedure might include physical restraint, multiple major survival surgery, food or fluid restriction , user edge ones , use of death has an end point , use of noxious stimuli, skin or corneal irritancy testing, allowance of excessive tumor burden, intracardiac or orbital - sinus blood sample, or the use of abnormal environmental conditions. Relevant objective information regarding the procedure and the purpose of the study should be sought from the literature, veterinarians, investigators, and other knowledgeable about the effects of animals. If the little is known regarding a specific procedure, limited pilot studies design to assess the effects of the procedure on animals, conducted under IACUC oversight, might be appropriate. General guidelines for evolution of some of those methods are provided in this section, but they might not apply in all instances.

1.2.7 Clinical Development

Clinical trial or study is any investigation in human subjects intended to discover or verify the clinical, pharmacological and the Pharmacodynamic effects of an investigational product and or identify any adverse reactions to investigational products or study ADME of an investigational product with the object of ascertaining its safety and/or efficacy.

Phases of clinical trials

Phase I: Human Pharmacology.

Phase II: Therapeutic Exploration.

Phase III: Therapeutic Confirmation.

Phase IV: Post Marketing Studies.

Phase I: Human Pharmacology

1st stage of testing in human subjects. Normally (20-80) group of healthy volunteers will be selected to participate in these studies. This phase includes trail designed to assess the safety, tolerability, Pharmacokinetic & Pharmacodynamic of drug.

Phase II: Therapeutic Exploration

Once the initial safety of study drug has been conformed in phase I trials, phase II trials are performed to assess how well the drug works (efficacy) require large group (200-300) of patient volunteers. Most of the development processes are failed in phase II only because of toxic effects (in 90% cases).

Phase III: Therapeutic Confirmation

They are performed after preliminary evidence suggestions effectiveness of the drug has been obtained in phase II. They are intended together additional information about effectiveness and safety that is needed to evaluate the overall benefit. Risk relationship of drug. Usually include several hundred to thousand patients. Data obtained from phase III is the major component of new drug application. It determines dosage schedule.

Phase IV: Post Marketing Studies

Those studies performed with drugs that have been granted marketing authorization.

1.2.8 Ethics in Preclinical Research

Monitoring the use of Animals Institutional animal care and use committee was present.

The responsible administrative official at each institution must appoint an IACUC, also referred to as "the committee" to oversee and evaluate the institution's animal program, procedures, and facilities to ensure that they are consistent with the recommendations is this guide, the AWRs [Animal Welfare and Regulations], and the PHS policy. It is the institution's responsibility to provide suitable orientation, background materials, access to appropriate resources, and, if necessary, specific training to assist IACUC members in understanding and evaluating issues brought before the committee.

Committee membership should include the following:

- A doctor of veterinary medicine, who is certified (see American College Of Laboratory Animal Medicine, ACLAM, appendix B) or has training or experienced in laboratory animal science and medicine or in the use of spices in question.

- At least one practicing scientist experienced in research involving animals.
- At least one public member to represent general community interests in the proper care and use of animals. Public members should not be laboratory animal users, be affiliated with the institution, or be members of the immediate family of a person who is affiliated with the institution.

The size of the institution and the nature and extent of the research, testing, and educational programs will determine the number of members of committee and their terms of appointment. Additional information about committee composition can be found in the PHS policy and the AWRS.

The committee responsible for oversight and evolution of the animal care and use program and its components described in this guide. In functions include inspection of facilities; evolution of programs animal activity areas; submissions of reports to responsible institutional officials; review of proposed uses if animals in research testing or educational (i.e., protocols); and establishment of a mechanism for receipt and review of corners involving the care and use if animals at the institutions.

The IACUC must meets as often as necessary to fulfill its responsibilities, but it should meet at least ones every 6 months. Records of committee meetings and results of deliberations should be maintained. The committee should review the animal-care program and inspect the animal facilities, activity areas at least once every 6 months. After review and inspection, a written report, signed by a majority of the IACUC, should be made to the responsible administrative officials of the institution on the status of the animal care and use program and other activities as stated herein and as required by federal, state, or local regulations and policies, protocols should be reviewed in accord with the AWRS, the PHS policy, U.S. government principles for utilization and care of vertebrate animals used in testing, research, and training (IRAC 1985; see appendix D), and this guide (see foot note,p.2).

1.3 HIGH THROUGHPUT SCREENING

Traditional drug discovery research (TDDR) has been revolutionized and every day new assay and techniques are being developed to make DDR a success and to cut down the loss incurred by the failing molecule in clinical trials.

This revolution considerably reduces the time and expenses involved in DDR by setting the process on fast tract. New drug discovery0020 (NDD) for oval therapeutic targets is thus an amalgamated process of various steps in today's modern pharmaceutical research. This process is used for developing new leads for the new targets with improved Pharmacokinetics/ Pharmacodynamic or finding utility for novel compounds obtained from diverse resources.

In the domain of drug research target identification, purification and assay development constitute the initial step. Then they screened for identify targets. It needs huge investment of manpower, time and money.

It has so many steps

- Like centrifugation, phase extraction, filtration, precipitation and subsequent signal amplification and detection, evaluation of few hundred compounds might take weeks and months. Conventional drug discovery program has been called slow process.

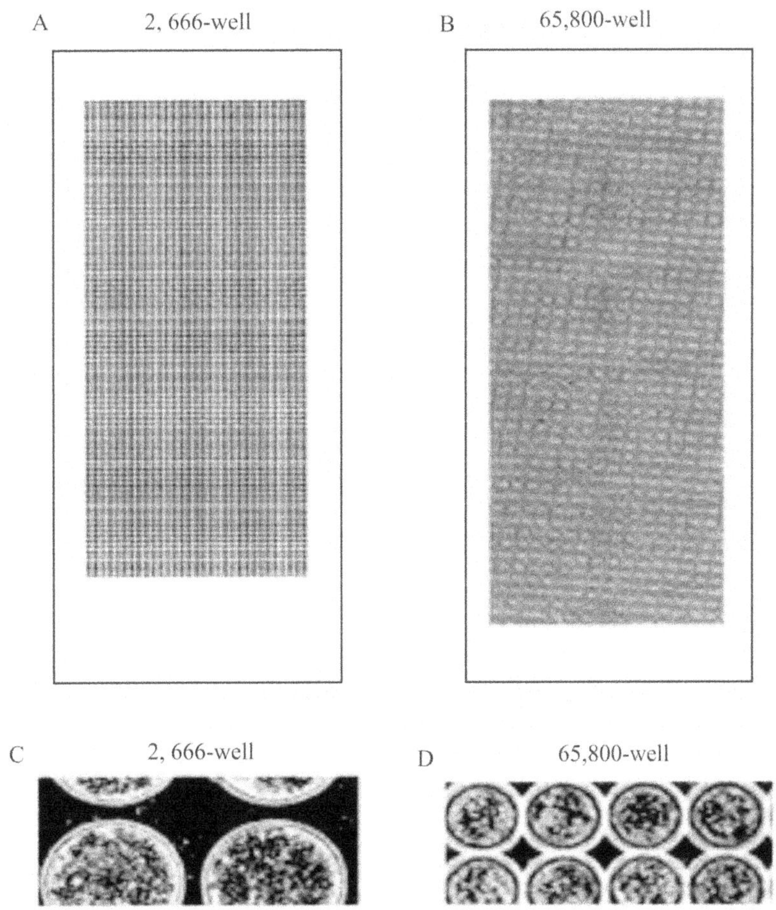

Fig. 1.1 Wells of highthroughput screening.

- The last 2 decades have seen astonishing innovation in technology that have helped the manual low speed screening to evolve into an automated, microprocessor controlled robotic process called "HIGH THROUGH PUT SCREENING". This recent process is synergy of chemistry, biology, engineering and informatics.

  HTS has helped to speed up conventional languid process and now over 50,000-1,00,000 compounds can be screened per week.
- Further advancements are making it possible to screen 10,000-1,00,000 compounds within 24 hours. This process is called "ULTRA HIGH THROUGHPUT SCREENING" (uHTS).
- HTS of large no. of test compounds in a lesser time is also reality now.
- It is also useful in other areas as drug synthesis; toxicity screening, drug metabolism and pharmacokinetics (DM&PK) are helping the process to achieve its ultimate speed in NDD.

1.3.1 *In vitro* Matrix-Ligand Interactions Studies

They are two types

1. Heterogeneous assays.
2. Homogeneous assays.

These Assays are carried to evaluate

- Protein-Protein interactions.
- Receptor-ligand interaction.
- Enzyme-ligand interactions.

Heterogeneous assays include

Nonradio active assay: ELISA (Enzyme linked immunosorbent assays).

Radioactive assay: Such as filtration, adsorption, Precipitation and Radio immune Assay (RIA).

Heterogeneous assays are laborious and require multiple steps like addition, incubation, washing, transfer, filtration and etc., mainly final reading based on color produced or the remaining radioactivity measurement. In contrast heterogeneous assay, homogeneous assays offer a unique advantages by drastically reducing the number of steps involved in analysis and by integrating or sequencing them.

Homogeneous assays include

Nonradioactive assays:

- Chromogenic assays.

- Absorbance-based assay.
- Fluorescence- based assay.
- Luminescence-based assay.
- Bead-based assay.

Radioactive assays:

- Scintillation proximity assay (SPA).
- Scintillation plate assay.

1.3.2 HTS Binding Assay

In HTS the interaction of ligand with the biological compartment is elucidated by luminescence based binding assay. In this manner several thousands of compounds from chemical library can be assessed for their binding in a few days period.

Various florescence techniques

- Fluorescence anisotropy (FA).
- Fluorescence correlation spectroscopy (FCS).
- Fluorescence Intensity Assay (FIA).
- Fluorescence life time Imaging Microscopy (FLIM).
- Fluorescence Resonance energy Transfer (FRET).
- Total Internal reflection Fluorescence (TIRE).
- Time resolved resonance Anisotropy (TRRA).

And NANO based techniques are there

- Scintillation proximity assay (SPA).
- Amplified Luminescence proximity Homogeneous assay (ALPHA).

Fluroscence techniques in drug screening: The recently developed fluorescence based assays are good enough to elucidate the molecular mechanism of receptor function and signal transduction process, as well as for applications in field of screening for novel therapeutic compounds and homogeneous assay there by used. Fluorescent labels are their inherent property of shifting the emission wavelength from the exciter wavelengths to differentiate minute information regarding binding.

(i) ***Fluorescence Intensity Assay (FIA):*** Flurogenic assay is production of property of fluorescence from non fluorescence reagent. And quench is decrease in fluorescence intensity up to cleavage of substrate.

(ii) ***Fluorescence Anisotropy (FA):*** It is suitable to detect receptor ligand binding reactions used to conventional biophysical laboratories. Low polarization observed when ligand is free in solution. Plane polarized light to excite the fluroprobe and emission is recorded perpendicular and parallel to plane of polarization.

(iii) ***In Vivo Imaging of Drug Action (Near Infrared Imaging):*** It is a newly added method to evaluate the drug action and quantification without killing the animal. Rapid development in this technology is accepted to revolutionize *in vivo* studies that warrant the killing of experimental animals. Fundamental of technique is using molecules capable of emitting light in higher wavelength near IR region there by, it gains the capability of crossing biological membrane and to be detected by sensitive camera turned for near IR region.

1.4 PHARMACOGENOMICS, PROTEOMICS AND ARRAY TECHNOLOGY

1.4.1 Pharmacogenomics

Pharmacogenomics is one of the important branches in new drug development process. In these approaches newly developed drugs leads to advent of "Personalized medicine" in which drugs for each individual's unique genetic makeup. Individual variability in drug efficacy and drug safety is a major challenge in current clinical practice, drug development and drug regulation. In recent studies also Pharmacogenomics have provided examples of causal relations between genotypes and drug responses to account for phenotypic variations of clinical importance in drug therapy. In recent progress the understanding of genetic contributions to major individual variability in drug therapy with focus on genetic variations of drug target, drug metabolism, drug transport, disease susceptibility and drug safety. Pharmacogenomics is the technology that analyses how genetic makeup affects an individual's response to drugs. It deals with the influence of genetic variation on drug responses in patients by correlation gene expression or single nucleotide polymorphisms with a drug's efficacy or toxicity. The main aim of Pharmacogenomics is to develop rational means to optimize drug therapy, with respect to patient's genotype, to ensure maximum efficacy with minimal adverse effects.

In a large patient population, a medication that is proven efficacious in many patients often fails to work in some other patients. Furthermore, when it does work, it may cause serious side effects, even death, in a small number of patients. Although large individual variability in drug efficacy and safety has been known to exist since the beginning of human medicine, understanding the origin of individual variation in drug responses has proven difficulty. On the other hand, the demand to overcome such variation has received more attention now than ever before. It is well documented that large variability of drug efficacy and adverse drug reaction in patients is a major determinant of the clinical use, regulation, and withdrawal from market of lineal drugs and a bottleneck in the development of new therapeutic agents.

Pharmacogenomics and individualized drug therapy are increasingly influencing medicine and biomedical research in many areas, including clinical medicine, drug development, drug regulation, pharmacology and toxicology, a thematic reflexation of the post genomic era of today's medicine. This article is intended to provide a comprehensive review of recent progress in the understanding of the basis of individual variability of drug efficacy and adverse drug reaction with focus on genetic polymorphisms of drug targets, drug-metabolizing enzymes, drug transporters and targets of drug toxicity.

(i) Some individual drug responses

- *Individual variability in drug therapy:* Drug efficacy and adverse drug reactions dose dependently determine the clinical outcome of a medication. A higher dose boosts drug therapeutic effect but simultaneously increases the propensity for new or greater undesirable side effects. The drug dosage between its therapeutic effect and apparent adverse reaction, define therapeutic window. For many drugs the optimum dose required for effective and safe therapy varies significantly from patient to patient. A drug dose within the therapeutic window for the majority of a patient population can be too low or too high for a small number of patients who have an atypical dose response curve for a drug therapeutic effect, toxicity or both resulting in unexpected undesirable outcomes in the patients. Individual variability generally has a larger impact on drugs that have a narrow therapeutic widow than those with a wide one.

(ii) Factors affecting individual drug response

- Genetic and nongenetic factors affect individual variability of a drug response by modulating the dose response curves of drug efficacy and drug toxicity of patients. Genetic factors generally cause permanent changes in protein functions, whereas environmental and physiological factors and their impact on drug response are transient in most cases.
- Genetic polymorphisms of proteins involved in drug targeting and drug metabolism and transport are likely to be the most important sources of individual variability in drug efficacy. Drug target responsible for an adverse drug reaction can be the same as or different from the therapeutic target of the drug resulting in on target or off target side effect.

- At the molecular level genetic variations can change the structure of a target protein via mutation in the coding region of the gene or the amount of the protein expressed by modulating gene regulation both of which ultimately alter the function of the protein or the rate and kinetic constants in the cases of an enzyme. Mutations can also modulate gene expression by way of epigenetic regulation.
- Genetic polymorphisms of drug metabolizing enzymes and transporters can affect the absorption, distribution, metabolism and elimination of drugs and thereby modulate their plasma and target tissue concentrations. Defective DNA repair enzymes reduce the ability of cells to repair mutations induced by alkylating chemotherapeutic agents. Mutations that alter the structure or reduce the amount of the enzymes involved in the biosynthesis of glutathione are likely to reduce the intracellular content of glutathione, which is critical in protecting cells from oxidative stress and reactive intermediates commonly encountered adverse drug reaction.
- Environmental chemicals co-administered drugs, dietary constituents, tobacco smoking and alcohol use are all known to induce or inhibit Cytochrome P450 other drug metabolizing enzymes and drug transporters to alter drug efficacy and to induce drug-drug and drug chemical interactions and drug side effects.
- Physiological factors including age, sex, disease states, pregnancy, exercise, starvation and circadian rhythm can also contribute significantly to individual variations of the pharmacokinetic and pharmacodynamic properties of administered drugs. Some physiological traits are also genetic generally polygenic in nature such as sex, body weight and chronic diseases.
- *Human genetics in drug response:* Genetic influence on drug response involved variations in single genes (monogenic inheritance) in which polymorphisms of a single gene encoding a drug metabolizing enzyme responsible for the metabolism and disposition of a substrate drug caused aberrant response to the drug.
- Traditional approach was used to establish a genotype-phenotype connection in three steps: Identify individual phenotypes (normal or extensive metabolizers versus poor or slow metabolizers) by measuring drug levels in the urine or plasma before the genetic mechanism was known, establishing a correlation between drug pharmacokinetics and drug response (efficacy or toxicity) and

finally identifying the genetic defects that account for the low or lack of the enzyme activity later.

- Genetic variations can result from single nucleotide polymorphism (SNP) insertion, deletion or duplication of DNA sequences. SNP is probably the most common variation. More than 90% of human genes contain at least one SNP and nearly every human gene is marked by a sequence variation. More than 14 million SNPs have been identified in the human genomes.

(iii) Genetic polymorphisms of drug targets

- Polymorphism in genes encoding drug targets directly affect target protein function, drug target interaction or both to produce profound effects on drug response.
- ***Example:*** Warfarin is most commonly used oral anticoagulant. The main target of Warfarin is vitamin K epoxide reductase (VKOR), (especially VKOR complex subunit 1- VKORC1). VKOR catalyzes the conversion of vitamin K epoxide to reduced vitamin K, which is required for post translational γ carboxylation of the glutamic acid residues of coagulation factors II,VII,IX and X and the anticoagulant proteins C, S and Z by γ-glutamyl carboxylase (GGCX). Warfarin acts by inhibiting VKORC1, it leads to depletion of reduced vitamin K and consequently it leads to production of hypofunctional coagulation factors resulting in anticoagulation. In case of Warfarin dose determination depends on inhibition capacity of Warfarin on VKOR. But VKOR is exposes in so many types of polymorphic forms (like A41S, V45A, R58G, V66M and L128R etc.,) but these mutations are rare in human population (<0.1%) but influences the dose determination. Overall, polymorphisms of VKORC1 were estimated to account for 25% of the variation in Warfarin dose.

(iv) Genetic polymorphism of drug metabolizing enzyme

- Most of all clinical drugs are metabolized by one or more microsomal cytochrome P450 enzymes. P450 catalyzes the mono oxygenation of lipophilic drugs to give rise to metabolites with altered water solubility or metabolites more suitable to further metabolism by other enzymes. In many cases P450 polymorphism is a major variable affecting drug plasma concentration, drug detoxification and drug activation.

  Example: CYPED6 polymorphism is one of the important example for understanding of genetic polymorphism role in new drug discovery, by mutation of metabolizing enzymes may lose their metabolizing capacity. Sometimes it leads to toxicity of those particular drugs. CYP2D6 is responsible for the metabolism of approximately 20 to 25% of all marked drugs like β adrenergic receptor blockers, antidepressants, antiarrhythmics and antipsychotics. CYP2D6 is highly polymorphic, variant alleles of CYP2D6 are classified on the basis of enzymatic activities. If CYP2D6 is mainly responsible for the metabolism of any drug it leads to high blood levels of that drug by polymorphic form. So by knowing of phenotype of an individual patient would allow physician to prescribe a safe and effective dose of the drug.

- Many non P450 drug metabolizing enzymes also play critical roles in the metabolism of a variety of drugs. Polymorphisms of these enzymes influence the metabolism and therapeutic effect of the drugs, some of them are clinically significant.

  Example: Thiopurine methyltransferase (TPMT) catalyzes the S-methylation of 6-mercaptopurine, azathiopurine and thioguanine, which are used for treatment of leukemia and autoimmune diseases. More than 20 variant alleles of the TPMT gene have been identified (like TPMT*2, TPMT*3A, TPMT*3C etc.,) they produce poor enzymatic activities. Approximately 90% of white persons inherit high enzyme activity, 10% inherit intermediate activity (heterozygous) and 0.3% inherit low or no activity. The persons carrying defective TPMT alleles accumulate higher levels of cytotoxic thiopurine nucleotides than those with the wild type alleles after receiving a standard dose of the drug, leading to severe hematological toxicity by the parent drugs. In these scenarios, a reduced drug dose should be prescribed.

(v) Genetic polymorphism of drug transporters

- Drug transporters modulate the absorption, distribution and elimination of drugs by controlling of influx and efflux in cells. With genetic polymorphism of transporters can have impact on drug disposition, drug efficacy and drug safety.

  Example: TheABCB1 gene encodes the P-glycoprotein (Pgp, ABCB1, multidrug resistance that transports many important drugs out of cells, ABCB1 is highly polymorphic, and some allelic variants exhibits ethnic-dependent distribution. The SNP C3435T of ABCB1 occurs with high frequencies in many populations (20-60%), it leads to disposition of digoxin (a substrate of Pgp). In some individuals it raises the serum digoxin concentration and in some others it may decreases serum dioxin levels, all these differences because of different polymorphic forms of ABCB1.

(vi) Genetic variables indirectly affecting drug response

- Many genetic variables affect drug response by modulating the functions of proteins that are not direct drug targets, drug metabolizing enzymes or drug transporters but influence the biological context of a drug response.

(vii) Genetic variables affecting adverse drug reaction

- Adverse drug reactions are highly variable in many cases and thus represent a major limiting factor in drug therapy and drug development. Idiosyncratic adverse drug reactions characterized by rare occurrence of multiple exposures are the most extreme cases of individual variability in drug safety. Drug safety issues are to understand the mechanism of adverse drug response, determine the gene or genes responsible for the adverse events and develop reliable biomarkers for screening sensitive individuals. Illustrate the utility of this Pharmacogenomics approach and bring the hope that drug dose or alternative drugs can be chosen according to individual genotypes and phenotypes to minimize adverse drug reactions in patients.
- Drug toxicity a result from the inhibition or activity of a therapeutic target by a drug or from an interaction between a drug and a target protein different from the therapeutic target of the drug. In some cases "on target" (such as excessive bleeding from high doses of Warfarin) is observed, in other cases "off target" toxicity (such as statin induced myopathy) may observed. All genetic factors that influence drug response-drug targets, drug-metabolizing enzymes, drug transporters and genes indirectly affecting drug action can modulate drug toxicity and contribute to its individual variability.
- The statins–simvastatin, pravastatin and rosuvastatin inhibit HMG-CoA reductase to reduce LDL cholesterol levels, which reduces the incidence of heart attacks, strokes and revascularization procedure by approximately one fifth for each reduction of 40 mg/dl in the LDL cholesterol level. On the other hand statins cause myopathy (muscle pain and weakness associated with elevated creatine kinase levels) in a small number of patients receiving statin therapy. Statin induced myopathy occasionally develops into rhabdomyolysis (muscle breakdown and myoglobin release) that may cause renal failure and death. The mechanism of statin is unclear. In study of healthy volunteers, a common polymorphism of SLCO1B1 (C.5211>c, V174A, or rs4149056) was shown to

markedly affect individual variations of statin pharmacokinetics. The plasma $AUC_{0-\infty}$ of simvastatin acid (but not simvastatin) was increased more than 2 or 3 folds in persons with the homozygous C. 521CC genotype compared with the TC heterozygous or the TT homozygous genotypes respectively as a result of reduced uptake of simvastatin acid into hepatocytes via OATP1B1 in the later genotypes. Increased plasma concentrations of simvastatin aid in patients carrying the C.521C variant allele may have increased risk of systemic adverse effects and reduced cholesterol-lowering efficacy as a result of reduced intracellular simvastatin acid for inhibition f HMG-CoA reductase in hepatocytes.

- Drug Hypersensitivity Reactions (DHRs) are the effective of drugs that occurs at a dose tolerated by typical subjects and clinically resemble allergy. DHRs may represent up to one third of adverse reactions and concern more than 7% of the general population. DHRs can be life threatening, require or prolong hospitalization or entail change in drug prescription. The pathogenic mechanisms of many DHRs remain unclear. Although DHRs are unpredictable for most part genetic polymorphisms of certain genes can predispose patients to drug allergy.

  Example: The use of abacavir a potent HIV-1 nucleoside analogue reverse-transcriptase inhibitor is complicated by a potentially life threatening hypersensitivity syndrome, Abacavir hypersensitivity occurs in approximately 5 to 9% of the patients receiving abacavir treatment and is characterized by multisystem involvement. The hypersensitivity was strongly associated with the HLA polymorphism HLA-B*5701 and its combination with a haplotypie polymorphism of Hsp70-Hom (M493T).

- Carbamazepine (CBZ) a commonly prescribed first line anticonvulsant for the treatment of seizures, frequently cutaneous DHRs including maculopapular eruption, hypersensitivity syndrome, Stevens Johnson syndrome (SJS) and toxic epidermal necrosis (TEN). CBZ- induced SJS/TEN was strongly associated with a HLA polymorphism HLA-B*1502 in Han Chinese.
- The Warfarin story reveals that prospective clinical trials demonstrating that incorporation of genetic testing can induced benefit the selection of appropriate therapeutic agent and drug dose for individual patients to improve therapeutic response, reduce adverse drug effects and reduce overall healthcare cost are critical for wide clinical acceptance of Pharmacogenomic testing.

Pharmacogenomics in drug development

Pharmacogenomics can be used to improve drug discovery and drug development in at least two ways: development of new drugs to overcome drug resistance or target new drug targets, and optimization of drug metabolism and pharmacokinetics (DMPK) to minimize variation in drug levels.

- A major challenge in targeted cancer therapy is the rapid development of resistance to targeted anticancer agent as a result of frequent mutation of drug targets in cancer cells.

Applications of Pharmacogenomics

Pharmacogenomics has applications in illnesses like cancer, cardiovascular disorders, depression, bipolar disorders attention deficit disorders, HIV, Tuberculosis, asthma and diabetes etc.

Toxicogenomics

Toxicogenomics is a field of science that deals with the collection, interpretation and storage of information about gene and protein activity within particular cell or tissue of an organism, in response to toxic substances.

- In pharmaceutical research toxicogenomics is defined as the study of structure and function of the genome as it responds to adverse renobiotic exposure.
- Toxicogenomics combines toxicology with genomics or other high throughout molecular profiling technologies such as transcriptiomics, proteomics and metabolism.
- It is also defined as study of inter-individual variations in whole – genome or candidate gene single-nucleotide polymorphism maps, haplotype markers and alternations in gene expression that might correlate with drug responses.

Clinomics

- Clinomics is the study of omics data along with its associated clinical data. The term - omis generally refers to a study of biology.
- Clinomics will be a bridge between basic biological data and its effect on human health.
- Clinomics takes the next step by looking at not only the genetics of the patient and proteins associated with a patient and a disease.

Genetic Engineering

- Genetic engineering also called genetic modification is the direct manipulation of an organism's genome using biotechnology.

- A new DNA may be inserted in the host genome by first isolating and copying in genetic material of interest using molecular cloning methods to generate a DNA sequence or by synthesizing the DNA and then inserting this construct into the host organism. Genes may be removed or "knocked out" using a nuclease. Gene targeting is a different technique that uses homologous recombination to change an endogenous gene and can be used to delete a gene, remove exons, add a gene or introduce point mutations.
- An organism that is generated through genetic engineering is considered to be a genetically modified organism (GMO).
- Genetic engineering techniques have been applied in numerous fields including research, agriculture industrial biotechnology and medicine.
- Enzymes used in some medicines such as insulin and human growth hormones are now manufactured in GM cells, experimental GM cell lines and GM animals such as mice or Zebra fish are being used for research purposes and genetically modified crops have been commercialized.
- **Genome editing:** Genome editing is a type of genetic engineering in which DNA is inserted, replaced or removed from a genome using artificially engineered nucleases or "molecular scissors". The nucleases created specific double standed break (DSBs) at desired locations in the genome and harness the cell's endogenous mechanisms to repair the induced break by natural process of homologous recombination (HR) and non homologous and joining (NHJ).

1.4.2 Proteomics

Proteomics has been said to be the next step from genomics. Proteomics is the study of the proteome. The proteome is the complete complement of proteins found in a complete genome or specific tissue.

Proteomics and genomics are inter dependent

The main aims of proteomics

- Detect the different proteins expressed by tissue, cell culture or organism using 2-dimensional gel electrophoresis.
- Store that information in a data base.
- Compare expression profiles between healthy cells versus a diseased cell.
- That data comparison can then be used for testing and rational drug design.
- Protein identification
- Protein expression studies

- Protein function
- Protein post-translational modification
- Protein localization and compartmentalization
- Protein-protein interactions.
- Proteomics is very important study because possibility of parallel analysis of multiple proteins including their post translational modifications. Discovery of disease specific proteins is possible in this technique, by targeting to specific candidate.

Mainly 3 types of proteomics are important

1. **Functional proteomics:** This type of proteomics used for identification of protein functions, activities or interactions at a global or organism wide scale.
2. **Expressional proteomics:** This type of proteomics used for analysis of global or organism wide changes in proteins.
3. **Structural proteomics:** This type of proteomics used for high through put or high volume expression and structure determination of proteins by X ray, NMR or computer based methods.

Roles of proteins

- Proteins are the instruments through which the genetic potential of an organism are expressed. And these are active biological agents in cells.
- Proteins are involved in almost all cellular processes and fulfil many functions.

Some functions of proteins:

- Enzyme catalysis, transporters, mechanical support organelle constituents, storage reservoirs, metabolic control, protection mechanisms toxins and osmotic pressure.
- Proteome is a protein compliment of genome. Proteomics is study of proteome.

Transcriptiomics is often insufficient to study functional aspects of genomics

DNA	– RNA	– Proteins
Genome	– Transcriptome	– Proteome
DNA Sequencing	– DNA arrays	– 2D-PAGE

- Some post translational modification of proteins are chemically modified or regulated after synthesis.

  Those are identified by proteomics.

Table 1.3 Some covalent post translational modifications.

Modification	Residues	Role
Cleavage	Various	Activation of proenzymes and precursors
Glycosylations	Asn, ser, thr	Molecular targeting, cell-cell recognition etc.
Phosphorylation	Ser, thr, tyr	Control metabolic processes & signaling
Hydroxylation	Pro, Lys	Increase H-bonding & glycosylation sits.
Acetylation	Lys	Alter charge & weaken interactions with DNA
Methylation	Lys	Alter interactions with other molecules.
Carboxylation	Glu	More negative charge, e.g., to bind calcium
Transmidation	Gln, Lys	Formation of crosslinks in fibrin

Different approaches for proteome purification and protein separation for identifications by MS (Mass Spectrometer)

1. Separation of individual proteins by 2 - DE (2 dimensional proteins electrophoresis)
2. Separation of protein complexes by non-denaturing 2 - DE
3. Purification of protein complexes by affinity chromatography +SDS - PAGE
4. Fractionate by organic solvent
5. Separate complex protein mix
6. Hydrophobic membrane proteins.

2-dimensional protein electrophoresis: This method is useful to purify proteins from desired organelles, cell or tissue.

In this method first proteins are separated by 1 D, after that separated in 2 D by using stain gel and data analysis processes.

In first dimension separation, IPG (immobilized pH gradients) method allows the generation pH gradients of any desired range between pH 3 and 12. In this method sample loading capacity is much higher.

This method is useful for micro preparative separation or spot identification.

In second dimension separation (SDS - PAGE) method pour linear or gradient standards are present to separate proteins visualized gels are recorded by scanning or CD cameras.

Mass spectrometer is containing some basic components. Variations of instrument components typically used in protein sequencing and identifying experiments.

Instrument components

Sample inlet: Direct probe or stage, Capillary column liquid chromatography

Ion Source: Electrospray, Matrix assisted laser desorption

Mass analyzer: Quadrupole mass filter, Ion trap mass analyzer, Time of – flight mass analyzer

Detector

In Data System

Instrument contract system

Types of mass spectrometery

1. Maldi – TOF
2. ESI tandem mass spec instruments
   - Quodropole mass analyzers
   - Ion trap mass analyzers
   - TOF Mass analyzers

1. **Maldi – TOF MS**
   - In these instruments samples are placed on slide, spectra generate masses of peptide ions.
   - Protein identified by peptide mass fingerprinting
   - But this instruments are expensive
   - These are good for sequenced genomes.
2. **Tandem MS (Mass Spectrometer)**
   - In these instruments samples are placed as solution form
   - Proteins identified by cross correlation algorithms
   - These also very expensive
   - These are good for unsequenced genomes.

Proteomis applications: Differential display proteomics

- DIGE difference gel electrophoresis
- MP – Multiplexed proteomics
- ICAT – Isotope coded affinity tagging.
- 2 DE is a powerful technique to separate of coulees protein mixtures and analyze proteomes.

- Mass spectrometry microsequencing an identify proteins from 2DE gels and other samples.
- There are multiple databases and computer programmes available to analyze MS data for protein identification.
- Proteomics approach can be used to identify all proteins in particular sample, elucidate additional components of biochemical pathways or analyze post translational modifications at a small or a large scale.

1.4.3 Array Technology

Micro array technology is revolutionizing current drug development. Gene expression micro-array technology is benefiting all phases of the discovery, development and subsequent use of new cancer therapeutic.

Micro arrays measure the gene expression profiles of the cell. These profiles provide clues to the cells genetic makeup and response to the environment. They are unique signatures that biochemical pathways and broader cellular functions.

For example studding the signatures of tumors and normal cells may pinpoint differences that can be exploited in drug development. Genes associated with failure to treatment or poor outcome can be identified. 'metagenes' a combination of individual genes that describes a particular pathway or gene activity, can also be generated providing additional therapeutic targets.

This technology is used as a complement to other genetic methods. "The development of safe and effective drugs remains challenging". These new technologies will improve the rate at which novel molecular therapeutics are developed and evaluated and provided wealth of information.

This technology generally consists 4 phases.

1. Fabrication of the array
2. RNA isolation and labelling
3. Application of the labelled sample to the array and measurement of hybridization.
4. Data analysis and interpretation.

CHAPTER 2

LABORATORY ANIMALS

2.1 LABORATORY ANIMALS CARE

Laboratory animal care facilities are intended according to **CPCSEA guidelines (Committee for Purpose of Control and Supervision of Experimental Animals)**

Goal

The goal of these guidelines is to promote the human care towards animals used in biomedical and behavioral research and testing with the basic objective of providing specifications that will enhance animal well being, quality in the advancement of biological knowledge that is relevant to humans and animals.

The *Guide* plays an important role in decision making regarding the use of vertebrate laboratory animals because it establishes the minimum ethical, practice, and care standards for researchers and their institutions. The use of laboratory animals in research, teaching, testing, and production is also governed or affected by various federal and local laws, regulations, and standards; for example, in the United States the Animal Welfare Act (AWR 1990) and Regulations (PL 89-544; USDA 1985) and/or Public Health Service (PHS) Policy (PHS 2002) may apply.

Taken together, the practical effect of these laws, regulations, and policies is to establish a system of self-regulation and regulatory oversight that binds researchers and institutions using animals. Both researchers and institutions have affirmative duties of human care and use that are supported by practical, ethical, and scientific principles. This system of self-regulation establishes a rigorous program of animal care and use and provides flexibility in fulfilling the responsibility to provide humane care.

The specific scope and nature of this responsibility can vary based on the scientific discipline, nature of the animal use, and species involved, but because it affects animal care and uses in every situation this responsibility requires that producers, teachers, researchers, and institutions carry out purposeful analyses of proposed uses of laboratory animals. The *Guide* is central to these analyses and to the development of a program in which humane care is incorporated into all aspects of laboratory animal care and use.

Intended audiences and uses of the *guide*

The *Guide* is intended for a wide and diverse audience, including

- The scientific community
- Administrators
- IACUCs
- Veterinarians
- Educators and trainers
- Producers of laboratory animals
- Accreditation bodies
- Regulators
- The public

Ethics and animal use

The decision to use animals in research requires critical thought, judgment, and analysis. Using animals in research is a privilege granted by society to the research community with the expectation that such use will provide either significant new knowledge or lead to improvement in human and/or animal well-being (McCarthy 1999; Perry 2007). It is a trust that mandates responsible and humane care and use of these animals. The *Guide* endorses the responsibilities of investigators as stated in the *U.S. Government Principles for Utilization and Care of Vertebrate Animals Used in Testing, Research, and Training* (IRAC 1985; see Appendix B). These principles direct the research community to accept responsibility for the care and use of animals during all phases of the research effort. Other government agencies and professional organizations have published similar principles (NASA 2008; NCB 2005; NIH 2006, 2007; for additional references see Appendix A). Ethical considerations discussed here and in other sections of the *Guide* should serve as a starting point; readers are encouraged to go beyond these provisions. In certain situations, special considerations will arise during protocol review and planning.

Humane care

Humane care means those actions taken to ensure that laboratory animals are treated according to high ethical and scientific standards. Implementation of a humane care program, creation of a laboratory environment in which humane care and respect for animals are valued and encouraged, underlies the core requirements of the *Guide* and the system of self-regulation it supports (Klein and Bayne 2007).

Animal care and use program

The *animal care and use program* (the Program) means the policies, procedures, standards, organizational structure, staffing, facilities, and practices put into place by an institution to achieve the humane care and use of animals in the laboratory and throughout the institution. It includes the establishment and support of an IACUC or equivalent ethical oversight committee and the maintenance of an environment in which the IACUC can function successfully to carry out its responsibilities under the *Guide* and applicable laws and policies.

Regulations, policies, and principles

The use of laboratory animals is governed by an interrelated, dynamic system of regulations, policies, guidelines, and procedures. The *Guide* takes into consideration regulatory requirements relevant to many US-based activities, including the Animal Welfare Regulations (USDA 1985; US Code, 42 USC § 289d) and the Public Health Service Policy on Humane Care and Use of Laboratory Animals (PHS 2002). The use of the *Guide* by non-US entities also presumes adherence to all regulations relevant to the humane care and use of laboratory animals applicable in those locations. The *Guide* also takes into account the U.S. Government principles for utilization and care of vertebrate animals used in testing, research, and training (IRAC 1985; see Appendix B) and endorses the following principles:

- Consideration of alternatives *(in vitro* systems, computer simulations, and/or mathematical models) to reduce or replace the use of animals
- Design and performance of procedures on the basis of relevance to human or animal health, advancement of knowledge, or the good of society
- Use of appropriate species, quality, and number of animals
- Avoidance or minimization of discomfort, distress, and pain
- Use of appropriate sedation, analgesia, and anesthesia
- Establishment of humane endpoints
- Provision of adequate veterinary care
- Provision of appropriate animal transportation and husbandry directed and performed by qualified persons

- Conduct of experimentation on living animals exclusively by and/or under the close supervision of qualified and experienced personnel.

2.2 EXPERIMENTAL ANIMALS

Veterinary care

Veterinary care is essential for laboratory animals. A person who has training or experience in laboratory animals sciences and medicine should be present. Daily observation of animal can be accomplished by someone other than veterinarian for animal well being and healing behavior and also for animal husbandry and animal welfare.

Animal procurement

Animals must be acquired lawfully as per the CPCSEA guidelines.

Quarantine

Quarantine is the separation of newly received animals from those already in the facility until the health and possibly the microbial status of newly received animals.

Stabilization

Newly received animals should be given a period for physiological and nutritional stabilization before their use.

Separation

Physical separation of animals by species to avoid interspecies disease transmission and eliminate anxiety and possible physiological and behavioral changes due to interspecies conflict. Separate rooms also provides in cubical shape with laminar air flow units, cages have filtered air or separate ventilation. All animals should be observed for signs of illness, injury or abnormal behavior by animal house staff. Animals that show signs of contagious disease should be isolated from healthy animals in the colony. Survivelance of animals is very important thing.

Animal care

Animal house require technical and husbandry support.

Personal hygiene

It is essential that the animal care staff maintain a high standard of personal cleanliness. Example: Showers, change of uniforms, foot wears etc.

Animal experimentation involving hazardous agents

Institutional Bio safety committees whose members are knowledgeable about hazardous agents are in place in most of the higher level education, research institutes and many pharmaceutical industries for safety issues. Animals used for some special consideration need both institutional bio safety committee and Institutional Animal Ethics Committee (IAEC).

Multiple surgical procedures on single animal

For any testing or experiment are not to be practiced unless specified in a protocol only approved by IAEC.

Physical relationship of animal facilities to laboratories

Laboratory animals are very sensitive to their living conditions. They should be housed in an isolated building located as far away from human and not exposed to dust, smoke, noise, wild rodents, insects and birds. Building, cages and environment of animal rooms are the major factors, which affect the quality of animals. Planning an animal facility the space should be well divided for various activities – 50-60% area for rooms, remaining area – for stores, washing, office & staff, machine rooms, quarantine and corridors.

Functional areas

Special laboratories are required. Individual areas for surgery, intensive area, and necropsy, and radiography, preparation of special diets, experimental manipulation, treatment and diagnostic laboratory procedures are required. Equipments, hazardous biological, physical or chemical agents also required. Receiving and storage areas for food and bedding also required. However, sinks, lockers and toilets for persons (who are working in that animal house) also required. Washing, sterilization areas also required. Autoclave also required. The area is required for solid and cleaned equipments. The area to store prior to incineration or removal also required.

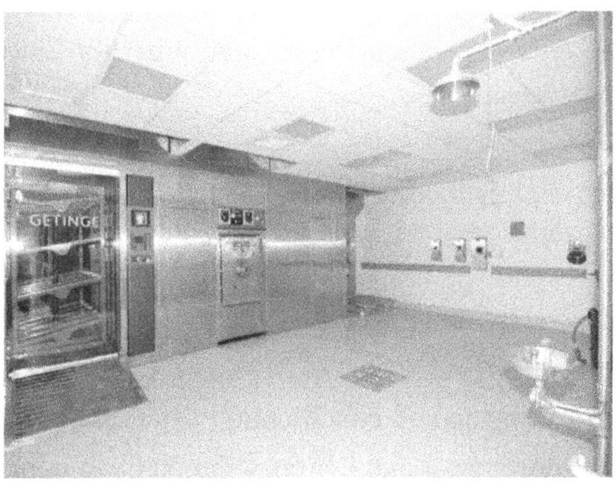

Fig. 2.1 Functional area and physical facilities.

- Building materials should be selected to facilitate efficient and hygienic operation of animal facilities.
- Durable, moisture proof, fire resistant, seamless materials require for interior surfaces.
- Corridors should be wide enough to facilitate movement of personnel as well as equipment.
- Utilities such as water lines drain pipes and electrical connections should preferable.
- Animal room doors should be run, vermin and dust proof and convenient to animal's movement.
- Exterior windows not recommended for small animals.
- Floors should be smooth, moisture proof, non absorbent, skid proof, resistant to wear acid, solvents, adverse effects of detergents and disinfectants.
- Drains essential in all rooms, where floor drains are used, the floors should be sloped and drain taps kept filled with water or corrosion free mesh to prevent high humidity.
- Walls and ceilings should be free of cracks, unsealed utility penetrations or imperfect junctions with doors, ceilings, floors and concern.
- Storage areas designed for feed, bedding, cages and materials not in use.
- Facilities for sanitizing equipment and supplies are essential with adequate water supply.
- Experimental area for small animals same area where they housed for large animals required aseptic surgery area need surgical support area. Preparation area, operation room and area for intensive care also required.

Environment

- Temperature and Humidity control maintenance is very important to prevent variations due to changes in climatic conditions in different rooms.
- Normal temperature range 18 to 29 °C (64.4 to 84.2 °F).
- Humidity range (30% to 90%).
- Ventilation, heating and air conditioning system should be designed.
- Electrical system (power and lighting) should be safe, presents of number of power outlets should be important.
- Noise control should be require, noise free environment is required.

- Concrete walls are more effective than metal or plastic walls they reduce sound transmission.

Animal husbandry

Caging and housing system is very important element for animal well being. Housing system should provide following requirements:-

- Provide space, permit freedom of movement.
- Provide comfortable environment.
- Escape proof enclosures.
- Provide easy access food and water.
- Provide adequate ventilation.
- Meet the biological needs of animals. Maintenance of body temperature, urination, defecation, reproduction.
- Keep animals dry and clean.
- Maintaining good health.
- Sheltered or outdoor housing is also required for when animals are maintained in outdoor runs, pens or other large enclosures.

Social environment

All interactions among individuals of a group or among those able to communicate.

Activity

Provision should be made for animals with specialized locomotors to express these patterns.

Food

Animals should be fed palatable, no contaminated and nutritionally adequate food daily.

- Feeders should allow access to avoid contamination by urine and faeces.
- Animal's food should be available in amounts sufficient to ensure normal growth, maintenance of normal body weight, reproduction and lactation in adults.

Bedding

- Bedding should be absorbent, free of toxic chemicals or other substances which cause injure animals.
- Bedding should be removed and replaced with fresh material to keep animal clean and dry (twice a week).

- Nesting materials for newly delivered pups where ever can be provided (Example: Paper, tissue paper, cotton).

Water

- Ordinary animals should have continuous access to fresh, potable, uncontaminated water, according to their particular requirements.
- Watery devices such as drinking tubes and automatic waters if used should be examined.
- It is better to replace water bottles than to refill them.

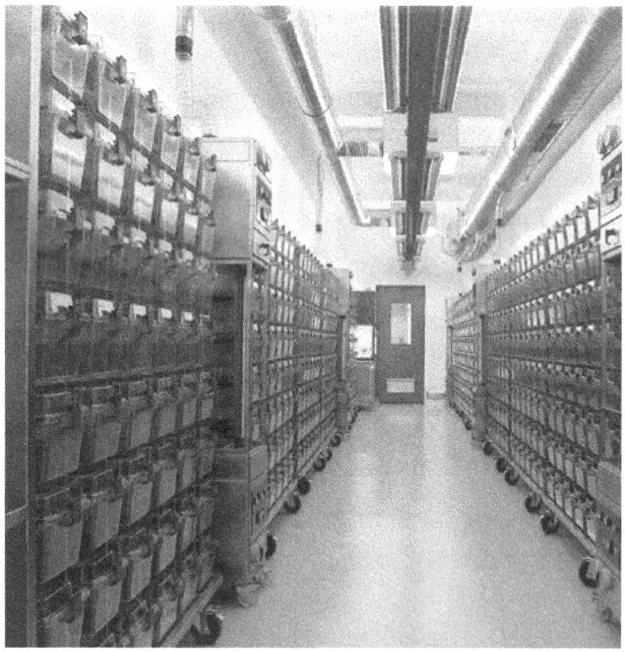

Fig. 2.2 Animal cages in animal house.

Sanitation and cleanliness

- Sanitation is essential in animal facility. Animal rooms, corridors, storage spaces and other areas should be cleaned with appropriate detergent and disinfectants as often as necessary to keep them free of dirt, debris and harmful contamination.
- Animal waste is removed by hosting or flushing should be done at least twice a day.
- Water bottles, sipper tubes, stoppers and other watering equipment should be washed and then sanitized by rinsing with water of at least 82.2 °C (180 °F) or appropriated chemical agents.

Waste disposal

- Waste should be removed regularly and frequently. All waste should be collected and deposited off in a safe and sanitary manner. Pest control programs designed to prevent, control or eliminate the presence of or infestation by pests are essential in an animal environment.
- Emergency care need with qualified personal every day.
- Weekend and holiday care including emergency veterinary care in the event of an emergency.

Record keeping

- Animal house plant, which includes typical floor plan.
- Both technical and non technical.
- Health record of staff/animals.
- All standard operating procedures (SOPs) relevant to the animals.
- Breeding, stock, purchase and sale records.
- Minutes of institutional animal ethics committee meeting.
- Records of experiments conducted with number of animals used.
- Death records.
- Clinical record of sick animals.
- Training record of staff involved in animal activities.
- Water analysis report.

SOPs (Standard Operating Procedures/guidelines)

The institute shall maintain SOPs describing procedures. Those methods adopted with regard to animal husbandry, maintenance, breeding, animal house microbial analysis.

SOPs should contain:

- Name of author.
- Title of SOP.
- Date of preparation.
- Reference of previous SOP in the same subject and date.
- Location and distribution of SOPs with sign of each recipient.
- Objectives.
- Detailed information of instrument.

- Name of manufacturer of reagent.
- Normal value of all parameters.
- Hazard identification and risk assessment.

Transport of laboratory animals

Transport of animals from one place to another place is very important and must be undertaken with care. Main consideration is about containers and animal density in cage. Food and water during transport is very important. Protection is important from transit infections, injuries and stress.

Anaesthesia

- Unless contrary to the achievement of result of study sedatives, analgesics, anaesthetics should be used to control pain or distress under experiment.
- Anaesthetic agents generally effect cardiovascular, respiratory and thermo regulatory mechanism in addition to central nervous system.
- With anaesthesia animals also should fasted by overnight and using pre anaesthetics to block parasympathetic system (reduce salivary secretions) and cardio pulmonary system.
- Local anaesthetics also useful.

Euthanasia

- This is resorted to events where an animal is required to be sacrificed on termination of an experiment or otherwise for ethical reason.
- The procedure should be carried out quickly and painless in an atmosphere free from fear of anxiety.
- Death without causing anxiety, pain or distress with minimum time log phase.
- Minimum physiological and psychological disturbances.
- Compatibility with the purpose of study and minimum emotional effect on the apparatus.
- Location should be separate from animal rooms and free from environment contaminants.
- Tranquilizers have to be administered to large species such as monkey, dogs and cats before euthanasia procedure.

2.3 COLLECTION OF BLOOD FROM LABORATORY ANIMALS

Collection of blood from different animals is in different types.

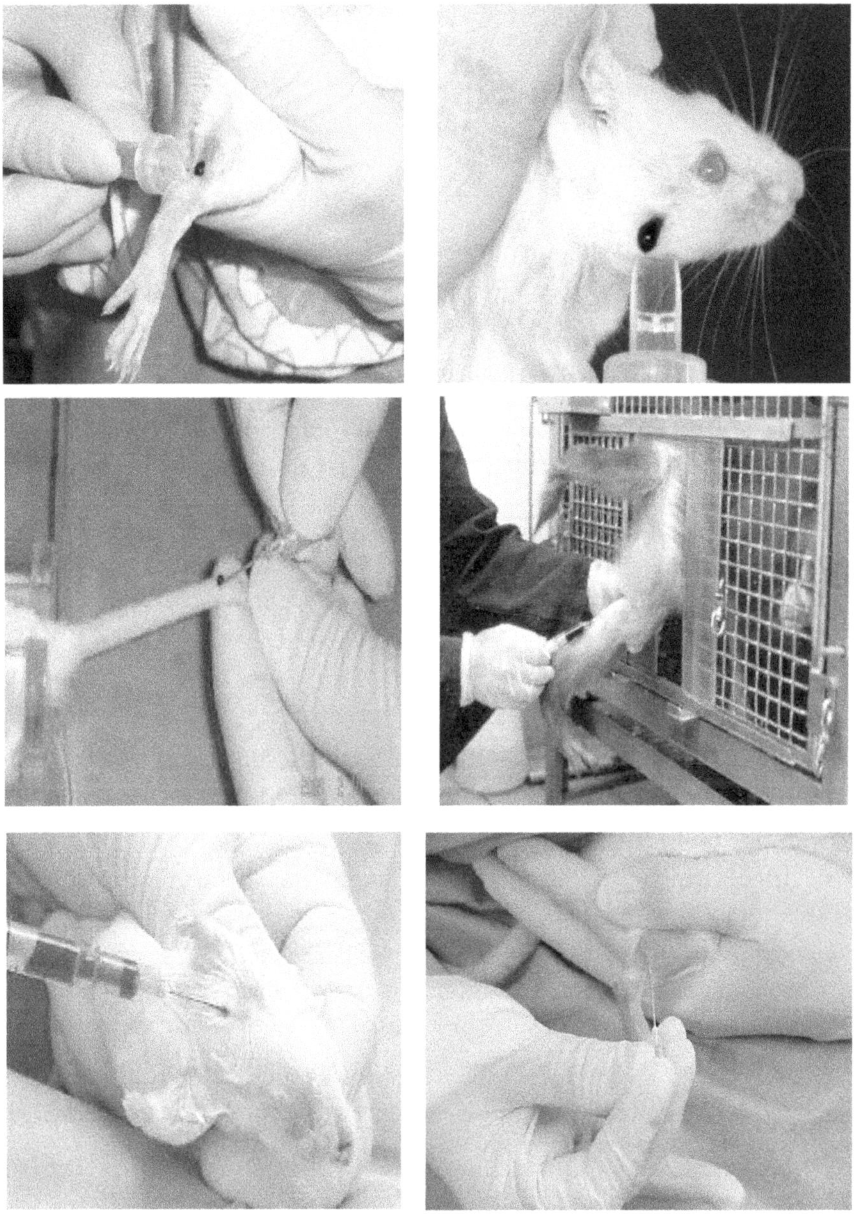

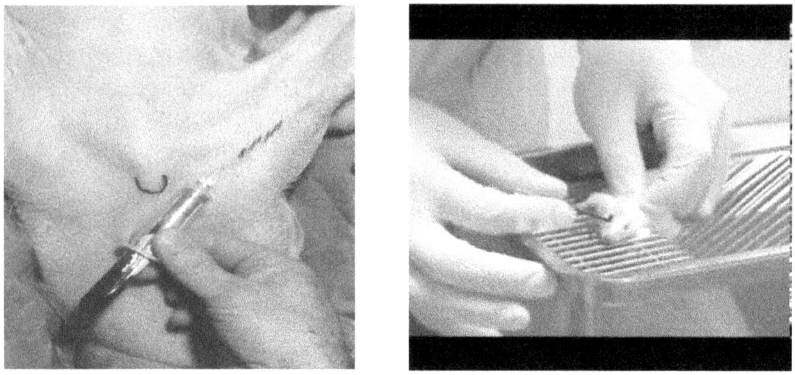

Fig. 2.3 Various types of blood collection techniques.

Number of efficient methods available for collection of blood from small laboratory animals. These methods should be least stressful while blood sample collection in experimental animals. Because stress will affect the outcome of the study. Various guidelines and regulatory agencies have restricted the use of animals and techniques used for blood collection techniques for laboratory animals (like rodents, lagomorphs and nonrodents). For animal studies permission of Institutional Animal Ethics Committee is necessary for use of animals for demonstrating the techniques.

General principles of blood collection in animals

- The method of blood collection should be described in the protocol approved by the Institutional Animal Ethics Committee (IAEC).
- It should be least painful and stressful.
- Blood sample collection from animals may be under anaesthesia or without anaesthesia.
- Some preanesthetic medication for all species is necessary to reduce salivation, bronchial secretion and protect heart from vagal stimulus. Atropine (0.02 mg/kg s.c./i.m.) is used as preanesthetic medication.
- Adequate training is required for blood collection.
- In general blood sample is withdrawn from venous, arterial blood vessels or heart chambers.
- Frequency of blood collection is very important. Once in two weeks is ideal for nonrodents. Sometimes study need multiple blood samples lagomorphs (Examples: Hares and Rabbits).
- All nonterminal blood collection without replacement of fluids is limited up to 10% of total circulating blood volume in healthy, normal, adult animals on a single occasion and collection may be repeated after

3 to 4 weeks. Sometimes in particular cases repeated blood samples are required at short intervals, a maximum of 0.6 ml/kg/day or 1.0% of an animal's total blood volume can be removed in every 24 hours.

- If the study involves repeated blood sample collection the samples can be withdrawn through a temporary cannula, this may reduce pain and stress in the experimental animals.
- Care should be taken in older and obese animals. The estimated blood volume in adult animals is 55 to 70 ml/kg body weight. Sometimes blood collection volume exceeds more than 10% of total blood volume. So fluid replacement may be required Located Ringer's Solution (LRS) is recommended as the best fluid replacement by National Institutes of Health (NIH). If the volume of blood collection exceeds more than 30% of the total circulatory blood volume, adequate care should be taken so that the animal does not suffer from hypovolemia.

Table 2.1 Commonly recommended anesthetic agents for laboratory animal experiment.

Animal species	Short anesthesia	Medium anesthesia	Long anesthesia
Mice	Isoflurane (inhalation)	Xylazine + ketamine (5 mg + 100 mg i.m.)	Xylazine + ketamine (16 mg + 60 mg i. m. i.p)
	Halothane (inhalation)	Xylazine + ketamine (5 mg + 100 mg i.m.)	Xylazine + ketamine (16 mg + 60 mg i.p.) or Urethane (1200 mg/kg i.p.)
Guinea pig	Isoflurane (inhalation)	Xylazine + ketamine (2 mg + 80 mg i.m.)	Xylazine + ketamine (4 mg + 100 mg)

General methods for blood collection: Blood samples are collected using the following techniques:

- Blood collection not requiring anaesthesia
  - (i) Saphenous vein (rat, mice, guinea pig)
  - (ii) Dorsal pedal vein (rat, mice)
- Blood collection requiring anaesthesia(local/general anaesthesia)
  - (i) Tail vein (rat, mice)
  - (ii) Tail snip (rat, mice)
  - (iii) Orbital sinus (rat, mice)
  - (iv) Jugular vein (rat, mice)
  - (v) Temporary cannula (rat, mice)
  - (vi) Blood vessel cannulation (rat, guinea pig, ferret)

(vii) Tarsal vein (guinea pig)
(viii) Marginal ear vein/artery (rabbit)

- Terminal procedure
  (i) Cardiac puncture (rat, mice, guinea pig, rabbit, ferret)
  (ii) Orbital sinus
  (iii) Posterior vena cava (rat, mice)

(i) ***Procedure for saphenous vein blood sample collection:*** For this type of collection requires rodent handling gloves, towel, cotton, sample collection tubes and 20G needle.

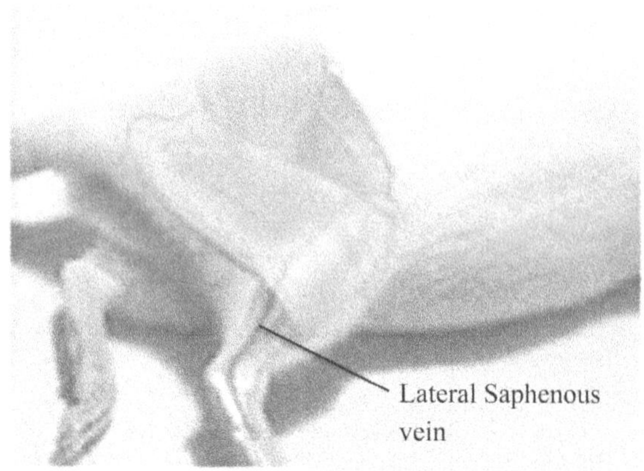

Fig. 2.4 Blood collection from lateral saphenous vein.

- While collection of blood from saphenous vein aseptic precautions are necessary.
- Hair removal cream can be used at the back of hind leg. Otherwise hind leg shaved with electric trimmer until saphenous vein is visible.
- If the animal is strained, the animal should be restrained manually or by using a suitable animal restrainers.
- Hind leg is immobilized and slight pressure may apply gently above the knee joint.
- 20G needle is used to puncturing of vein. After puncturing, syringe with a needle or capillary is used to collect blood from that animal.
- At the time of puncturing and collection of blood animal may get lot of pain, to avoid that pain local anaesthetic cream is apply on collection site.

- Continuous sampling should be avoided and not more than three attempts are made.
- Colleting more than four samples in a day (24 hour period) is not advisable.

(ii) ***Procedure for blood sample collection from dorsal pedal vein:*** For collection of blood sample from dorsal pedal vein requires animal (rat or mice), rodent handling gloves, cotton, capillary tube and 23G/27G needle and blood sample collection tubes.

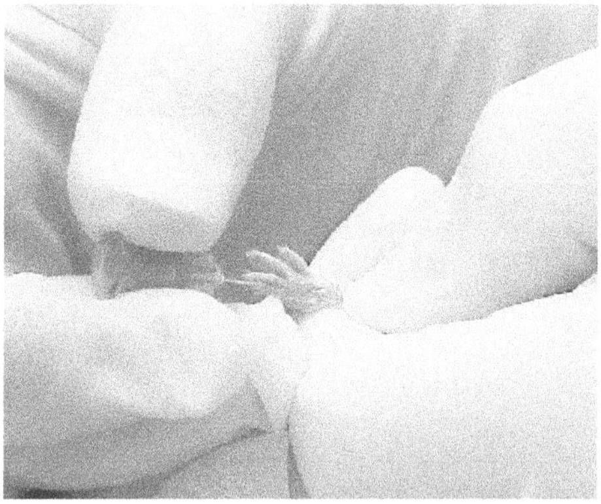

Fig. 2.5 Blood sample collection from dorsal pedal vein.

- The animal is kept in restrainers.
- Medical dorsal pedal vessels are located on top of the foot so hind foot around ankle is held for that.
- The foot is cleaned with absolute alcohol and dorsal pedal vein is punctured with 23G/27G needle.
- Then the drops of blood that would appear on skin surface are collected in a capillary tube and a little pressure is applied to stop the bleeding.

(iii) ***Procedure for blood sample collection from tail vein:*** For collection of blood sample from tail vein requires animal, rodent handling gloves, towel, cotton, sample collection tube and animal warming chamber.

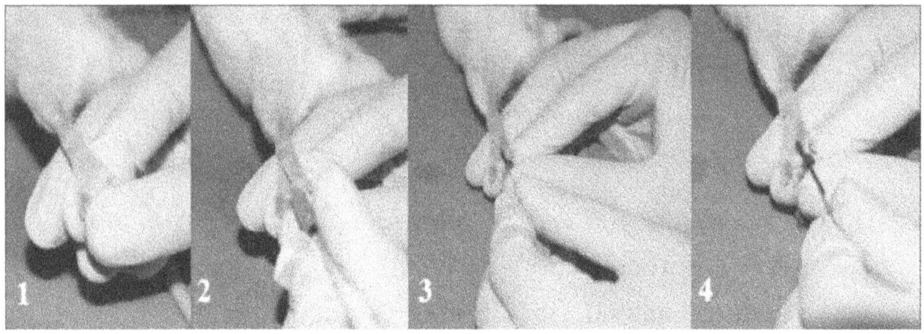

Fig. 2.6 Blood collection from tail vein.

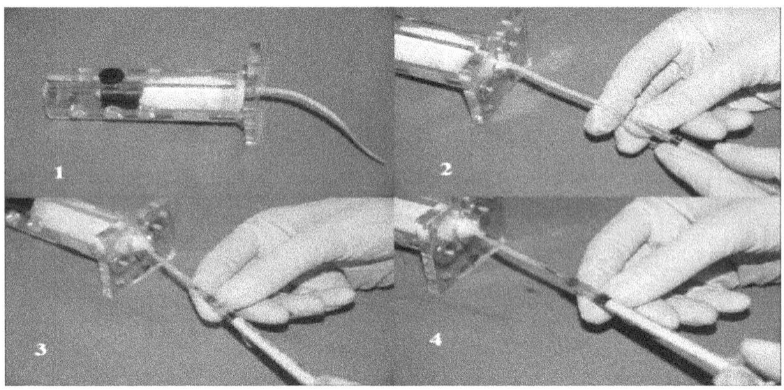

Fig. 2.7 Blood sample collection from tail vein of mouse.

- Whenever large volume of blood sample is required (up to 2 ml/withdrawal) this method is recommended.
- While maintaining the temperature around at 24 to 27 °C, animal is made comfortable in restrainers.
- If the vein is not visible, the tail is dipped into warm water (40 °C), the tail should not be rubbed from the base to tip, as it will result in leukocytosis.
- To avoid pain of tail, local anaesthetic cream must be applied on surface of tail 30 min before the experiment.
- For collection of blood first a 23G needle inserted into blood vessel with the help of capillary tube or syringe with needle blood sample collected.
- In some cases blood collection is very difficult for those animals 0.5 to 1 cm of surface of skin is cut open & the vein is pricked with blood lancet or needle and the blood is collected with capillary tube or a syringe with a needle.

- For that animal after collection of blood lot of bleeding will occurs. Pressure will applies or silver nitrate ointment or solution applied to stop the bleeding.
- If multiple samples are needed, temporary surgical Cannula may be used.
- To avoid or prevent pheromonally induced stress or cross infection, restrainers is washed frequently (Fig. 2.5, 2.6).

(iv) ***Procedure for blood sample collection from tail snip:*** For collection of blood sample from tail snip it requires animal, anesthetic agent, cotton, surgical blade and blood sample collection tubes.

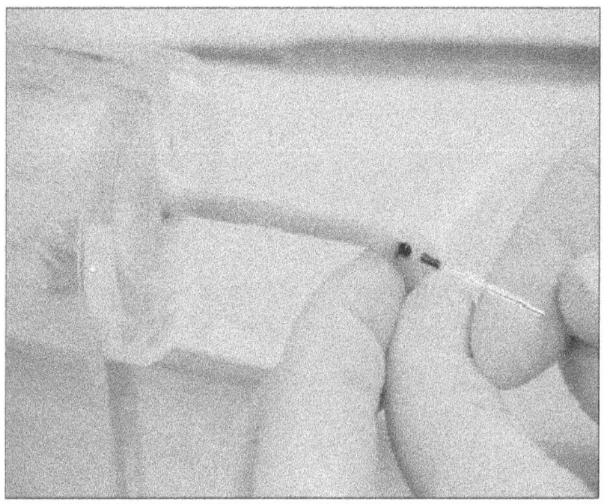

Fig. 2.8 Blood sample collection from tail snip.

- For collection of blood from mice this method is recommended.
- This method can cause potential permanent damage on animal tail, so this method should be avoided as far as possible. If this method is needed it should be done under terminal anaesthesia only.
- Local anaesthetic is applied on tail before collecting the blood by using scalped blade a cut is made 1 mm from the tip of the tail. After collection of blood, blood flow is stopped by dabbing the tail tip.

(v) ***Procedure for blood collection from orbital sinus:*** For collection of blood sample from orbital it requires animal, anesthetic agent, cotton, capillary tube and blood sample collection tube.

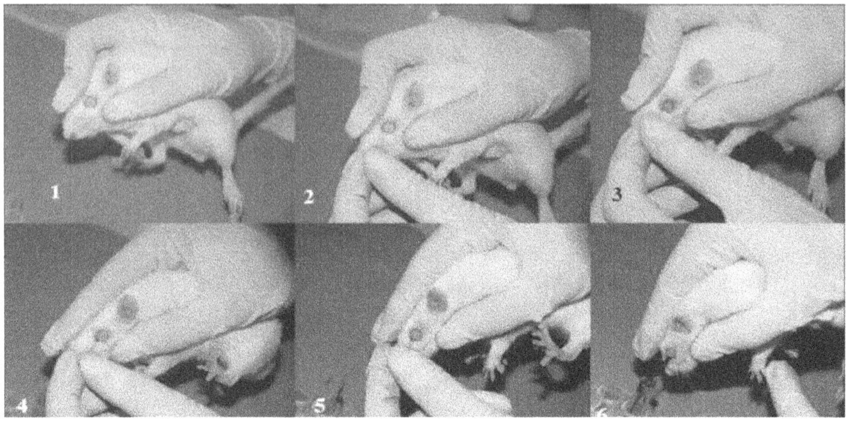

Fig. 2.9 Blood sample collection from orbital sinus.

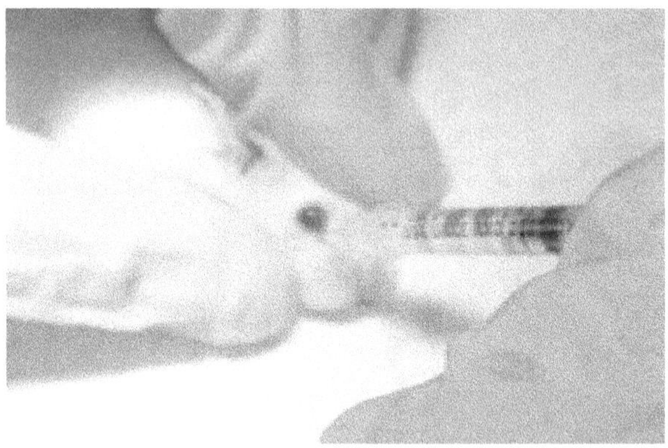

Fig. 2.10 Blood sample collection from orbital vein.

- This method is also called periorbital, posterior orbital and orbital venous plexus bleeding. This technique is used with recovery in experimental circumstances.
- Topical ophthalmic anaesthetic agent is applied to the eye before bleeding.
- The animal skin around the eye is pulled taut and scuffed with thumb and fore finger of the nondominant hand.
- A capillary is inserted into 30 degree angle to nose at the medial canthus of the eye.
- To puncture the tissue slight thumb pressure is enough and enter the plexus or sinus.

- Blood will come through the capillary tube after puncture of plexus or sinus.
- Capillary tube gently removed after required volume of blood is collected from plexus. Bleeding can be stopped by wiping with sterile cotton by applying gentle finger pressure.
- 30 min after blood collection animal is checked for periorbital postoperative lesions.

Caution

- For collection of blood in this method lot of skill is required.
- Repeated blood sampling is not recommended.
- Eyes may damage even by minor mistake also.
- Time requires between two collection is two weeks.
- So many adverse effects reported by this method, which includes hematoma, corneal ulceration, keratitis, pannus formation, rupture of the globe, damage of optic nerve and the intra orbital structures and neroti dacryoadenitis of harderian gland.

(vi) ***Procedure for blood collection from jugular vein:*** For collection of blood in this method requires animal, anesthetic agent, cotton, 25G needle and blood sample collection tubes.

- This method is useful while collecting micro volumes to 1 ml of blood sample. In this method warming of animals is not required.
- In this method 2 persons are needed to collect blood sample from the animal. This method has to be carried out under general or inhalation anaesthesia.
- One person has to restrain the animal and monitor the animal. Another person is required to collect the blood sample from the animal.
- The jugular veins appear blue in colour and is found 2 to 4 mm lateral to sternoclavicular junction. The neck region of animal is shaved and kept in hyper extended position.
- A 25G needle is inserted in the caudocephalic direction (back to front) and blood is withdrawn slowly to avoid collapse of these small blood vessels.
- Animal has to be handled carefully and not more than 3 to 4 mm of needle is to be inserted into the blood vessel.

- If the attempt to collect fails, one more attempt can be made if there is no bleeding otherwise the needle is slowly removed and the site is monitored for bleeding.
- Further attempts should be avoided in case of bleeding as it may collapse the view.
- To stop bleeding finger pressure is applied.
- Number of attempts is limited to three.
- Apply local anaesthetic cream 30 minutes prior to sampling.

(vii) ***Procedure for blood sample collection with temporary cannula:*** For blood collection in this method requires animals, anaesthetic agent, cotton, 25G needle, animal warming chamber and blood sample collection tubes.

- Usually this method, cannulation is made in the tail vein and used for a few hours.
- Local anaesthetic cream is applied on the tail (1.2 cm above the tail tip) the animal is restrained after collection.
- The tail is either cannulated or a 25G needle is used.
- Normally animal to be warmed for tail bleeding in order to dilate the blood vessels (37-39 °C for 5-15 min).
- After cannulation, in large cages animal has to be housed individually.

(viii) ***Procedure for blood vessel cannulation:*** For collection of blood by this method requires animal, anesthetic agent, cotton, 25G needle, i.v. cannula, surgical blade, heparin (or any anticoagulant) and blood sample collection tubes.

- If experiment needs continuous is done in any part of animal like femoral artery, femoral veins, carotid artery, femoral viens, arotid, artery jugular vein, vena cava and dorsal aorta.
- After giving of appropriate anaesthesia only cannula is inserted by surgery. Analgesics should be used to minimize the pain.
- Animal should be housed singly in a large and spacious cage after surgical cannulation.
- Blood sample may be collected over 24 hour at the volume of 0.1 of 0.2 ml per every sample.

- After withdrawing the blood, the cannula is flushed with anti coagulant and withdrawn volume of blood may be replaced if required Cannula should be close tightly. [Fig. 2.11].

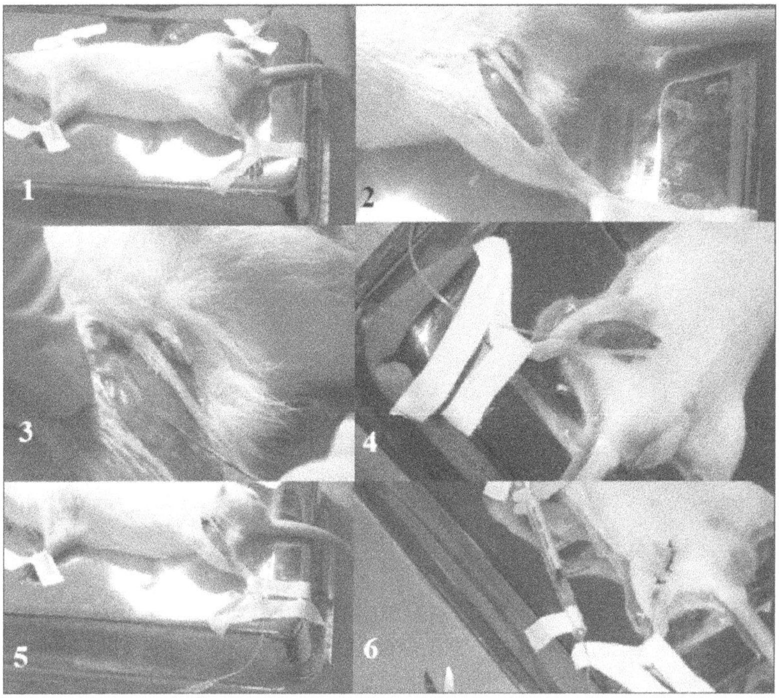

Fig. 2.11 Blood vessel cannulation of rat femoral vein.

- The experiment has to be conducted fully under aseptic precounting only. Sometimes there is a chance of infections, haemorrhage, blockage of cannula and swelling around the cannulation site may happens precautions should be taken to avoid these problems.

The needle size and maximum blood volume to be collected are also important factors in blood sample collection process.

Table 2.2 Needle size and maximum collection volume in different species.

Species	Needle to be used	Max collection vol.
Mice	23-25G	1 ml
Rat	19-21G	10-15 ml
Rabbit	19-21G	60-200 ml
Guinea pig	20-21G	1-25 ml

(ix) ***Procedure for blood sample collection from tarsal vein:*** For collection of blood sample in this method required animal, anaesthetic agent, cotton, 22G needle, hair remover and blood sample collection tubes.

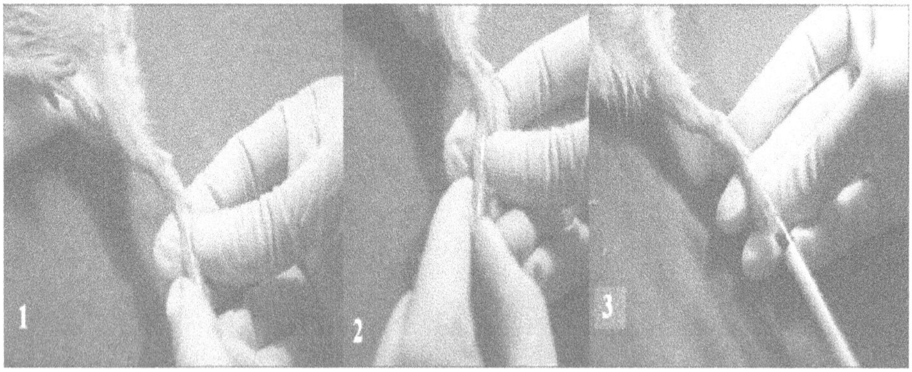

Fig. 2.12 Blood sample collection from guinea pig tarsal vein.

- This method is commonly recommended for guinea pigs. Tarsal vein is identified in one of the hind legs of large animal.
- 2 persons requires for blood collection in this method. One person has to restrain the animal properly. 2nd person has to be collect blood sample.
- By applying of suitable hair remover, surface hairy are removed. Local anaesthetic cream is applied on collection site. After 20 to 25 minutes of local anaesthetic, blood sample is collected slowly by using 22G needle.
- 0.1 to 0.3 ml of blood can be collected per sample, maximum three samples can be taken per leg. After the sample collection gentle pressure is applied with finger for 2 minutes to stop bleeding [Fig 2.11].
- Caution to be taken when blood collection by this method, not more than six samples from both hind legs are taken. The number of attempts is three or less.

(x) ***Procedure for marginal ear vein or artery blood sample collection:*** For blood collection in this method requires animals, anaesthetic agent, cotton 26G needle, 95% v/v alcohol, o-xylen, surgical blade and blood sample collection tube.

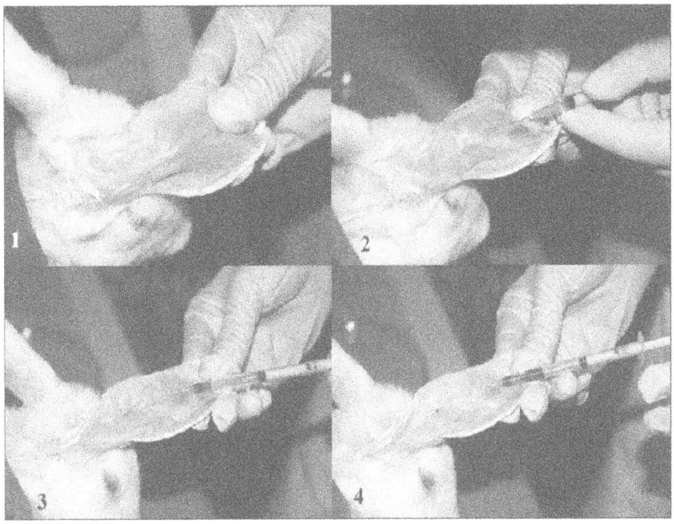

Fig. 2.13 Blood sample collection from rabbit marginal ear vein using 26G needle.

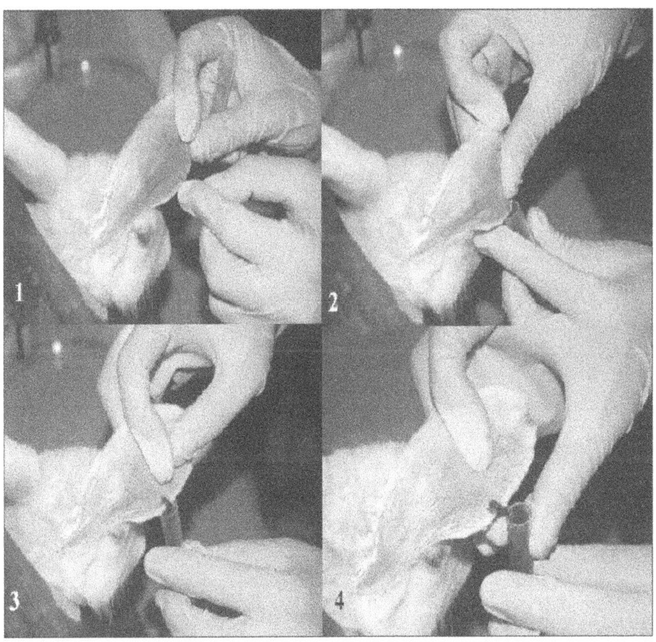

Fig. 2.14 Blood sample collection from rabbit marginal ear vein using incision method.

- For blood sample collection from rabbits this method is adopted.
- The animals should be placed in a restrainer.

- Ear is cleaned with 95% v/v alcohol and local anaesthetic cream is applied on collection site 10 min prior to sampling. If requires vasodilators also applies to dilate the blood vessels (like o-xylene, topical vasodilators).
- 26G needle may be used to collect blood from animal marginal vein. Sometimes size 11 surgical blade is used to cut the marginal ear vein and then blood is collected in colleting tube.
- Sterile cotton is kept on the collection site, after collecting blood and finger pressure is applied to stop the bleeding.

(xi) ***Procedure for cardiac puncture:*** For blood collection in this method required animal, anaesthetic agent, towel, and cotton, 19-25 G needle with 1 to 5 ml syringe, surgical blade, tube (internal diameter of 0.1 to 0.3 mm) for thoracotomy, plastic disposable bag and blood sample collection tubes.

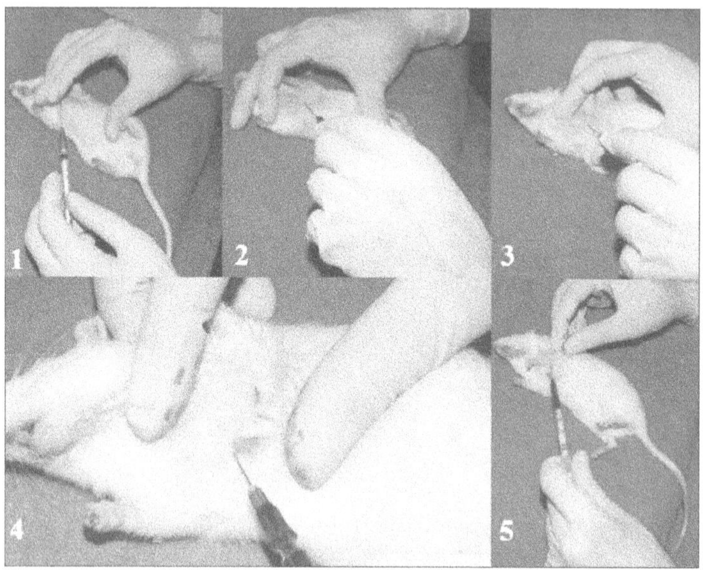

Fig. 2.15 Blood sample collection through cardiac puncture in rat.

- In this method blood sample will be taken directly from the heart. Preferable from the ventricle slowly to avoid collapsing of heart.
- Normally, cordial puncture is recommended for terminal stage of the study to collect single, good quality and large volume of blood from the experimental animals.

- During blood sample collection, animal will be in terminal anaesthesia.
- For blood sample collection appropriate needle is used, with or without thoracotomy.
- If animal has dextrocardia, sampling may fail.

(xii) ***Procedure for blood sample collection through posterior vena cava:*** For blood collection by this method requires animal, anaesthetic agent, surgical blade, small glass rods, surgical scissors, 21 to 25G needle with 1 or 5 ml syringe and blood sample collection tube.

- In terminal stage of study, posterior vena cava blood sample method is recommended.
- Animal have to be anesthetized and 'Y' or 'V' shaped cut in the abdomen is mad and the intestine are gently removed.
- The liver is pushed forward and the posterior vena cava. (Between the kidneys) is identified.
- 21 to 25G needle is inserted to collect blood from the posterior vena cava.
- This procedure will be repeated 3 to 4 times to collect more volume of blood sample.

Blood collection from the experimental animals is one of the important procedures in biomedical research. Even a small error in the collection procedure may lead to a lot of variation in the results. Before starting any kind of blood sample collection, it must be ensured that all chemical, surgical, fluid requirements are available in the working site. Not more than two to three attempts should be made to collect any kind of *in vitro* biological sample (excluding biological secretion). The blood collection tube must be labeled before starting the experiment and blood sample collected in the appropriately labeled collection tube.

2.4 LABORATORY ANIMALS

2.4.1 Breeding Techniques

The most important species of laboratory animals-Tests performed

- ***Mouse:*** Most frequently used. Pharmacology, genetics of mammals, virology, models of human diseases (mutant strains, transgenic and knock-out mice)
- ***Rat:*** Physiology of cognitive processes, behaviour, models of diabetes
- ***Rabbit:*** Serology, insulin quantification, pyrogens quantification, tests of irritable effect of chemical substances on the cornea

- ***Cat:*** Study of CNS and respiratory system
- ***Dog:*** E.g., beagle, use in electrophysiology, neurophysiology
- ***Guinea-pig:*** In microbiology and serology, physiology of the auditory system
- ***Hamster:*** Genetics
- ***Pig:*** Training of surgical techniques, temporary covering of burns with porcine skin
- ***Primates:*** Rhesus monkey, baboon, chimpanzee – use in neurology, virology, behaviour
- ***Frog:*** Physiology of blood circulation, electrophysiology
- Fish, molluscs, insects etc.

Animal laws: Cruelty – wild life – control

The constitution of India

The Indian penal code, 1860

The criminal procedure code, 1973

The prevention of Cruelty to Animals Act, 1960

The wild life Protection Act, 1972

The Policy Acts

The Municipal Corporation Acts

Animal regulations: Animal Welfare Act (AWA) (Public Law 89-544, 1966) is the principal Federal statute governing the sale, handling, transport and use of animals.

The AWA applies to all species of warm blooded vertebrate animals used to research, testing, or teaching, except for mice, rats, birds and farm animals.

Animal regulation – AWA: The United States Department of Agriculture (USDA), Animal and Plant Health Inspection Service (APHIS)/Animal Care (AC) implements the AWA through the Animal Welfare Regulations (AWR) codified at the code of Federal Regulations, title 9, Chapter 1, Sub chapter A, Parts 1, 2 and 3.

Animal regulation – PHS: Health Research Extension Act of 1985.

(Public Law 99-158) provides the Public Health Service (PHS) Policy on Humane Care and use of Laboratory Animals (PHS Policy).

- PHS Policy mandates that institutions use the Guide as a basis for developing and implementing an animal care and use program.
- The *Guide* for the care and use of laboratory animals (GUIDE) prepared by the institute for laboratory animal research, National Academy of Sciences

is a widely accepted primary reference on animal care and use that offers guidance throughout these principles.

- Office of Laboratory Animal Welfare (OLAW) with the Department of Health and Human Services (DHHS) has the responsibility for the general administration and coordination of the PHS policy.
- PHS policy mandates that no activity involving animals may be conducted or supported until the institution conducting the activity has filled a written assurance with OLAW.

Genetics of laboratory animals

Laboratory animals are genetically 3 types

1. Isogenic [genetically defined strains].
2. Non-Isogenic [genetically undefined strains].
3. Genetically semi-defined strains.

1. ***Isogenic animals:*** These are the animals which are genetically defined as genetic uniformity of all individuals.
    - *Inbreed strains:* These strains obtained by close breeding for more than 20 generations (brother + sister or offspring + one of the parents).
    - Homozygosis higher than 98% (degree of homozygosis is expressed as a coefficient of in breeding).
    - The main features of these type of animals are isogenicity (genetic uniformity), phenotype uniformity (low variability of reactivity) usually low fertility, disposition to diseases.
    - Main advantage of this breed in experiment individuals is sufficient.
    - Main disadvantage of this breed in experiment is a risk that the findings are strain specific and are not valid for other strains, problematic generalization of the result.

    A. Coisogenic strains: (Mutant strains): In this type of breed, the animals are differing from the original strain only in one gene, in which a mutation occurred.

    B. Cogenic strains:
    - This type of strains originated by cross breeding of two strains and following back cross breeding with one of the original strains (at least 10 times, selection of some specific feature)
    - Presence of specific genes of one strain of genetically back ground of the second strains.

    C. Recombinant-inbred strains: Crossing of 2 strains, the hybrids give origin of new lines which are then crossed brother x sister, which leads to establish of a new strains.

D. Recombinant-Cogenic strains: In this type of breeding crossing of 2 strains followed with 3 back crosses to one of the original strains and inbreeding with crossing brother x sister (at least 14 times).

E. Consomic strains: This method is more complicated. A complete chromosome of one strain is transferred on the back ground of the second strain with back crosses.

2. ***Non isogenic strains:*** Out breed lines: In this type of breeding some level of phenotype variability (higher variability of reactivity) is possible and also highly fertility rate occurs.

   These animals are resistant to diseases.

   - Main advantage of these breed animals in experiments are cheaper, easier production, the finding have more general validity.
   - Main disadvantage of this breed animals in experiments are less homogeneous set, higher number of animals is necessary.

3. ***Genetically semi defined methods:*** In this method strains are prepared by genetically heterogenous lines and also by out bred selected lines.

   - Genetically heterogenous lines are originated by crossing of several inbred strains followed with breeding according to principles of outbred population.

Scheme of barrier facility

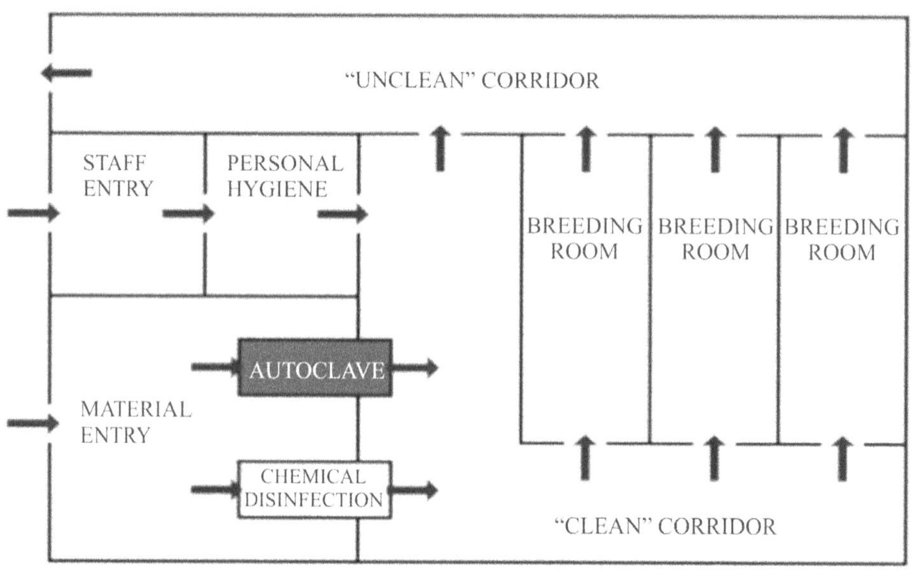

Fig. 2.16 Scheme of barrier facility.

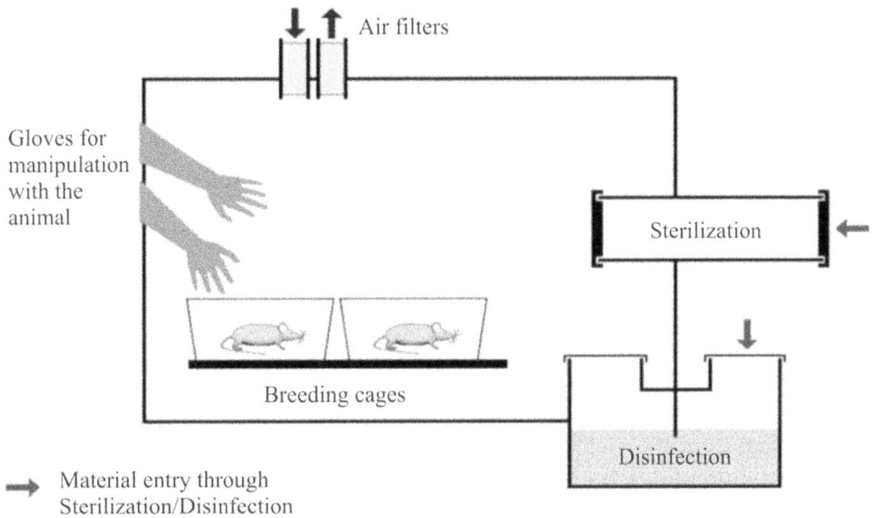

Fig. 2.17 Scheme of Isolator.

2.4.2 GLP (Good Laboratory Practices)

For animal facilities is intended to assure quality maintenance and safety of animals used in laboratory studies while conducting biochemical and behavioral research and testing of products.

The exact definition depends on who is defining it and for what purpose.

A broad definition encompasses such issues as

- Organization of the laboratory
- Management
- Personnel
- Facilities
- Equipments
- Operation
- Method validation
- Quality assurance and
- Record keeping

Good laboratory practices

The goal is to certify that every step of the analysis is valid. The aspects that need to be particularly addressed will vary by laboratory.

Good Laboratory practices can be defined as "a body of rules, operating procedures and practices established by a given organization that are considered to be mandatory with a view to ensuring quality and correctness in the results produced by a laboratory".

Good Laboratory Practices Established by worldwide bodies such as

- Organization for Economic Co-operation and Development (OECD)
- International Organization for Standardization (ISO)

2.5 TRANSGENIC ANIMALS

Transgenic animal is an animal whose gene composition has been altered by the addition of foreign (exogenous) DNA – is said to be transgenic animal. Using the recently introduced transgenic technology. Well defined tissue specific genetic alterations can be produced in animals that may result in specific pathological condition. These are useful tools in biomedical research. Thus a transgenic animal can be defined as "one whose genome has been altered in a heritable manner by introduction of a foreign DNA sequence into genome of its zygote or embryo". The foreign gene is constructed using recombinant DNA technology.

In addition to structured gene, the DNA usually includes other sequences to enable it.

- To be incorporated into the DNA of the host.
- To be expressed correctly by the cells of the host.

The DNA that is introduced is called transgenic and over all the process is called Transgenesis.

Advantages of transgenic animals

- Increased growth rate.
- Improved disease resistance.
- Improved food conversion rates.
- Leaner meat.
- Increased wool quality.

Disadvantages

- Inserted gene has more than one function.
- Breeding problems.
- Expensive.
- Sometime leads to mutagenesis and functional disorders.
- Low survival rate of transgenic animals.

Some of the goals of transgenic animal creation are

- Research into animal and human diseases.
- Improve lifetime of animals.
- Use of animals as bio reactors.
- The transgenic animals prove to be valuable sources of proteins for human therapy.

Example: Normal mice cannot be infected with poliovirus.

They had the cell surface molecule that, in humans serves as the receptor for the virus.

So normal mice cannot serves as easily manipulated model for studying the disease. Transgenic mice expressing the human gene for the poliovirus receptor.

The methods involve to produce or to make transgenic animals.

- The embryonic stem cell method (method 1)
- The pronuclear method (method 2)
- Retrovirus mediated gene transfer (method 3)

The embryonic stem cell method

Embryonic stem cell is harvested from the inner (1 cm) cell mass of mouse blast cysts. They can be grown in cell culture and retain their full potential to produce all cells of natural animal, including its gemmates after they are reintroduced into another blast cyst embryo. Such cells are called pluripotent embryonic stem cells.

- *Make the DNA using recombinant DNA methods:* Build the molecules of DNA containing a vector DNA to enable the molecules to be inserted into host DNA molecule
- *Transforming ES cells in culture:* Expose the cultured cells to the DNA so that some will re corporate it.
- Select for successfully transformed cells.
- Inject three cells into inner cell mass (1 cm) blast cysts.
- ES cells carrying an integrated transgenic can cultured and inserted into blast cyst stage embryo.
- *Embryo transfer:* Embryo can be implanted into pseudo pregnant foster mother. The stimulus of mating elicits the normal changes needed. Transfer the embryos into her uterus only. Hope that they implant successfully and develop into healthy pups.
- *Establish a transgenic strain:* Mate two heterozygous mice and screen their off spring for the 1:4 that will be homogenous for the transgenic.

Pronuclear method

- Prepare the DNA
- Transforming fertilized eggs. [Implant the embryos in a pseudo pregnant foster mother and produced as in method 1]. Establishing transgenic mice with genetically engineered ES cells. An ES cell culture is initiated from the inner cell mass of a mouse blast cyst.

The ES cells are transferred with a transgenic. After growth, the transfect cells are identified by either the positive – negative selection procedure or PCR analysis.

Retrovirus mediated gene transfer

Gene transfer is mediated by means of a carrier or vector, generally a virus or a plasmid. Retroviruses are commonly used as vectors. Normally killed virus has replication defective. The virus gene is replaced with transgene. The transgene is delivered to the host cell by transfection (gene therapy), it can be used to transfect a wide range of cells.

DNA micro injection method

Because of disadvantage of the retroviral vector method, micro injection of DNA is currently the preferred method for producing transgenic mice.

This Procedure involves following steps

- The number of available fertilized eggs that are to be inoculated by micro injection is increased by stimulating donor females to super ovulate.
- Female mice are given an initial injection of about 48 hours later, of human chronic gonadotropin.
- Super ovulated mouse produce about 35 eggs instead of the normal 5 -10.
- The super ovulated females are mated and then the fertilized eggs are flushed from their oviduct.
- Micro injection of fertilized eggs usually occurs immediately after their collection.
- The micro injected transgenic constant is often linear form and free of prokaryotic vector DNA sequences.
- In mammals, after the entry of sperm into egg, both the sperm nucleus (male nucleus) and formal nucleus are separate entities.
- Different models for transgenic animals are used for Alzheimer's disease, Atherosclerosis, Hypertension, Cardiac hyper trophy.

Different animals which can be genetically modified

- Mice
- Sheep
- Goat
- Chicken
- Pigs
- Fish
- Guinea pigs
- Rabbits
- Cows
- Rats
- Cats
- Dog
- Horse

Transgenic cows: Dairy cows carrying extra copies of two types of care in genes produce 13% more milk protein and also that milk more nutritious and contain more cheese [reviewed under FDA].

Transgenic microbes: Genetically modified bacteria are used to produce the protein insulin to treat diabetes. Similarly bacteria have been used to produce clotting factors to treat hemophilia and human growth hormone to treat various forms of diseases.

Transgenic sheep: The first transgenic animal to produce a recombinant protein in sheep milk. Uses of Transgenic and Genetically modified sheep are

- Has more immunity.
- Has human blood clotting factor.
- Used to transplantation.
- Used to hematology.
- Used to biological product manufacturing.
- Used to form recombinant DNA.
- More production of milk.

Transgenic rabbit: Used to Study

- Hemorrhagic disease
- Gene mutation
- Cell metabolism

- Eye disease
- Heart problems
- Atherosclerosis
- Retinal regeneration

Transgenic monkey: Similar to human so used in clinical trials.

Used for study of HIV, Huntington's disease

Disadvantage

- Expensive
- Difficult to handle
- Breeding problems

Transgenic fish: Most have extra copies of growth hormone can grow up to 6 times faster than wild type fish.

Transgenic pigs: The transgenic pigs expressing phytase production in the salivary glands to overcome nutritional deficiency

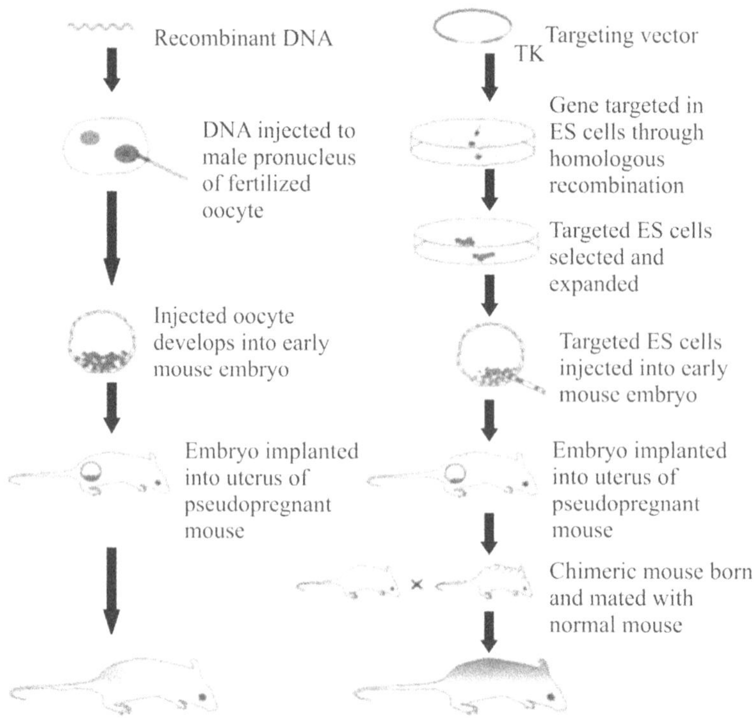

Fig. 2.18 Transgenic mouse and knockin or knockout mouse.

2.6 KNOCKOUT ANIMALS

Gene Knockout

A gene knockout is a genetic technique in which an organism is engineered to carry the genes that have been made inoperative (have been knock out of the organism). Also known as knock out organisms or simply knockouts. They are used in learning about a gene that has been sequenced, but which has an unknown incompletely known action.

- Knocking out 2 genes simultaneously in organisms is known as a double knock out (DKO). Similarly the term Triple Knockout (TKO) and Quadra pole Knockouts (QKO) are used to describe 3/4 knocked out genes.
- Knock out is accomplished through a combination of techniques being in the test tube with a plasmid bacterial artificial chromosomes or DNA construct. Individual's cells are genetically transformed with DNA construct. The Goal is to create transgenic animal that has the altered genes.

Knockin

- Knockin is similar to knockout, but instead it replace a gene with another instead of deleting it means replace of the mouse own gene with a new gene.
- The first knockout mice were created by Mario R.Capechi, Mratin Evans and Oliver smithies in 1989. For which they were awarded the noble prize for medicine in 2007.

Knockout Mouse

- A knockout mouse is a genetically engineered mouse in which one or more genes have been turned off through a targeted mutation.
- Knockout mice are important animal models for studying of the role of the geneses which have been sequenced.
- By causing a specific gene to be inactive in the mouse, and observing a difference from normal behaviors or condition.
- *For Example:* A laboratory mouse in which a gene affecting hair growth has been knockout. So, it becomes hairless.
- Knockout is the activity of a gene provides information about what the gene normally does. So that the information can be used to understand how a similar gene may cause disease in humans.

Knockout mice application

Examples of research in which knockout mice have been useful include studying and modeling different kinds of diseases like

Cancer

Obesity

Heart Disease

Diabetes

Arthritis

Substance abuse

Anxiety

Aging

Parkinson's disease

Different strains of knockout mice

Many models are named after the gene that has been inactivated for example.

P^{53} Knockout mice: It is named after the P^{53} gene which codes for a protein that normally suppressed growth of tumors by arresting cell division. Human born with mutations that deactivates the P^{53} gene from **Li-Fraumeni** syndrome, a condition that dramatically increase the risk of developing bone cancers, breast cancer, blood cancer at an early stage.

Rhodopsin knockout mice

- Inactivation of the mouse Rhodopsin gene by targeted gene disruption lead to deterioration of the rod cells in retinitis pigmentosa. Thus, the progression of retinal degeneration and the effects of possible therapeutic agents that might either delay or block the genetically induced retinopathy can be studied by using the Rhodopsin Knockout mice.
- **Cre – LoxP** recombination system for inactivating a gene in specified cell.
- The **cre gene** is isolated and place under the control of a tissue specific promoter (P^{53}).
- Transgenic mice with the cre gene construct are established, and the tissue specificity of the cre gene activity is confirmed.
- Lox P sites with repeat sequences in the same direction are inserted on either of a clone DNA sequences.
- A segment of DNA that is flanked by lox P site is set to be floxed.
- The construct with lox P site is introduced into a chromosome site of embryonic stem cells by hologus recombination.
- So these cells are selected, cultured and established a transgenic mice line.

- Then, the two transgenic lines are crossed.
- In cells, where both construct are present the cre recombination's is synthesized, and 2 cre gene molecules bind to each lox P site.
- The lox P site undergo recombination leading to the excision and circularization of lox P site and an exon (2) that is eventually degraded and the formation of a inactivated gene that is retained in the chromosomes.

Advantages

- The Cre – LoxP technology has been extensively to study the biological consequences of tissue specific gene inactivation with the goals of establishing models for human disease.

Example

- Selective removal of the kinsen II gene which is expressed exclusively in retinal photoreceptor cells, leads to an accumulation of opsin and arrest in and eventually to cell death.
- It can be used for detailed studies of the pathophysiological effects on the retina.

Nude mice: Nude mice is a laboratory animal, it is wildly useful to screening the drugs used to treat tumours. The nude mouse is very valuable animal to research because it can receive many different types of tissue and tumor grafts, at the same time it has no rejection response. Nude mouse is a laboratory mouse from a strain with a genetic mutation that causes a deteriorated or absent thymus. In absence of thymus animal gets inhibited immune system due to greatly reduced number of T cells. It leads to main changes in outside appearance of mouse as lack of body hair. The main genetic basis of the mouse mutation is a disruption of the FOXNI gene.

Nomenclature for the nude mouse has changed several times since their discovery. When the time of discovery it is discredited as nu

- After that it is updated to HFHIINU when the mutated gene was identified as mutation in the HNF – 3/forehead handing II gene.
- After this in 2000 it is updated as FOXNINU mutation was identified as member of Fox gene family. Because of lack a thymus, nude mice cannot generate mature T lymphocytes. So they are unable to mount most types of immune responses like,
  - ➢ Antibody formation (that requires CD4 + helper T cells)

- Cell mediated immune responses, (which requires CD4+ and/or CD8+ Tells)
- Delayed type hypersensitivity responses (which requires CD4+ T cells)
- Graft rejection (which requires both CD4+ and CD8+ T cells).

Because of these features, nude mice have served in laboratory screening of drugs used to treat leukemia, solid tumors, AIDS and other forms of immune deficiency as well as leprosy.

These nude mice cannot reject grafts, not even reject Xenografts (that is grats of tissue from and other species). This features of nude mice because of absence of functioning T cells.

- For this reason, nude mice are slightly "leaky" and do have a few T ells, especially as their age about this reason nude mice are less popular in research today, since knockout mice complete defects in the immune system have been constructed (E.g., RAG I and RAG II Knockout mice).

Life span: The life span of nude mice is normally 6 months to a year.

NIH Swiss Athymic nude mice are bred and maintained under strict environmental conditions. The NU mutation was first reported in 1966 in a lab in Glasgow, Scotland. But it was two years later that it was discovered that a homozygous nude mouse also for studying allograft, xenografts, tumorogenicity and cancer metastasis.

Although the nude mouse lacks T cells, it has a normal complement of a bone dependent B cells. Nude mice also have elevated levels of both macrophages and NK cells; their macrophages are also more potent than those from mice with a normal functioning thymus.

Some other characteristics include

- A high incidence of glomerulonephritis by three months of age. This includes higher than normal deposits of IgG, IgM and IgA.
- Have normal hair growth cycles despite a hairless state.
- Have a low incidence of nonsuppurative dermatitis.
- Low incidence of Keratoacanthoma and Squamous carcinoma.
- Very high incidence of corneal vasculrization.

Table 2.3 Applications of gene knockout animals.

Sr. No.	Different Strains	Research Applications
1.	The pound mouse mutation was mapped to a region with less than 2 cm of the leptin on chromosome 4	Obesity, hyper insulinaemia, insulin resistance dyslipidaemia, fatty liver disease
2.	NU/NU Nude mouse	Tumour biology and Xeno graft Research
3.	NIH-III Nude mouse	Tumour biology and Xeno graft research
4.	PGP mouse (p- Glycoprotein deficient)	PGP deficient BBB multi drug sensitive for neuro biology, chemotherapy, toxicology, transport excretion involving methods
5.	CD-1-E Mouse	Pseudo Pregnancy Safety and efficacy rating
6.	CD2,F1 (CDF1) Mouse	Transplanting research
7.	CD-1-E Mouse Lacks thymus T-cells	Tumour biology Xenon graft research
8.	BALB/C Mouse	Hybridoma development monoclonal antibody production infectious disease.
9.	SJL-E Mouse FVB Mouse	Immunology, Retinal infectious disease
10.	NOBLE Rat	Prostate carcinoma model
11.	OPCD Rat (Observe Prone CD rat)	Obesity metabolic syndrome
12.	SHR Rat (Spontaneous Hypertensive)	Genetic hypertension model
13.	PCK Rat	Polycystic kidney disease.
14.	ZDF Rat (Zucker Diabetic Fatty)	Glucose intolerance hyper insulinaemia.
15.	FHH Rat	Pulmonary hypertension
16.	Long Evans rat	Behavioral research
17.	Copenhagen rat	Carcinogenesis research
18.	Buffalo Rat	Carcinogenesis
19.	Guinea Pig IAF hairless Guinea Pig	Dermatology
20.	Rabbit LVG Golden Syrian hamster	General multipurpose model

CHAPTER 3

ALTERNATIVE TO ANIMALS

3.1 INTRODUCTION

Toxicity studies are generally performed to determine drug related effects that cannot be evaluated to standard pharmacology profile.

They are occurring only after repeated administration of the drug on animals. To perform toxicity studies rodents and non rodents are preferable to evaluate, then so many unexpected adverse effects are possible. During the last 100 years these were largely depended on research with animals. So use of animals in scientific research and testing has raised controversy and criticism for long.

The scientific and legislative authorities and animal right activity throughout the world have been demanding the abolition of the animal experiments in the laboratory advocating the development of some alternatives. The use of animals to test drug is unfortunately necessary to safe guard human health.

Striking a balance between these two views RUSSELL & BURCH in 1959 developed the concept of 3R's alternatives that can minimize to a great extent the use of animals in the area of drug development and testing.

3R's are as follows

- Refinement
- Reduction
- Replacement

Refinement

- To minimize the incidence or severity of in human procedures
- To decrease potential pain or distress to animals

Reduction

- To reduce the number of animals used in study.
- In past large number of animals required for regular requirements of vaccine control. By following the principle of 3 R's, there has been significant reduction in the animal use.

Replacement

- Substitution of insentient material in place of conscious higher animals i.e., experiment should not be performed in animals if suitable and scientifically proven non animal method is available.
- *In vitro* studies like perfused organs

  Tissue slices

  Tissue culture

  Cellular and sub cellular fractions.
- To avoid the animal usage in new drug discovery these alternative to animal studies were developed.
- It is not possible to replace whole animal model with *in vitro* systems to evaluate drug effects on major organ systems. However techniques can greatly reduce the number of animals needed and refined protocols can improve the design efficiency and quality of studies and lessen stress and discomfort experienced by lab animals.

Definition of alternatives technique

- The term alternative is used to refer to those techniques or method that replace the use of laboratory animals altogether. Reduce the number of animals required or refine an existing procedure or technique to minimize the level of stress endured by the animals.
- This concept now wide spread throughout the scientific community.
- The JOHNS HOPKINS Center for Alternatives to Animal Testing (CAAT) was founded in 1981 and is structured to support four core programmes.

Those methods are

- *In vitro* methods [Full thickness skin model].
- *In silico* methods.
- Cell line techniques.
- Patch clamp techniques.
- Computer aid drug designing methods.

Bio technology department is very broad sense to make useful products. Particularly gene technology is especially important to pharmaceuticals in the manufacturing of vaccines, development of more diagnostic aids and therapeutic agents and ultimately in gene dosing and expression of genes. Peptide engineering generation and use of various antibodies, mammalian cell cultures and transgenic techniques.

3.1.1 *In vitro* Methods

Instead of using animals, cell and tissue culture can be used to test drugs.

3.1.2 *In silico* Methods

Substance with similar chemical structures often has similar properties. The required calculations are performed using specially developed computer programs.

3.1.3 Cell Line Techniques

The term cell line refers to the propagation of culture after the first sub culture. Once the primary culture is sub cultured it becomes cell line. A cell line derived by selection or cloning is referred to as cell strain. Cell strain does not have infinite life, as they die after some divisions.

Types of cell lines

- Finite cell line.
- Continuous cell line.

Applications of cell lines

- Screening of anti cancer drugs.
- Cell based bioassay.
- To determine the cytotoxicity.
- *In vitro* screening of several drugs.
- Production of anti viral vaccines.
- Cell fusion technique.
- Genetic manipulation.
- Gene therapy.
- Recombinant DNA therapy.
- Molecular biology etc.

3.1.4 Patch Clamp Technique

The technique developed by Erwin Nether and Bert Sakmann. Patch clamp technique is a technique in electrophysiology that allows the study of individual ion channels in cells.

Use a pipette to pinch off a small region of membrane.

Types of patch clamp

- Inside out.
- Whole cell.
- Outside out.

Applications of patch clamp technique

- For evaluation of anti arrhythmic agents in kidney cell.
- In CVS drugs evaluation.
- To identify multiple types of calcium channels.
- Used in molecular biology.
- Voltage clamp studies on sodium channels.
- Used to investigate a wide range of electro physical cell properties.
- Measurement of all membrane conductance.

3.1.5 Computer Aid Drug Designing

- Computers are an essential tool in modern medicinal chemistry and are important in both drug discovery and drug development.
- Rapid advances in computer hardware and software have meant that many of the operations.

Uses in various operations

- Molecular modeling's – which calculate structure and property results from bond stretching, angle bonding and non bonded interactions and torsinal energies. Quantum physics used to calculate the properties of molecule.
- Drawing chemical structure – some drawing packages linked with the software's which allow quick calculations. IUPAC name, molecular formula, molecular weight, exact mass are calculated. NMR, chemical shifts, melting points, freezing point, log P value, molar refractivity is also measured.
- 3D structures of molecule are possible to see in some packages like chem-3D, Sibyl, Alchemy, Hyper chem.
- Possible to automatically convert of a 2 D drawing into a 3 D structure.
- Energy minimization is also possible after 3D structure is built. This calculates the energy of starting molecule varied the bond lengths, bond angles and torsion angles to create a new structure.
- Molecular dimension is possible after 3D structure constructed by measuring all of its bond length, bond angles and torsion angles.

- Various molecular properties of 3D Structure calculated like bond stretching, bond comparison, deformation bond angles, deformed tension angles and also measurement of predicted heat of formulation, dipole movement, electrostatic potential, electric spin density, partial charges.
- Conformational analysis used to identification of most stable conformations and may lead to identification of global minimum.
- X-ray crystallography and comparison or rigid and non rigid liquids methods are used to identify the active conformation.
- Docking procedures are useful to dock or fit a molecule into a model of its binding site.

3.2 CELL LINE TECHNIQUES

The term cell line refers to propagation of culture after the first sub culture. In other words, once the primary culture is sub cultured it becomes cell line.

Such a cell line derived by selection or cloning is referred to as cell strain. Cell strain does not have infinite life, as they die after some divisions.

3.2.1 Types of Cells used in Cell Line

- Precursor/stem cells/master cells.
- Undifferentiated but committed precursor cells.
- Mature differentiated cells.

Animal cell culture technology was first successfully undertaken by – HARRSION in 1907 in order to study behavior of animal cell. He preferred to select frog as source of tissue for his studies

1907	–	Rass Harrison	–	Frog tissue culture Technique
1940	–	R.H.	–	Chick embryo
1950	–	Hela	–	Human Tumor cells

Cell culture is very important to grow cell lines.

3.2.2 Characteristics of Cell Culture

- Cells can be isolated by grading the tissue and subsequent treatment with trypsin.
- Cell line can be obtained by culturing isolated cell.
- Such culture consisting of differentiated cell types are known as primary culture.
- A secondary culture can be established from primary culture by culturing and repeated sub culture.

3.2.3 Requirements

- Clean and quite sterile area.
- Predation facilities.
- Animal house.
- Microbiology laboratory.
- Storage facilities.

3.2.4 Equipments Required

Laminar air flow, sterilizers, incubators, refrigerators, Hemocytometer, fluorometer, microscope, centrifuge, freezer, Balance etc.

3.2.5 Culture Vessels

In tissue culture technology, the cells attach to the surface of a vessel and it serves as a substrate and grows.

3.2.6 Materials used for Culture Vessels

- Glass
- Disposable plastics
- Palladium

3.2.7 Types of Culture Vessels

- Multi well plates.
- Petri dish.
- Flasks.
- Stirrer bottles.

Non adhesive substrates used like Agar, Agarose and Methyl Cellulose.

3.2.8 Culture Media used in Cell Line Technique

The nutrient media used for culture of animal cells tissues must be able to support their survival as well as growth.

A. Natural media
B. Artificial media

A. Natural Media

This is nutrient for perforation and grows of animal cell or tissue.

It contains:

- ***Clots:*** Plasma clots [Prepared from blood of male fowl].
- ***Biological fluids:*** Plasma, serum, lymph, amniotic fluid, ascetic, aqueous humor from eyes.

- *Tissue extracts:* Chick embryo extract most commonly used, other extracts of spleen, liver, bone narrow etc., generally used for organ culture.

B. Artificial Media

- It has been in use since 1950.
- Different artificial media have been devised to serve one of the following purposes.
  1. Immediate survival [balanced salt solution].
  2. Prolonged survival [BSS with serum, organic compound].
  3. Indefinite growth.
  4. Specialized functions.
- Different types of artificial mediums
  (i) Serum containing media
  (ii) Serum free media
  (iii) Chemically defined media
  (iv) Protein free media

(i) Serum containing media:

Example: EMEM

- It supplemented with 5-10% serum culture of most type of cells
- It contains plasma proteins, lipids, carbohydrates, minerals, enzymes
- Hormones – Insulin, cortisone, testosterone, prostaglandins (PG)
- Growth factors – PDGF, TGFβ, Endothelial Growth factor, Fibroblast Growth factor etc.
  - PDGF – Platelet Derived Growth Factor
  - TGFβ – Tissue Growth Factor
- Supply proteins: Fibrotic, Attachment of cell of substrate
- To increase viscosity of medium – Protection from mechanical damage
- Protease inhibitors in serum, protect cells from proteolysis.
- Provide minerals – Na^+, k^+, Fe^{2+}, Cu^{2+}, Zn^{2+}

(ii) Serum free media: Serum replaced with mixture of amino acids with organic compounds. Growth factors proteins supplemented when required. DEM [Dulbecco's Enriched Modification], Ham's F12, RPMI 1640, GMEM [Glasgow's Modification of Eagle's medium].

3.2.9 Physicochemical Properties of Culture Media

- ***pH:*** Normal pH of Culture Media is 7-7.4.

  Phenol Red – Used to detection of pH media.

pH value	Indicating color
6.5	Yellow.
7.0	Orange.
7.4	Red.
7.8	Purple.

- ***CO_2, Bicarbonate, Buffering:*** Increases atmospheric CO_2 – reduce pH acidic

  $$CO_2 + H_2O \rightarrow HCO_3^- + H^+ \text{ ions.}$$

- ***Oxygen:*** Regular and adequate supply required.

  High supply – Generates free radicals.

  Glutathione – Toxicity.

- ***Temperature:*** Warm Blooded animals is 37 °C ± 0.05 °C

  Birds is 38.5 °C

  Cold blooded animals are 15 °C to 25 °C.

- ***Osmolality:*** Human plasma– 290 mosm/kg.

  Cultured cells – 260-320 mosm/kg.

  C.S = calf serum

  F.B = fetal bovine

Table 3.1 Various cell line mediums.

Cell or Cell lines	Medium	Serum
Chick Embryo Fibroblasts	EMEM	C.S.
Chinese Hamster	EMEM	C.S.
Hela cells	EMEM	C.S.
Human Leukemia	RPMI 1640	F.B.
Mouse leukemia	Fisher's medium, RPMI 1640	F.B.
Neurons	DMEM	F.B.
Skeletal Muscle	DMEM,F 12	F.B.
Hematopoietic Cells	RPMI 1640, Fisher's medium	F.B.

3.2.10 Types of Cell Culture

- Monolayer Culture.
- Suspension Culture.
- Immobilized Cell System.

  In laboratories cell culture technique is carried out by these methods only.

- **Monolayer Culture**

  (a) ***Roux bottle:*** Commonly used in laboratory. Only a portion of its internal surface available for cell.

  175 – 200 cm^2 – cell attachment.

  750 – 1000 cm^2 – total surface.

  Roux Bottle

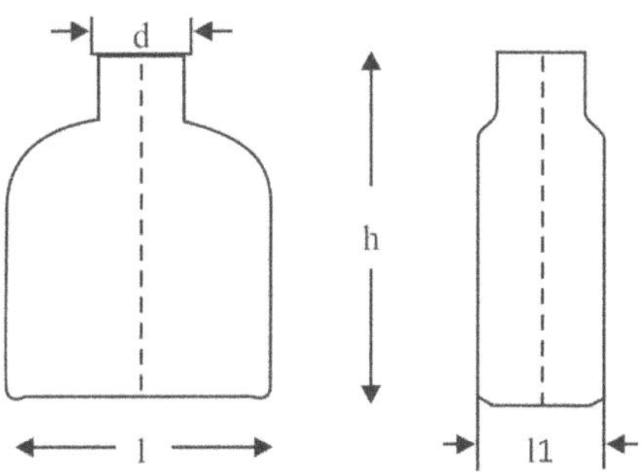

Fig. 3.1 Roux culture bottle central neck.

  (b) ***Roller bottle:*** It is rolled, so that increase internal surface area available for cells.

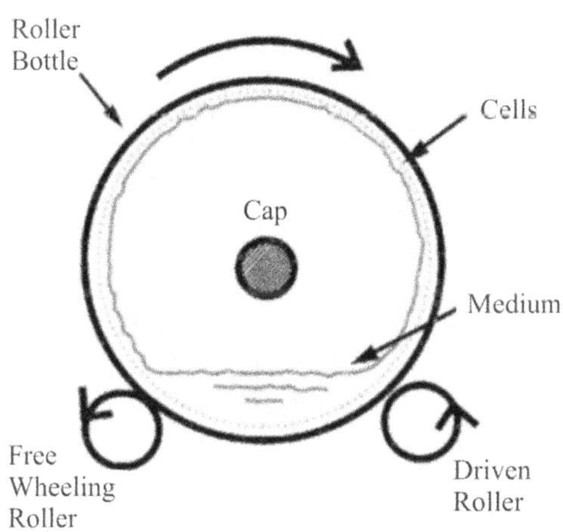

Fig. 3.2 Roller bottle.

  (c) ***Multi surface culture:*** Commonly used multi surface propagation rectangular petri dish like units huge surface area (1000-25000 cm^2).

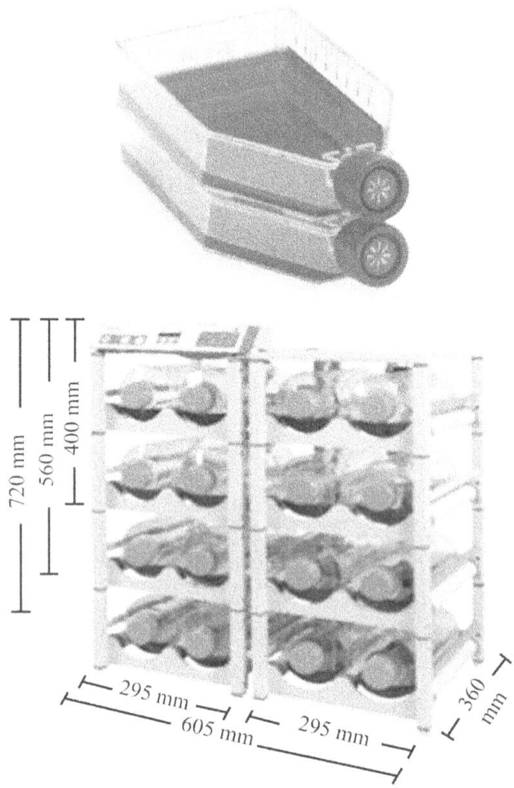

Fig. 3.3 Suspension culture vessels.

- **Suspension Culture**
  - Preferred method
  - Increase volume of culture

  (a) ***Stirred suspension culture:*** Strains maintain in stirred suspension. E.g., Stirrer flask.

  (b) ***Continuous flow culture:*** Keep the cells at a desired and set concentration.

  Removal and replacement easy. Stirred Suspension Culture Flow of medium regulated by peristaltic pump. Example: Biostatic.

  (c) ***Air lift fermented culture:*** The maximum movement of liquid or medium achieved.

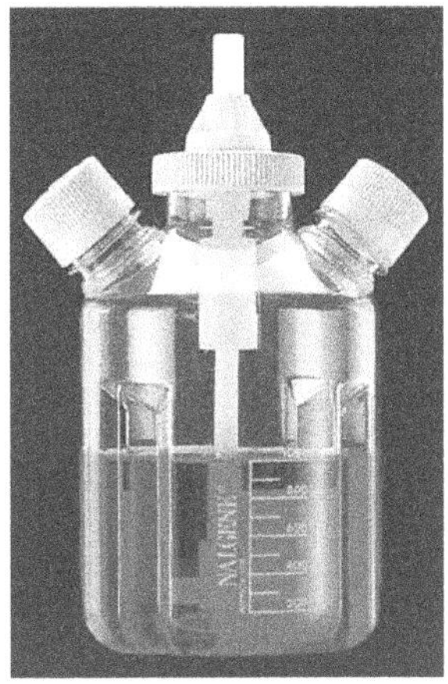

Fig. 3.4 Stirrer flask.

3.2.11 Source of Explants Tissue

- Cells or tissues are collected from the lab animals like mice, rabbits and guinea pig etc.
- Enough amount of food is given to lab animals.
- Animals are transported to operation room and killed and sterilized. These cells are main source of explants tissues.

3.2.11.1 Cell line is 2 types

1. Finite cell lines.
2. Continuous cell lines.

1. ***Finite cell lines:*** The cells in culture divided only a lintier number of times, before their growth rate declines and they eventually die. The cell lines with limited culture life spans are referred to as finite cell line. The cell normally divided 20 to 100 times cell lines. The cells normally divided 20 to 100 times before extinction.

   The actual number of doublings depends on Species:

   - Human cells generally divide 50-100 times.
   - Marine cells generally divide 30-50 times.

2. ***Continuous cell lines:*** A few cells in culture may acquire a different morphology and get altered. Such cells are capable of growing faster resulting in an independent culture. The progeny derived from these altered cells has unlimited life. They are designed as continuous cell line. The continuous cell lines are transformed, immortal and tumorigenic. The transformed cells for continuous cell line may be obtained from normal primary cell cultures by treating them with chemical carcinogens or by infecting with oncogenic viruses.

Table 3.2 Primary explant technique for primary cultivation.

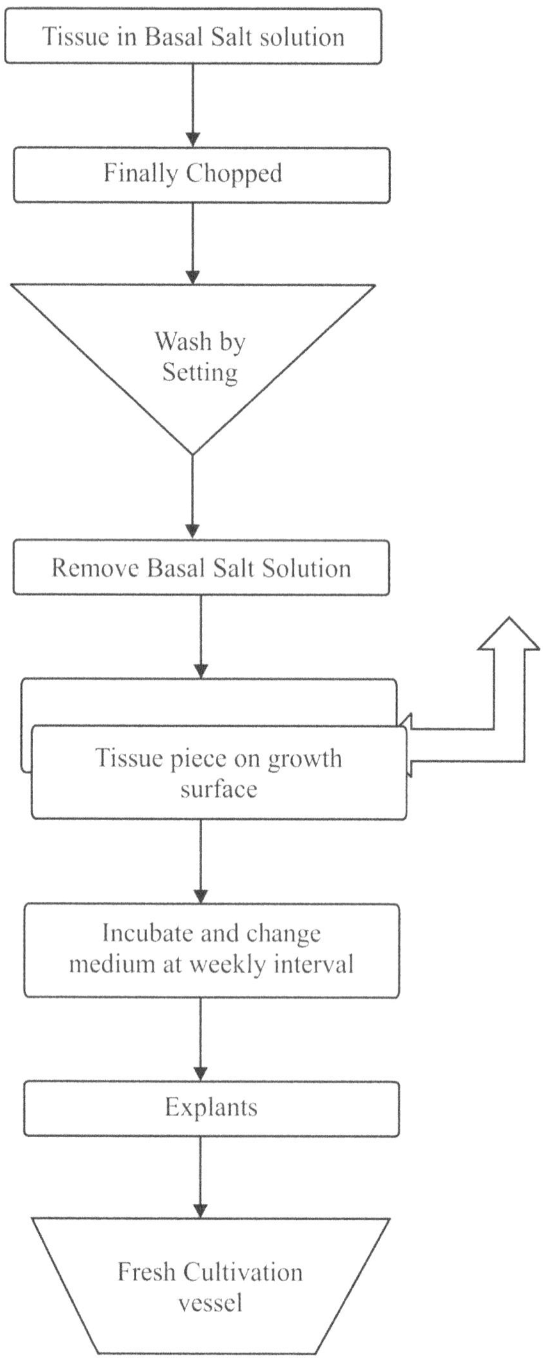

Table 3.3 Properties of finite cell line, continuous cell lines.

Property	Finite Cell Line	Continuous Cell Line
Growth Rate	Slow	Fast
Mode of Growth	Monolayer	Suspension/Monolayer
Yield	Low	High
Transformation	Normal	Immortal
Ploidy	Euploidy	Aneuploidy
Anchorage Dependence	Yes	No
Contact Inhibition	Yes	No
Cloning Efficacy	Low	High
Serum Requirement	High	Low
Markers	Tissues specific	Chromosomal Antigenic

3.2.12 Sub Culturing

The cells in culture cannot remain viable for long time because the cell utilizes all nutrients in the medium. Substructure need to be done. Cells are diluted with fresh medium and passed into fresh culture flask.

3.2.13 Applications of Cell Line Techniques

- Production of therapeutically significant biological compounds like hormones and proteins.
- Research on animal virus.
- Production of wide range of biological products.
- Monoclonal antibodies.
- Viral vaccines.
- For study of biochemistry and bio physics of cell growth and division.
- Screening of anti cancer drugs.
- Cell based bioassay.
- To determine the cytotoxicity.
- *In vitro* screening of several drugs.
- Cell fusion technique.
- Genetic manipulation, Gene therapy.
- Recombinant DNA therapy.
- Molecular biology etc.

3.2.14 List of some Vaccines Prepared by Cell Culture are

- Measles – chick embryo fibroblast.

- Polio – monkey kidney cells.
- Rabies – human diploid cells.
- In Drug Discovery process the drug must pass many phases the testing of test drug on animals in harmful or fatal this can be minimizes if the drug is tested of cell line [Sacrifice one life to save many].
- Reduce probability death of test animals.

3.3 PATCH CLAMP TECHNIQUE

The Patch Clamp Technique is a laboratory technique in electrophysiology that allows the study of single or multiple ion channels in cells. The technique can be applied to wide variety of cells, but is especially useful in the study of excitable cells such as neurons, cardiomyocytes, muscle fibers and pancreatic beta cells. It can also be applied to the study of bacterial ion channels in specially prepared giant spheroplasts. The patch clamp technique is a refinement of the voltage clamp.

Erwin Neher and Bert Sakmann

[Received Nobel Prize in 1991 for this topic]

- He developed the patch clamp technique in the late 1970s and early 1980s this discovery made it possible to record the current of single ion channel for the first time, proving their fundamental cell process such as action potential conduction.
- Patch clamp recording uses, as an electrode a glass micropipette that has an open tip diameter of about one micro meter, a size enclosing a membrane surface area or patch that often contains just one or a few ions channel molecules.
- This type of electrode is distinct from the sharp micro electrode used to impale cells in traditional intra cellular recordings in that it is sealed on to the surface of the cell membrane rather than inserted through it.
- In some experiments the micropipette tip is heated in a micro forge to produce a smooth surface that assist in forming a high resistance seal with the cell membrane. The interior of the pipette is filled with a solution matching the ionic composition of the bath solution as in the case of cell attached recording or the cytoplasm for whole cell recording.
- Chloride silver curve is placed in contact with this solution and conducts electrical current to the amplifier.
- This investigation can change the composition of this solution or add drugs to study the ion channels under different conditions.

3.3.1 Variations in Patch Clamp Techniques

There are several variant techniques; they are called as "Excised patch" techniques. They are called like that because the patch is excised (removed) from main body of the cell.

Some types of variations:

- On cell patch or cell attached
- Whole cell patch
- Out side out patch
- Inside out patch
- Perforated patch
- Loose patch

3.3.1.1 On cell patch or cell attached

- It allows for recording of currents without disruption inside the cell. This recording occurs through single ion channels.
- The electrode is sealed to patch of membrane.
- In pipette solution only neurotransmitter or drug to be studied is added, it is in contact with external surface of membrane.
- The technique is limited to at one site in dose response curve per patch. Usually dose response is accomplished using several cells and patches.
- Voltage gated ion channels can be lamped different membrane potentials using the same patch.

3.3.1.2 Whole cell patch

- This method is useful for recording current through multiple channels at once on entire cell.
- It has larger opening at the tip of cell through sharp microelectrode recording this is the advantage of this method.
- The soluble contents of cells interior will slowly be replaced by contents of electrode because of volume of electrode is larger than the cell, this is the disadvantage of this method.
- The electrode is left in place on the cell but more suction is applied to rupture the membrane patch thus providing access to the intracellular space of the cell. The high potassium solution is used as pipette solution.

3.3.1.3 Outside-out patch

- The electrode can be slowly withdrawn from the cell, after the whole cell patch is formed, this allows a bulb of membrane to bleb out from cell. (bleb: a large blister filled with serous fluid or out patching of any kind).
- This experiment can perfuse same patch with different solutions. The dose response curve can be obtained, if the channel is activated from extracellular face.

3.3.1.4 Inside-out patch

- This method is useful when an experiment wants to manipulate the environment at the intracellular surface of ion channel.
- Micropipette is quickly withdrawn from cell after the gigaseals are formed, that leads to ripping the patch of membrane of the cell, then the intracellular surface of membrane is exposed to external media.
- ***Example:*** Channels are activated by nitrocellulose ligands studed through a range of ligand concentration.

3.3.1.5 Perforated patch

In this variation of whole-cell recording the experimental forms the ohm seal, but does not use suction to rupture the patch membrane. Instead the electrode solution contains small amounts of an antibiotic, such as amphoterician-B or Gramicidin.

3.3.1.6 Loose patch

It is different in that it employs a loose seal rather than the right giga seal used in the conventional technique.

Advantage: Pipette used can be repeatedly removed from the membrane after recording, and the membrane will remain intact.

Disadvantage: Possibility of leak.

3.3.2 Patch–Clamp Technique in Kidney Cells

In the different parts of the kidney fluid is reabsorbed and substance may be transported either from the tubule lumen to the blood side (re-absorption) or vice versa.

Besides active transport and coupled transport systems, ion channel play an important role in the function of kidney cells. Various modes of patch clamp technique [cell attached, cell – excised, whole-cell mode] allow the investigation of ion channels.

Procedure:

- The patch clamp technique can be applied to cultured kidney cells or freshly isolated kidney cells or to cells of isolated perfused kidney tubules.
- The non – cannulated end of the tubules of rabbit kidney are dissected and per fused kidney tubules.
- Segments of late superficial proximal tubules of rabbit kidney are dissected and per fused from one end with a perfusion system.
- The non – cannulated end of the tubules is freely accessible to patch pipette.
- Under optical controls the patch pipette can be moved through the open end into the tubule lumen and is brought in contact with the brush border membrane.
- Alter slight section of the patch electrode, giga seals form instantaneously and single potassium or sodium channels can be recorded in the cell attached or inside – out cell – excised mode.
- In order to obtain exposed lateral cell membranes suitable to the application of the patch clamp method.
- Pieces of the tubule are turnoff by means of a glass pipette 40 μm.
- To facilitate the tearing off the tubules are inoculated for about 5 min in 0.5 gm/l collagens at room temperature.
- After tearing off part of the cannulated tubule clean lateral cell membranes are exposed at the conculated end.
- The patch pipette can be moved to the lateral cell membrane and giga seal can be obtained. It was possible, to investigate potassium channels and non selective action channels in these membranes.

Conclusion: In isolated perfuse renal tubules, concentration response curves of drugs which inhibit ion channels can be obtained with the patch clamp technique. In isolated cells of the proximal tubule, the whole- cell mode of the patch clamp technique enables the investigating of the sodium – almandine co transport system.

3.3.3 Applications of Patch Clamp Technique

- For the evaluation of anti arrhythmic agents.
- In kidney cells.
- Used for isolated ventricular myocytes from guinea pigs to study a cardio selective inhibition of the ATP sensitive potassium channel.
- To identify multiple types of calcium channel.
- To measure the effect of potassium channel openers.
- Used in the molecular biology.

- Voltage clamp studies on sodium channels.
- Used to investigate a wide range of electrophysiological cell properties.
- Measurement of all membrane conductance.

3.4 *IN VITRO* MODELS

In vitro testing is one of the major types of alternative to animal studies to minimize animal utilization. *In vitro* testing includes a battery of living system. Bacteria, cultured human and animal cells, fertilized chicken eggs, frog embryos. That can be employed to evaluate the toxicity of chemical in human beings. Ultimately workers hope to able to test chemical in cultures of human cells from various organs and tissues so that the question of human toxicity can be answered more directly.

3.4.1 Advantages of *In vitro* Studies

- Controlled testing conditions.
- Lack of system effects.
- Reduction of variability between experiments .
- Testing is fast and cheap.
- Small amount of test material is required.
- Limited amount of toxic waste is produced.
- Human cells and tissue can be used.
- Transgenic cells carrying human genes can be used.
- Reduction of testing in animals.
- No interactions with other organs.
- Increased sensitivity.
- Experiment is done in lander controlled condition.
- Better experimental flexibility.

3.4.2 Disadvantages of *In vitro* Studies

- *Invivo*-dose response not available.
- No systemic effect could be studied.
- Organ specificity lacking.
- Chronic and long term effects could not be studied.
- Transportation of material not easy.
- Possible change of properties.
- More difficult extrapolation.
- pK values cannot be evaluated.

3.4.3 *In vitro* Models are 3 Types that include

1. Replacement.
2. Reduction.
3. Refinement.

1. **Replacement:** Alternatives that replace animal models can be classified into.
   (a) Use of living system.
   (b) Use of non-living system and
   (c) Physical and mechanical system.

   (a) ***The use of living system:***
   - In this method isolated organs, tissue and cell culture are used.
   - This system works on providing of correct combination of atmosphere, humidity, temperature, pH and nutrient are provided.
   - Main examples are cell culture techniques, monoclonal antibody production, virus vaccine production, vaccine potency testing, screening for the cytopathic effects of various compounds.

   In vertebrate animals these are other type of living system, which can be used to replace more commonly used laboratory animals.

   Example: Fruit fly, Drophila, Melanogaster and also for Mutagenicity, Teratogenicity and Reproductive Toxicity.

   Marine species - For study of Nervous System.
   - ***Micro Organisms:*** The Ames Mutagenicity/carcinogenicity test uses *Salmonella Typhimurium* cultures to screen compounds that formerly required the use of animals. Plants also offer other alternative living systems.

   (b) ***Use of Non-Living system:*** Chemical techniques: Immuno-chemical techniques are used to detect the binding capacity of highly specific anti bodies to seek out minute quantities of antigen.

   E.g.: ELISA [Enzyme Linked Immuno Sorbent Assay]

   Available test kit used to Pregnancy detection.

   (c) ***Physical and Mechanical System:*** Computer linked mannequins in teaching basic principles of medicine.

2. **Reduction:** Four broad categories for reducing number of animals used are
   (a) Animal Sharing.
   (b) Improved Statistical Design.
   (c) Phylogenetic Reduction.
   (d) Better Quality Animals.
   (a) ***Animal sharing:*** Significantly reduce the number of animals use within a given Institution.

   Example: If 2 studies involve the need to use of standard control diets or the need to condition animals to particular environment, control animals could be shared with in the institution.

   (b) ***Improved statistical design***

   Example: Group Sequential Testing, Cross Over Design, can significantly reduce the numbers of animals required.

   (c) ***Phylogenetic reduction:*** Myriads of invertebrate species used instead of Non-Human Primate Species - useful to reduce the number of animals used

   (d) ***Better quality animals:*** While purchasing laboratory animals, keep in mind that cost and quality usually directly correlated. Choose the best quality and consistency of animals from study to study.

3. **Refinement:** Technique which reduce the pain and distress to which an animal is subjected. They are
   (a) Decreased invasiveness.
   (b) Improved instrumentation.
   (c) Improved control of pain.
   (d) Improved control of techniques.
   (a) ***Decreased invasiveness:*** Magnetic Resonance Imaging [MRI] for results that formerly required euthanasia of multiple animals along a time curve to obtain assay tissue. One animal can provide all the information along all part of its body.

   Now a day it is available in almost every area of biomedical research and project design.

   (b) ***Improved instrumentation:*** For Monitoring of animals - Micro Electronics, Fiber Optics, *Laser Instrumentation* is very useful. Improved instrumentation can minimize animal distress.

   Analyzing samples: Once obtained samples can be analyzed in very small volumes for multitude of parameters.

Example: Commercially available diagnostic laboratory equipments.

(c) ***Improved control of pain:*** The animal welfare act requires. Doctor of veterinary medicine is consulted in the planning of such pain producing drugs usage.

E.g., Tranquilizers, Analgesic, Anaesthetic.

3.4.4 Some of the Alternatives to Animal Tests are as Follows

(i) *In vitro* pyrogen test

(ii) Embryonic stem cell test (EST)

(iii) Local lymph node assay (LLNA) for skin sensitization

(iv) Clinical skin patch test on human volunteers

(v) Neutral red uptake (NRU) assay

(vi) Carcinogenicity test

(vii) Acute toxicity test

(viii) Repeated dose toxicity test

(i) ***In vitro pyrogen test:*** To replace the rabbit pyrogen test - number of alternative cellular assays. In that

- LAL test [Limulus Amebocyte Lysate Test].
- MAT test [Monocyte Activation Test].

All test systems are based on the response of Human Leukocytes [Primarily Monocots] that release of inflammatory mediators [Endogenous Pyrogens] in response to contamination [Exogenous Pyrogens].

Principle of LAL test: Lipo Polysaccharide (LPS) causes extra cellular coagulation of the blood (haemolymph) of the horse shoe crab. LAL test is more sensitive than rabbit test. But gives false negative results with certain products and does not detect pyrogens other than bacterial (gram negative) endotoxins viruses and fungi

(MAT) Monocyte Activation Test: Performed with human mononuclear cells and better than LAL and Rabbit test.

(ii) ***Embryonic Stem Cell Test (EST):*** Used for Detection of any embryonic toxicity. The EST develops spontaneously into contracting myocardium.

Different end points in the assay

- Inhibition of differentiation of ES into cardio myocytes.
- Cytotoxicity effects on the ES cell.
- Cytotoxicity effects on 3T3 fibroblasts.

In vitro Metabolism studies using human microsomal enzymes or cell lines provide information on whether a non toxic chemical is likely to metabolize to toxic form or vice versa.

- Positive result in EST is sufficient evidence of embryo toxicity.
- Negative results will be subjected to further assays if necessary.

(iii) *Local Lymph Node Assay (LLNA) for skin sensitization:*

Principle: When drug is applied in the skin, lymph node draining the site of chemical application reveals a primary proliferation of lymphocytes as measured by the radioactive labelling - It is considered as sensitizer.

This proliferation is proportional to the dose applied. So lymphocyte proliferation is the index for skin sensitization, stimulation index is calculated before and after application of the chemical. The index must be at least 3 before the substance is further evaluated as potential skin sensitizer.

(iv) *Clinical skin patch test on human volunteers:* First it should be tested with non animal *in vitro* mutagenicity test and corrosive nature. Then it is allowed to take it into human volunteers. It is beneficial as it directly relevant to the humans.

(v) *Neutral Red Uptake [NRU] assay*

- *In vitro* epidermal keratinocytes test for eye irritation alternative to the Draize test (the rabbit eye test).
- Cells are derived from BALB/c, 3T3 mouse fibroblasts, human epidermal keratinocytes and SIR cell line from rabbit cornea.
- The NRU assay measure the ability of a text substance to inhibit the uptake of neutral red dye, a marker for cell viability.
- Assay is conducted in primary cell lines with different concentrations.
- 50% inhibition of NRU is indication of toxicity. So these values are called as NRU50 and serves as toxicological end point.

(vi) *Carcinogenicity test*

- It is a cell transformation assay to identify the carcinogenicity potential *in vitro* method.
- BLAB/c, 3T3 or Syrian Hamster Embryo (SHE) assay.
- SHE assay is found to be more sensitive to wide range is found of both genotoxic and non-genotoxic. Carcinogens with 96% of know human carcinogens being detected.
- This assay is faster (6 weeks) and less expensive than rodent bioassay and transgenic mouse models.

- It takes only fewer animals (maximum eight embryos against 800 or more animals in the standard bio-assay).

(vii) ***Acute toxicity test***

- Many non specific cell toxicity tests have been developed as potential replacement to acute lethality test on animals.
- In addition there are several computer software packages for predicting acute toxicity from the chemical structures.

(viii) ***Repeated dose toxicity test***

- ADME profile of a chemical is critical determining the nature and degree of toxicity.
- Computerized softwares are available to predict the tissue distribution of the chemical based on the structure.
- This will help in prediction to organ specific toxicity.
- This can be verified using of culture specific techniques.
- This will help in using non animal model along with software prediction to determine the organ specific toxicity.

3.5 MOLECULAR BIOLOGY TECHNIQUES

Molecular biology is the study of biology at a molecular level. The field overlaps with other areas of biology and chemistry, particularly genetics and biochemistry. Molecular biology chiefly concern itself with understanding the interactions between the various system of a cell, including the interrelationship of DNA, RNA and protein synthesis and learning how these interactions are regulated.

Relationship to other "molecular-scale" biological sciences:

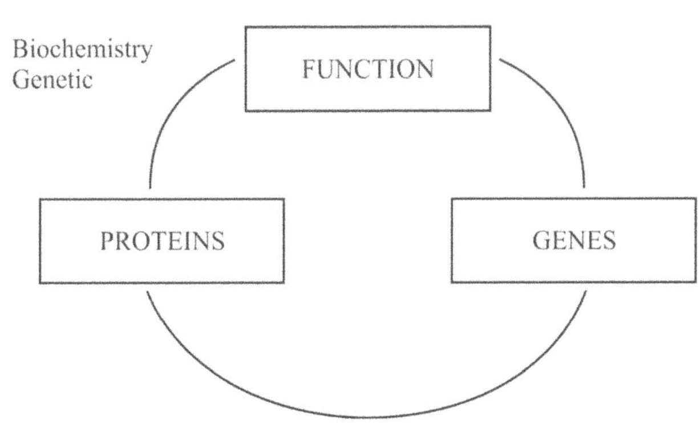

Fig. 3.5 Molecular scale.

Molecular biology

- Relationship between biochemistry, genetic and molecular biology.
- Researching in molecular biology use specific techniques native to molecular biology, but increasingly combine these with techniques and ideas from genetics and biochemistry. These are not a hard-line between these disciplines as there once was. Bio chemistry is the study of the chemical substances and vital process accruing in living organism.
- Molecular biology is the study of molecular under-pinning's of the process of replication, transcription, and translation of the genetic material. The central dogma of molecular biology where genetic material is transcribed into RNA and then translated into protein despite being on oversimplified picture of molecular biology still provides a good starting point for understanding the field. The picture however is understanding revision in light of emerging novel roles for RNA.
- The study of gene structure and function, molecular genetics, has been amongst the most prominent sub-field of molecular biology.

Techniques of molecular biology

The late 1950 and 1960s molecular biologists have learned to characterize, isolate and manipulate the molecular components of cells and organisms.

These components include DNA repository of genetic information RNA, a close relative of DNA whose function range from serving as a temporary working copy of DNA to actual structured and enzymatic function as well as a functional and structural part of the translation apparatus and proteins the major structural and enzymatic type of molecule in cells.

Expression cloning

One of the most basic techniques of molecular biology to study protein function is expression cloning.

In this technique, DNA coding for a protein of interest is cloned [using PCR or Restriction Enzymes] into a plasmid (know as an expression vector). Introducing DNA into eukaryotic cells, such as animal cells is called Transfecion.

Several different transfect ion techniques are available, including calcium phosphate transfect ion liposome transfection and proprietary transfection reagent such as fugene.

DNA can also be introduced into cells using viruses or pathogenic bacteria as carriers. In such cases and the cells are said to be transduced the technique is called viral/bacterial transduction.

Polymerase Chain Reaction (PCR)

The polymerase chain reaction is an extremely versatile technique for copying DNA. In brief, PCR allows a single DNA sequence to be copied (millions of times) and altered in predetermined ways. This reaction is done by biochemistry and molecular biology techniques for exponentially amplifying DNA *via* enzymatic replication.

PCR is commonly used in medical and biological research labs for a variety of tasks, such as the detection of hereditary diseases, the identification of genetic finger prints, and the diagnosis of infectious diseases, the cloning of genes, paternity testing and DNA computing.

PCR as currently practiced, required several basic components

These compounds are:

- DNA template that contains the region of the DNA fragment to be amplified.
- One or more primers, which are complementary to the DNA regions at the 5^1 and 3^1 ends of DNA region that is to be amplified.
- DNA polymerase used to synthesize a DNA copy of the region to be amplified.
- Deoxy Nucleotide Triphosphates, (d NTPs) from which the DNA polymerase builds the new DNA.
- Buffer solution, which provides a suitable chemical environment for optimum activity and stability of DNA polymerase.
- Divalent cation, magnesium or manganese ions generally Mg^{2+} is used, but Mn^{2+} can be utilized for PCR-mediated DNA mutagenesis. Monovalent cation potassium ions.

Use of PCR

PCR can be used for a broad variety of experiment and analyses, examples:

- Genetic finger printing is forensic technique used E_O identity a person by comparing his or her DNA with the DNA in given sample. Example: Blood from crime scene who's DNA is being genetically compared to DNA from a suspect.
- Detection of hereditary disease in a given genome is a long and difficult process, which can shorten signification by using PCR.
- Viral disease too can be detected by using PCR through amplification of the viral DNA.

Cloning genes

- Cloning a gene not to be confused with cloning a whole an organism, describe the process of isolating a gene from one organism and then inserting it into another organism [now termed a genetically modified organism (GMO)]. PCR is often used to amplify the gene, which can then be inserted into a vector (a vector is a piece of DNA which carries the transferred into an organism where the gene and its product can be studied more closely). Expression a cloned gene can also be a way of mass producing useful proteins.

Example: Medicines or enzymes in biological washing powders.

Mutagenesis: Mutagenesis is a way of introducing changes to the sequence of nucleotides in the DNA.

Analysis of ancient DNA: Using PCR, it becomes possible to analyze DNA that is of thousand years old. PCR techniques have been successfully used to detect an animal, such as a 40 thousand year old man, and also on human DNA.

Nucleic acids

In the case of nucleic acids, the direction of migration from negative to positive electrodes is due to the natural negative charge carried on their sugar phosphate backbone. Protein, on the other hand, can have different charges and complex shapes, they may not migrate into the gel at similar rates, or at all, where placing a negative to positive EMF on the sample. Proteins therefore, are usually denatured in the presence of a detergent such as Sodium Dodecyl/Sulfate. Dodecyl Phosphate that coats the protein with a negative charge.

Southern blotting

This method used for probing for presence of specific DNA sequence within DNA sample. Applications, such as measuring transgenic copy number in transgenic mice or in the engineering of gene knockout embryonic stem cell lines.

Northern blotting

It is used to expression patterns a specific type of RNA molecule as relative comparison among of a set of different sample of RNA.

Western blotting

In this method proteins are first separated by size, in thin gel sandwiched between 2 glass plates in technique known as SDS-PAGE.

In applications ranging from the analysis of Egyptian mummies to the identification of Russian Tsar.

Genotyping of specific mutations

This methodology has several applications, such as amplifying certain haplotypes [when certain alleles at 2 or more SNPs occur together on the same chromosome linkage disequilibrium] or detection of recombinant chromosomes and the study of miotic recombination.

Gel electrophoresis

Gel electrophoresis is one of the principal tools of molecular biology. The basic principle is that DNA, RNA and protein can all be separated using an electric field.

Applications

- Gel electrophoresis is used in forensics, molecular biology, genetics, microbiology and biochemistry.
- The results can be analyzed quantitatively by visualizing them with UV light and gel imaging device.
- The image is recorded with computer operated camera, and the intensity of the band or spot of interest is measured and loaded on the same gel. The measured and analysis are mostly done with specialized software.

Chapter 4

Bioassay

4.1 Introduction

Bioassay (commonly used in shorthand for biological assay), or biological standardization is a type of scientific experiment. Bioassays are typically conducted to measure the effects of a substance on a living organism and are essential in the development of new drugs and in monitoring environmental pollutants. Both are procedures by which the potency or the nature of a substance is estimated by studying its effects on living matter. Bioassay is a procedure for the determination of the concentration of a particular constitution of a mixture.

Bioassay also knows as Biological assay. Bioassay is defined as estimation of potency of an unknown concentration of a preparation using biological tissue or micro organisms.

Definition

"Estimation of the potency of an active principle in a unit quantity of preparation or detection and measurement of the concentration of substance in a preparation".

or

"The determination of the relative strength of a substance (as a drug) by comparing its effect on a test organism with that of a standard preparation".

By using biological method like observation of pharmacological effects on living tissues, micro organisms or immune cells or animals is known as "biological assays" or bioassay.

Principles of Bioassay

The basic principle of bioassay is to compare the test substance with the standard preparation of the same and to find out how much test substance is required to produce the same biological effect as product by the standard.

Burn & Dale enunciated certain principles for the conduction of bioassay procedures.

They are:

- All Bioassay must be comparative against standard drugs.
- The standard and new drugs should be as far as identical to each other.
- The method for comparing the unknown and the standard drugs should preferably (but not essential). Test the therapeutic property of the drug.
- The method should estimate as far as possible and allow an estimate of the error due to biological variation in different animals/persons at any one time and in the same animals/person at different times.

Advantages of Bioassays

Bioassay is the only method of assay if when

- Active principle of drug is unknown or cannot be isolated

  Example: Insulin, Posterior Pituitary Extract etc.
- Chemical method is either not available (or) If available it is too complex and insensitive (or) requires higher doses

  Example: Insulin, Acetyl choline.
- Chemical composition is not known

  Example: Long acting thyroid stimulants.
- Chemical composition of drug differs but have the same Pharmacological action and vice versa

  Example: Cardiac Glycosides, Catecholamine's etc.
- When the quantity of sample is too small.

  Example: Matching type of Bioassay.

Demerits

Bioassay as compared to other methods of Assays.

Examples

- Less accurate.
- Less elaborate.
- More laborious.
- More troublesome.
- More expensive.

Normally there are two types of Bioassays. They are:

(i) Qualitative Bioassay.

(ii) Quantities Bioassay.

(i) Qualitative bioassay: The objective is to determine what type of action a drug produces, by comparing its action with those of other substance of known activity. It can be used to detect small amounts of biologically active substance present at disease sites or released in pathology.

(ii) Quantitative bioassay: The objective is determined as the amount if active constituent present in the drug preparation, for this purpose another preparation containing a known amount of active constituents is used as standard.

Quantitative Bioassay is typically analyzed using the methods of biostatistics.

Methods of bioassays

(A) Direct methods:

1. Matching method
2. Bracket method

(B) Indirect methods:

1. Graphical or interpolation bioassay
2. Three point bioassay
3. Four point bioassay

(A) Direct methods:

1. ***Matching method:*** This test is performed by using fog's rectus abdominis muscle which placed in organ bath.
   - Main aim of this method is to find out potency (or concentration) of the test sample by comparing the doses of standard acetylcholine and test acetylcholine.

- In this type of bioassay, the test substance responses are obtained by adding different test solutions that responses are matched to standard responses.
- Main advantage of this method is it does not depend on this assumption of a dose response relationship.
- This method also has some disadvantages, like- it is purely subjective, experimental errors cannot be determined from assay itself, and qualitative differences are gives no indication of paralism of dose response curves of standard drug and test drug.
- This method has one limitation due to dilution of the factor by which test substance is diluted or concentrated in order to produce response that is equal to that of known amount of standard solution.
- In this method, Frog rectus abdominous muscle is placed in organ bath, with that DRC (Dose Response Curve) of drug (standard drug after that test drug) is carried out at various doses.
- The response standard, which matches with that of unknown, is determined and potency of test sample was calculated by this method.

2. **Bracket method:**
    - Bracketing Bioassay method is performed by selecting two standard doses, which will give a close bracket between lower dose and higher dose of standard when test dose is given.
    - The dose of standard drug is kept constant throughout the experiment, in order to check the sensitivity of the tissue with time. The response of test substance is bracketed between 2 standard responses, close bracketing gives more accurate results.
    - The method also carried out on frog rectus abdominous muscle, which is placed in organ both.
    - By taking of DRC of drug (for both standard and test) select two response of standard such that response to unknown dose is between these two responses.
    - After that titrate the doses of standard such that the bracket is as dose as possible with the standard and responses to the unknown.

The potency of drug is calculated by using following equation.

$$\text{Potency of drug} = \frac{S_1 + S_2}{2} \text{ mg/ml or µg/ml}$$

where S_1 = Standard dose of 1

S_2 = Standard dose of 2

In this method is calculating concentration of test solution is determining potency of test sample.

(B) Indirect methods:

1. ***Graphical/Interpolation bioassay:***

- This method is less time consuming and get reliable as compared to matching type of bioassay.
- Main advantage of this method is that the sensitivity of the tissue is determined by prior plotting of concentration response curve with known against as is the case with standard drug. If the linearity of curve is good on can do accurate estimate of test substance.
- The response of standard doses plotted and by interpolation.

2. ***Three point bioassay:***

- This method is performed on isolated frog rectus abdominous muscle.
- In this method two standard doses were selected which will give close bracket on either side of response produced by unknown. The response of 2 doses of standard (S_1, S_2) the test is obtained by changing the order in successive cycle.
- Three point bioassay is used when the active material is present in sufficient quantity. The potency of the substance is determined by using the following formula.

$$\text{Potency of test solution} = \text{S}\frac{n_1}{t}\,anti\log\left[\frac{(T_1 - S_1)}{S_2 - S_1}\right] \times \log\frac{n_2}{n_1}$$

where n_1 = Lower standard dose

n_2 = Higher standard dose

S_1 and S_2 = Standard responses

t = Test does (ml)

T_1 = Test response

- In this method 3 cycles of responses are taking as

S_1, T_1, S_2	1st cycle
T_1, S_2, S_1	2nd cycle
S_2, S_1, T_1	3rd cycle

The responses are not so rigidity selected as in case of bracketing assay except that the responses should lie between 20% and 80% of dose response curve. Then only potency is calculated for unknown sample by using formula.

3. ***Four point bioassay:*** This method incorporates the principles of interpolation and matching hence it is most accurate, precision and reliability is good. Since the sensitivity of tissue is tested at first by recording the dose response curve. In four point bioassay comprises are based on analysis of dose response curve and the matching dose of standard and unknown are calculated by following formula.

Potency ration: $$\frac{x_1}{y_1} \times anti\log\left[\frac{(T_1 - S_1) + (T_2 - S_2)}{(T_{2\_}T_1) + (S_2 - S_1)} \times \log\frac{x_2}{x_1}\right]$$

where x_1 = Lower dose of standard drug

x_2 = Higher dose of standard drug

y_1 = Lower volume of test

S_1, S_2, T_1, T_2 - mean responses of standard and test.

4.1.1 Bioassay of Vasopressin

Method – A

Aim: This is based on Anti diuretic activity of vasopressin.

Animals required	:	Male Albino rats (120 - 240 gm)
Chemicals required	:	Warm sterile distilled water
		Human albumin
		Citric acid
Equipments required	:	Measuring cylinder
		Metabolic cages

Standard Drug Preparation

The standard preparation of vasopressin consisting of freeze dried synthetic arginine vasopressin peptide acetate with human albumin and citric acid.

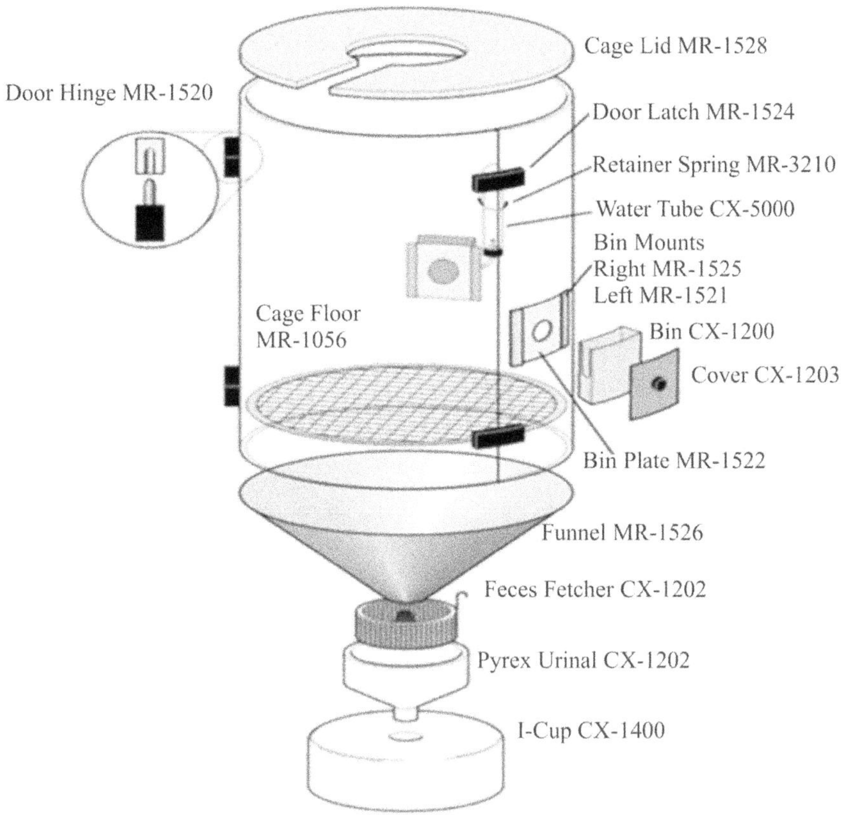

Fig. 4.1 Urine collection apparatus.

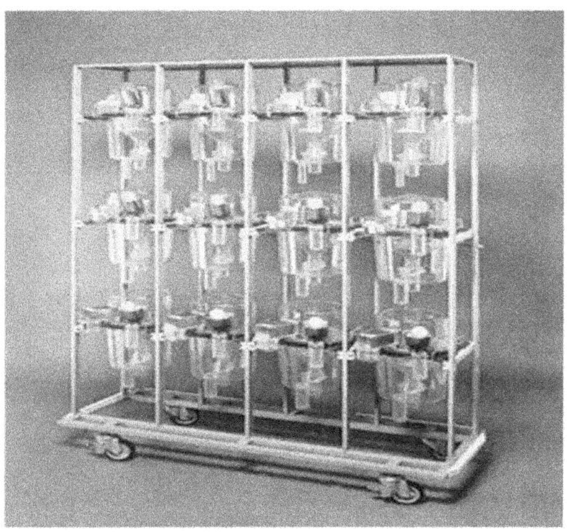

Fig. 4.2 Urine collection apparatus fixed to stand.

Procedure:

- This is based on anti diuretic activity of vasopressin. The experiment is conducted on 16 male albino rats weighting between 120-240 gm.
- Animals must be fasted over night.
- Warm sterile distilled water is given to them in the doses of 5 ml/100 gm of body weight.
- Animals divided as 2 groups (each group contain 8 rats).
- Vasopressin is administered through s.c. route.
- Rats are placed in metabolic cages and the urine sample is collected in a graduated measuring cylinder.
- The urine sample is first collected in a cylinder from each group and there after volume is recorded at intervals of 15 min for 3-4 hr.
- After this period, when ever the urine flow stops then observation is discontinued.
- Time in minutes for excretion of the half the volume of urine is calculated for each group.
- After 24 hr– Cross over test is carried out.
- Those rats received the standard sample previously are now given the test sample and vice versa.
- The experiment is run on similar line to minimize errors due to animal variation.
- From the results of 2 parts of the test mean values are obtained. These mean values should be between 96 and 135 min.

Conclusion: If they are the same for the standard and the test, then both should contain the same units. If the times are different then the relative potency can be calculated by comparing with the standard.

Method – B

Aim: This method is based on the principle of vasopressin may give appropriate rise in B.P.

Animals required	:	Male Albino rats (250-300 gm)
Chemicals required	:	L-Adrenergic receptor blockers, anaesthetics, heparin
Equipments required	:	Cannula, blood pressure recorder

Procedure:

- Male albino rat weighing about 250-300 gm is taken.
- L-Adrenergic receptor blocker E.g.: Phenoxybenzamine 10 ml/kg is injected into the tail vein of rat.
- After 18 hr of this injection, rat is anaesthetized with anaesthetic– that can maintain a prolonged and uniform blood pressure.
- That rat is tied on table.
- Trachea is cannulated to maintain respiration and carotid artery is cannulated to record B.P.
- Premolar vein is also dissected out and cannulated for injection of standard and test vasopressin.
- 200 units of heparin are also injected to prevent clotting of blood.
- Responses to 2 doses of standard preparation and 2 doses of test preparation of vasopressin are taken.
- Usually 3-5 milli units of vasopressin may give appropriate rise in B.P.

Conclusion: Based on the response obtained [As per four point graphical method bio assay] concentration of vasopressin can be obtained is observed.

4.1.2 Bioassay of Oxytocin

Method A

Aim: This method is based on height of contraction that produced by test sample is measured.

Standard Preparation

It consists of freeze dried synthetic Oxytocin Peptide with human albumin and citric acid.

Animals required	:	Female Albino rats (120-200 gm)
Chemicals required	:	Estradiol, De Jalon
Equipments required	:	Frontal lever, organ bath

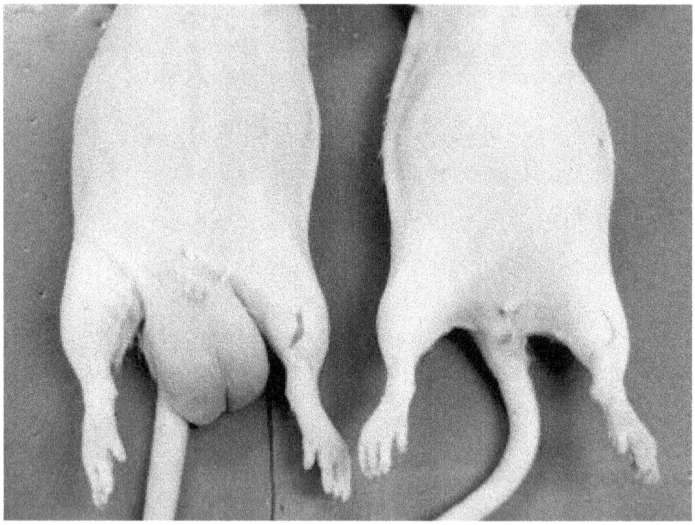

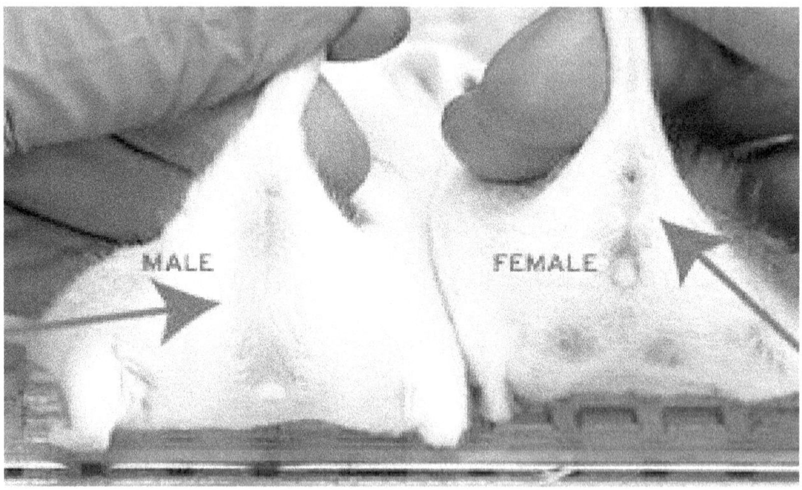

Fig. 4.3 Identification of male and female rats.

Procedure:

- As soon as female rats wean, they are separated from the males and used for test when they weighing between 120-200 gm.
- Before 18-24 hr of experiment [on the day of experiment] 100 μg/kg of Estradiol is injected through I.M.
- When estrous phase is confirmed by vaginal smear. The rat is sacrificed; uterine horns are isolated and mounted in organ bath containing De Jalon.
- Both maintained at temperature 32 °C and oxygenated.

- Contraction of uterine horn is recorded by frontal lever on surface of smoked paper fixed on slowly revolving drum.
- Standard Oxytocin Dose is 0.05 to 0.1 unit.
- This causes the uterus to contract and when contraction is complete, the solution of both is drained out and fresh solution is run in and the muscle is allowed to relax.
- Repeated additions of Oxytocin may be made at regular intervals.

Conclusion: The potency of test sample is calculated by comparing the height of contraction with that produced by standard sample. 3 or 4 Point Graphical method is recommended in IP1996.

Method B

Aim: This method citizen's property of oxytocin to depress blood Pressure in chicken.

Animals required	:	Chicken (12-23 gm)
Chemicals required	:	Anaesthetics (halothane), normal saline
Equipments required	:	Warm copper plate, venous cannula manometer (to record B.P.)

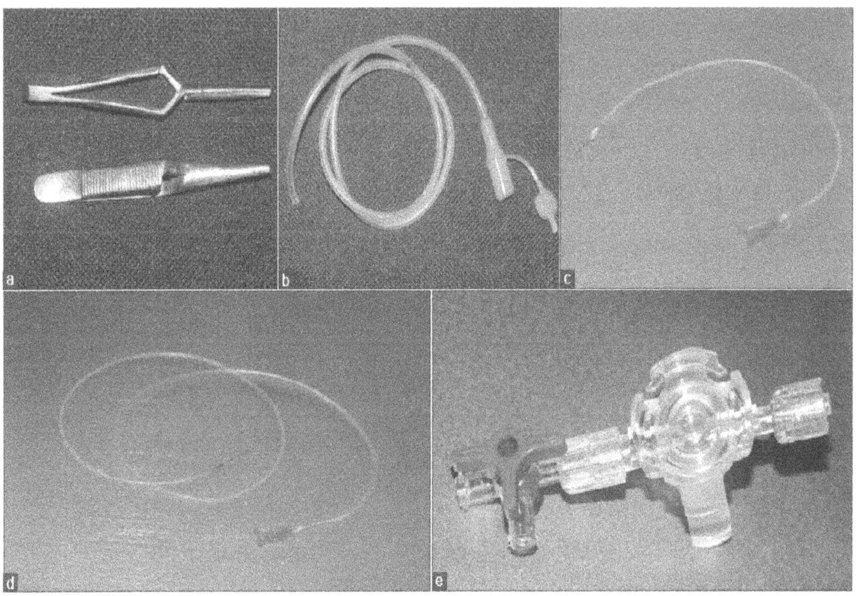

Fig. 4.4 Invasive B.P measuring apparatus.

Procedure:

- Healthy adult chicken weighing between 12-23 gm is anaesthetized with halothane.
- The temperature of animal is kept constant by means of warm copper plate.
- The rural vein is cannulated by means of venous cannula. Injections are made through the venous cannula only.
- The popliteal artery is cannulated by means of an arterial cannulated and then joined to monometer for recording arterial B.P. on the kymograph.
- First normal B.P. is recorded.
- Repeated injections of Oxytocin are made at regular intervals of time.
- A dose of 20-100 milli units at intervals of 30 min are given to get changes in B.P.
- The fixed volume of normal saline is passed to push the extract towards the heart and to maintain blood volume.
- The doses of standard extract and test sample are adjusted until the produce an equal fall in B.P. alternatively with varying doses of test sample.
- Till both produce the same rise in B.P.
- Four point bioassay is recommended in IP-1996 and activity is expressed in units/ml.

Conclusion: The Potency of test sample is calculated by comparing the rise in B.P. with that produced by standard sample.

4.1.3 Bioassay of Insulin

1. Rabbit method.
2. Mouse method.

Standard Solution Preparation

- It is pure, dry, crystalline insulin.
- 20 Units of Insulin are accurately weighed and dissolved in normal saline solution.
- It is acidified with HCl to make pH 2.5 and 0.5% phenol, 1.8% Glycerin added as preservative.
- Final volume should contain 20 Units/ml.
- Store the solution in cool place and use it within 6 months.

- Sample diluting was freshly prepared by diluting with normal saline solution. So they contain.
  1. Units/ml (Standard Dilution – I)
  2. Units/ml (Standard Dilution – II)

Test Sample Solution Preparation

The solution of test sample is prepared in the same way as the standard solution as described above.

Method A

Rabbit Method

Principle is based on potency of test sample that is estimated by comparing the hypoglycemic effect of the sample with that of the standard preparation of insulin.

Selection of Rabbits

- They should be healthy, Weight about 1.8-3.6 kg each.
- Maintained of uniform diet and fasted for 18 hr before assay.
- Water is withdrawn during the experiment.

Procedure:

- Animals are divided into four groups of three rabbits each.
- Then rabbits are put into an animal shoulder. They should be handled with care to avoid experimental errors.
- The first part of the test – a sample of blood is taken from marginal ear vein of each rabbit.
- Presence of reducing sugar is estimated per 100 ml of blood by suitable chemical method.
- This concentration is called "Initial Blood Sugar Level".

The four groups of rabbits are S.C. injection of insulin as follows.

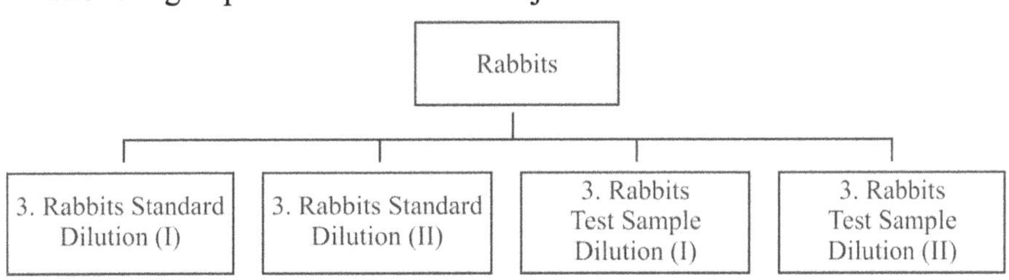

- From each rabbit a sample of blood is withdrawn up to 5 hr at the interval of 1 hr each.
- Blood sugar is determined again. This is known as "Final Blood Sugar Level".
- In second part of test – same animals are used for "Cross Over test" is carried out. Experiment is carried out after one week again the animals are fasted and initial blood sugar is determined.
- Grouping is reversed.
- Those which received test are now giving the standard.

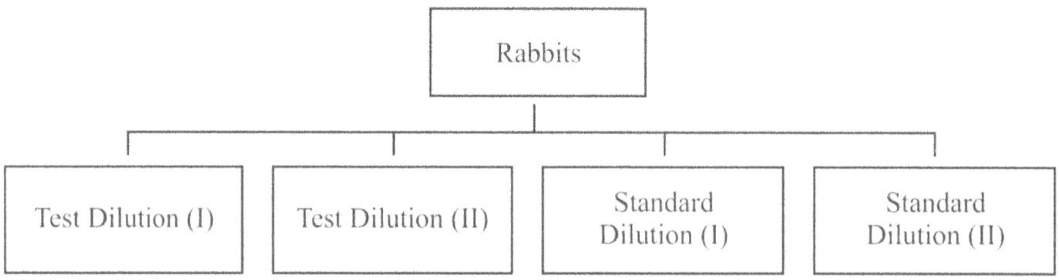

Conclusion: This test is known as "Twin Cross Over Test". Mean percentage decrease in blood sugar of first and second part is calculated.

Method B

Mouse Method

Aim: Principle based on characteristic conclusions after S.C. injection of insulin at elevated temperatures. Percentage produced by test and standard preparations is compared.

Animals required	:	100 mice of same strain (18-22 gm)
Chemicals required	:	Sterile saline solution
Equipments required	:	Air incubator boxes- made of perforated sheets of metal

Procedure: Mice are maintained on constant diet and fasted 18 hr prior to the experiment

- Standard dilutions are prepared with sterile saline solution
- 0.064 Units/ml (Standard Dilution – I)
- 0.096 Units/ml (Standard Dilution – II)
- First sample dilutions are also prepared in same manner
- Mice are divided into four groups. Each containing 25 mice. Insulin is injected S.C. as follows.

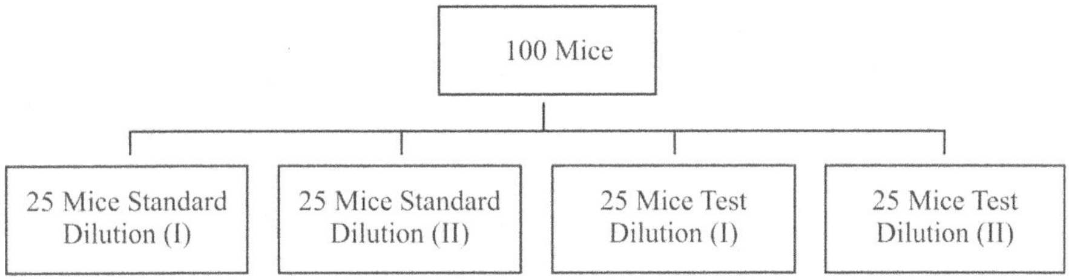

- Mice are put in an air incubator at 33 $^{\circ}$C and observed for half an hour. Air incubator with glass front provided with 6 shelves is used.
- Temperature is thermostatically controlled.
- Two mice are kept in each of the boxes made up of perforated sheets of metal.
- The mice which convulse or die are taken out of the incubator and observed. Conclusive mice may be saved by 0.5 ml of 5% dextrose injection.

Conclusion: Percentage convulsions produced by the test sample and standard sample are compared. Those animals which Survive may be used again for another experiment after an interval of 1 week.

4.1.4 Bioassay of D-Tubocurarine

D-Tubocurarine, a skeletal muscle relaxant acting on nicotine receptors produces a dose dependent competitive and reversible antagonism of acetylcholine. Thus graded responses of D-Tubocurarine in the form of inhibition of the fixed dose of acetylcholine can be determined.

Method A [Frog Method]

Aim: The response [% Inhibition] are plotted against Log dose of D-Tubocurarine and the concentration of unknown can be calculated by finding out the amount of standard solution of D-Tubocurarine producing the same response (Inhibition) as produced by unknown solutions

Animals required	:	Frogs
Chemicals required	:	Ringer solution, acetylcholine (Ach)
Equipments required	:	Organ bath, Kymograph

Procedure:

- Frog is sacrificed as per CPCSEA recommended guideline and rectus abdomens muscle is dissected out and mounted in the organ bath containing frog ringer solution.

- Preparation was stabilized for half an hour. Washout is given at every 10 min interval.
- Two responses to sub maximal dose of acetylcholine are recorded on kymograph place on drum.
- The drum is moved for 30 sec and lowest dose 0.1 ml of D-Tubocurarine is added in the bath.
- After two minutes response to same dose of Ach is taken in presence of D-Tubocurarine 5 min cycle is followed as usual.
- The responses to Ach are taken after every 5 minutes till the recovery to control height is achieved.
- The responses to D-Tubocurarine using different doses of standard and unknown are recorded in this manner.
- The graph is fixed and heights of control (H) and in the presence of antagonist (h) (D- Tubocurarine) are measured and the percentage inhibition is calculated as follows.
- Percentage = "H – h ÷ h × 100"
- Each time the height of response of Ach is taken just before addition of antagonist.

Conclusion: Percentage inhibition is plotted on semi log graph and the concentration of unknown is then calculated out from graph.

.... .No. of ml of Test = ...No. ml of Standard.

Concentration of test

$$x = \frac{\text{ml of standard}}{\text{ml of test}} \times \text{Concentration of standard}$$

Method B: (Rabbit Head – Drop Method)

Aim: D-Tubocurarine HCl is injected into marginal vein of the rabbit's ear till the rabbit's neck muscles are relaxed such that the animal cannot hold it head up.

The total amount if test sample required to produce the end point is compared with total amount of the standard sample required to produce similar end point.

Animals required	:	Rabbits (2 kg each animal)
Equipments required	:	Rabbit holders
Chemicals required	:	Neostigmine methyl sulphate Atropine sulphate

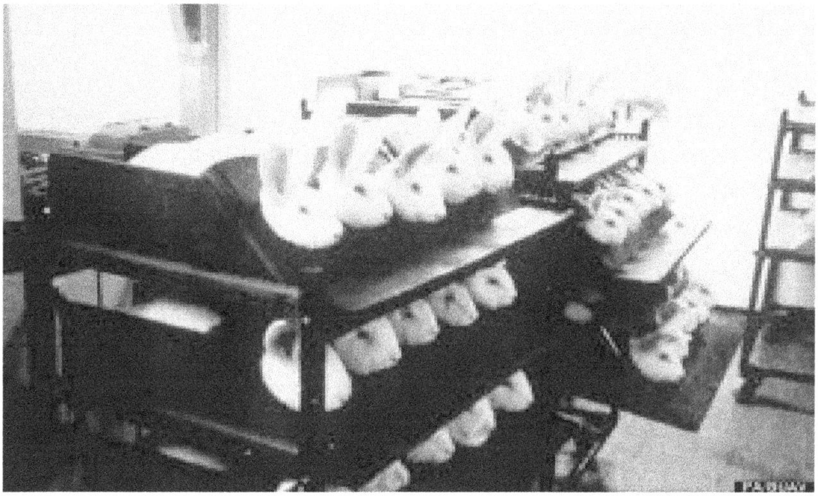

Fig. 4.5 Rabbit head drop method.

Procedure:

- 8 Rabbits- free from Disease.
- Obtained from a healthy colony should be chosen each rabbit placed in rabbit holder with its head protruding outside. Head should be freely movable then divided into 2 groups.
- D-Tubocurarine solution is injected at a constant speed by infusion apparatus through marginal vein.
- Injection given at rate of 0.4 ml/min and at 10 min interval. Infusion is continued till - rabbit will not be in a position to hold its head correct or there will be no response by focusing light on eyes and the neck gets elongated and toneless.
- Rabbits recover immediately from effect of curarization if any respiratory problem occurs treated by injection of neostigmine methyl sulphate by marginal-vein or atropine sulphate.
- Cross over test is carried out

Conclusion: Mean dose is – which produces head drop of test sample is compared with mean dose of standard preparation.

4.1.5 Bioassay of Acetylcholine

Acetylcholine produces a dose dependent contraction of rectus abdomen's muscle through the stimulation of nicotinic receptors. In the graphical method

4-6 responses to graded doses of Acetylcholine are obtained and then two equal responses to unknown sample are taken.

Method A [Frog Method]

Aim: The responses can be plotted against log – dose of standard and the amount of standard drug producing the same response as produced by unknown drug is directly.

Animals required	:	Frogs
Chemicals required	:	Ringer solution, Ach
Equipments required	:	Organ bath, frontal writing lever, Kymograph

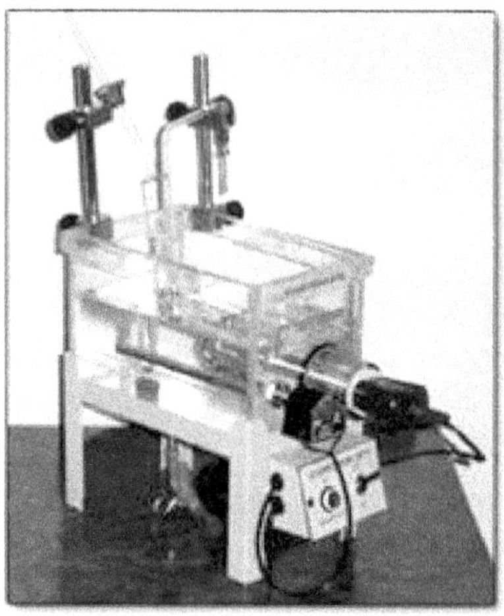

Fig. 4.6 Organ bath.

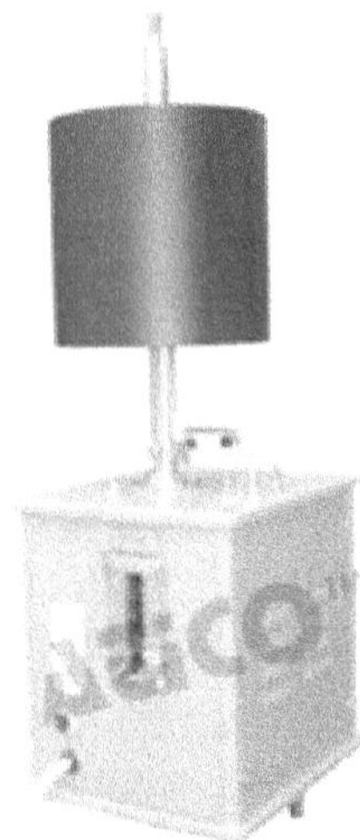

Fig. 4.7 Kymograph drum.

Procedure:

- A frog is sacrificed as per CPCSEA guidelines.
- The frog is placed in a tray with ventral side facing up. The skin is incised longitudinally in the midline of abdomen. Two rectal muscles are situated on the either sides of the midline. One rectus abdominus muscle is separated and mounted in the inner organ bath.
- One end of muscle is tied to aeration tube and the other is connected to isotonic frontal writing lever. The tissue is allowed to stabilize for half an hour.
- During this period the ringer solution is changed after every 10 min.

- Once the tissue is stabilized, graded doses of acetylcholine are added to obtain contractile responses. A five minutes time cycle is followed for each response.
- 5-6 responses of graded doses of standard are taken and then 2 Equities responses of the test sample are taken. The height of contraction is measured and plotted against the log- dose.

Conclusion: The dose of standard drug producing the same response is produced by the test drug is read directly from the graph and the concentration if test sample is determined.

$$\text{Concentration of test} = \frac{\text{...ml of Standard}}{\text{ml of test}} \times \text{Concentration of standard}$$

Method B: Rat Ileum

Aim: Acetylcholine produces a dose – dependent motility in rat ileum through the stimulation of cholinergic receptors.

Animals required	:	Rat
Chemicals required	:	Tyrode's solution, Acetyl choline
Equipments required	:	Pipette, Petridish, Isotonic frontal lever

Procedure:

- The animal kept for overnight fasting.
- After that sacrificed as per CPCSEA guidelines.
- The abdominal cavity is quickly opened and a piece of ileum is isolated.
- It is placcd in a pctridish containing tyrodc solution maintained at 37 °C.
- The mesentery of ileum is removed and the interior content is washed by blowing tyrode solution with the help of pipette and has to place in an organ both which is connected to isotonic frontal writing lever. The tissue is stabilized for 30 min.
- Then remaining experiment is same as previous method (frog method).

Conclusion: The responses of acetyl chorine are taken till the maximum effect is obtained.

Method C: Guinea Pig's Ileum (Same as Rat Ileum)

Aim: This method is carried out by measuring blood pressure.

Method D: Cat's Blood Pressure

Aim: This method is carried out by measuring blood pleasure.

- In this method – A cat is anaesthetized with suitable anaesthetic.

- The carotid artery is cannulated for recording B.P.
- Femoral vein is cannulated for injecting acetylcholine trachea is cannulated for artificial respiration.
- Acetylcholine produces a fall in blood pressure by dilating peripheral blood vessels.
- The extent which blood pressure falls due to the test sample is compared with the fall by the standard preparation.

4.1.6 Bioassay of Adrenaline

A. Rabbit ileum method.

B. Anaesthetized dog method.

C. Anaesthetized cat method.

D. De Jalon's method on rat's uterus

Method-A: Rabbit Ileum Method

Aim: Adrenaline is a sympathomimetic agent stimulates both (α and β) adrenergic receptors which are inhibitory in gastro intestinal muscle. Thus, it can produce a dose dependent relaxation of rabbit ileum.

Animals required	:	Rabbit
Chemicals required	:	Tyrode solution, Adrenaline
Equipments required	:	Pipette, isotonic frontal writing lever.

Procedure:

- Rabbits are kept for overnight fasting and sacrificed as per CPCSEA recommended guidelines.
- The abdominal cavity is quickly opened and piece of ileum is isolated and placed in tyrode solution maintained at 37 °C.
- The mesentery of ileum is removed and the interior content is washed by tyrode solution with the help of pipette. The tissue is mounted in the organ bath and connected to the isotonic frontal writing lever.
- It is allowed to stabilize till the spontaneous contractions become uniform for 5 min.
- Graded doses of adrenaline are added to the bath and the relaxant effect is recorded.
- 5-6 responses of graded doses of the standard are taken and then two equal active responses of the test sample are taken.
- The length of relaxation is measured and plotted against the log – dose *Vs* standard.

Conclusion: The dose of standard producing the same responses produced by the test is read directly from the graph and the concentration of test sample is determined.

$$\text{Concentration of test} = \frac{\text{ml of standard}}{\text{ml of test}} \times \text{Concentration of standard}$$

Method-B: Anaesthetized Dog Method

Aim: Based on that Adrenaline produces a dose dependent rise in Blood Pressure.

Animals required	:	Dog (10-13 kg)
Chemicals required	:	Pentobarbitone sodium, atropine sulphate
Equipments required	:	Mercury monometer, electrical stimulator

Procedure:

A medium size dog [10-13 kg] is anesthetized with Pentobarbitone sodium in the dose of 25 mg/kg i.e., 250-325 mg.

- Artificial respiration is given through tracheal tube; B.P. is recorded on a kymograph after cannulating carotid artery with arterial cannula and connecting the same with mercury monometer.
- The animal should be injected with 0.001-0.002 mg of atropine sulphate to paralyse the vagi.
- This paralysis is confirmed by stimulating vagi by electrical stimulation. There will be no fall in B.P. in atropinised animal after electrical stimulation.
- Adrenaline is injected into the femoral vein through venous cannula. Two successive responses (rise in B.P.) of the same dose of adrenaline are noted.
- The similar responses after the same dose of adrenaline are an indication that the animal is now ready for the assay.
- Then the test and the standard samples are given in alternate till both produce similar rise in B.P. injections are given at intervals of 5 min.

Conclusion: Potency of test sample is compared with that of the standard sample.

Method-C Anaesthetized Cat Method

Method is similar to that of dog. In this method chloralose (80 mg/kg) is used as anesthetic agent. [Instead of Atropinisation medulla oblongata is destroyed to prevent any reflex action].

Method D: De Jalon's Method on Rat's Uterus

Aim: This method used to determine % inhibition of contractions of adrenaline on rat uterus which is placed in De Jalon's solution.

Requirements:

Animals required	:	Female rats (100-150 gm)
Chemicals required	:	De Jalon's solution Frog Ringer solution Carbachol
Equipments required	:	Organ bath

Frog ringer solution composition	:	NaCl	- 9.0 grams
		$CaCl_2$	- 0.06 grams
		KCl	- 0.45 grams
		$NaHCO_3$	- 0.5 grams
		Dextrose	- 0.5 grams
		Distilled water	- 1000 ml
De Jalon's solution composition	:	NaCl	- 9.0 grams
		$CaCl_2$	- 0.06 grams
		KCl	- 0.42 grams
		$NaHCO_3$	- 0.5 grams
		Glucose	- 0.5 g/l

Procedure:

- A virgin female rat (100-150 grams) is used for this method.
- Rats are killed by head blow method, abdomen is opened after those uterine horns are isolated and placed in De Jalon's solution.
- After that uterine horns are ligated and suspended in mammalian organ bath containing modified ringer solution.
- Then by administration of carbachol (0.75 mg/ml) contractions of those uterine horns are recorded.
- Then the animals are divided into 2 groups.
- For one group 3 different doses of standard adrenaline is administered.
- For second group 3 different doses of test adrenaline is administered.

Conclusion: % reduction of carbachol induced contractions is recorded (While giving of adrenaline it reduces the contractions which are given by carbachol).

4.1.7 Bioassay of Autacoids

Aim: Based on histamine produces a dose dependent contraction of guinea pig ileum through the stimulation of H_1 receptor. Histamine is the main example of autacoid.

Animals required	:	Guinea pig (350- 450 gm)
Chemicals required	:	Tyrode solution, Histamine
Equipments required	:	Petridish, mammalian organ bath, isotonic frontal writing lever, pipette

Procedure:

- A guinea pig which is fasted overnight sacrificed as per CPCSEA recommended guidelines.
- The abdominal cavity is quickly opened and a piece of ileum is isolated. It is placed in a petridish containing tyrode solution maintained at 37 °C.
- The mesentery of ileum is removed and the lumen of ileum is cleaned by passing warm Tyrode solution through it from a pipette. The tissue is mounted in mammalian organ bath and connected to isotonic frontal writing lever.
- The tissue is allowed to stabilize for 30 min. The response of histamine is taken till the maximum effect is obtained.

Conclusion: Means DRC [Dose Response Curve] is observed.

Matching Method

Aim: Principle of this assay based on the test substance and the standard are applied and the responses obtained are matched by a trial and the error process until they produce equal effects. This test does not depend on assumptions of a dose response relationship.

Procedure:
Administer the smallest volume of unknown and keep increasing it till prominent responses are obtained. The response of standard which matches with that of unknown sample would be found by trial and error method.

……….. No. ml. of test =…….. No. ml. of standard is calculated.

Demerits

- It is purely subjected and experimental errors cannot be determined from the assay.

- Gives no indication or parallelism of the dose response curve of standard curves of standard drug and test substance have the qualitative difference as the effects are matched at only on dose level.

Three – point Method

Aim: Principle based on the potency of the substance is determined by using below formula

Three point Assay is used when the active material is present in sufficient Quantity.

Potency of test solution

$$\text{Potency of the test Solution} = \frac{n_1}{t} \text{anti log} \left\{ \frac{(t_1 - s_1)}{(s_2 - s_1)} \text{x log} + \frac{n_1}{n_2} \right\}$$

where

n_1 – Lower Standard Dose; n_2 – Higher Standard Dose; t – Test Dose.

The response of 2 doses of the standard (s_1, s_2) and the test are obtained by changing the order in successive cycles.

Procedure:

- Take the response with different volumes of unknown.
- Select two responses of standard (s_1, s_2) and the test administer them in cyclic manner.
- After selecting the (s_1, s_2) test administers them in cyclic manner.

Conclusion: Calculate Potency with above formula.

4.1.8 Bioassay of Corticotrophin

The potency of corticotrophin is determined by comparing its adrenal ascorbic acid depletion property with that of the standard preparation of corticotrophin under the conditions of a suitable method of assay.

Dry corticotrophin is taken as Standard Preparation.

Method –A

Animals required	:	Albino rats (100-200 gm)
Chemical required	:	5% solution of dextrose saline
Equipments required	:	Homogenizer

Procedure:

- Use rats of either sex weight between 100-200 gm and keep the rats under uniform condition for at least a week before the test.

- On the day before the test, weigh hypophysectomise the rats.
- After the operations allows access to a 5% solution of dextrose in saline solution in addition to rat diet and water and keep the animals at a constant temperature between 24 °C & 27 °C carry out the rest between 18 and 36 hr after hypophysectomise.
- On the day of experiment animals and assign them at random to 6 groups of 8-10 animals
- Choose 3 doses of standard and 3 doses of test being tested such that the smallest dose produces some depletion.
- Administer in random order by subcutaneous injection doses adjusted to the body weight of the animals.
- Doses of the order of 1.0, 0.5 & 0.25 units per 100 gm of body weight are usually suitable.
- 3 hr after injection remove both adrenal glands from anaesthetized rat, free from extraneous tissues and possible to avoid weight losses.
- Kill the rat and examine for completeness of hypophysectomy.
- Homogenize the pair of adrenal glands in a freshly prepared 2.5% w/v solution of meta phosphoric acid and adjust the volume to 10 ml with the same solution allow the homogenate to stand for 30 min and centrifuge.
- Add 7 ml of the clear supernatant liquid to a freshly prepared mixture of 7 ml of sodium acetate adjusted to pH-7.
- 30 sec after mixing, measure the extinction of the resulting at maximum at 520 nm

Conclusion: Calculate the weight of ascorbic acid from a standard curve prepared by L-ascorbic acid in a 25% w/v solution of meta phosphoric acid by the same process.

Method B

Follows method A with the following modifications

- Administer the standard preparation and preparation being tested by I.V. injection in saliva solution without the addition of gelatin.
- Remove the adrenal glands between 55 and 65 min after injection.
- Where in method A drug (sample) administered in S.C. or I.M.
- But in method B sample administered by I.V.

4.1.9 Bioassay of Pertussis Vaccine

The potency of pertussis vaccine is determined by comparison of dose necessary to protect mice against the effects of a measured dose of *Bordetella pertussis*.

[Challenge culture administered intra cerebrally]. With the dose of a reference preparation, required to same level of protection.

Method A

Reference preparation: It is an international standard of Pertussis vaccine, consisting of a freeze dried vaccine.

Animals required	:	Mice (13-16 gm)
Chemicals required	:	Liquid nitrogen, 1% w/v of casein hydrolysate, 0.85% w/v of NaCl
Equipments required	:	Cell line for subculture

Procedure:

- Healthy mice [between 13-16 gm] were selected. Distribute the mice randomly in 6-8 groups of not less than 16 and not more than 24 and 4 groups of 10 mice.
- The mice should all be of the same seized or the male and female should be distributed equally between the groups.
- Half of the groups of 16-24 should receive the reference preparation and the other half should receive the vaccine under examination.
- The 4 groups of 10 each should be used for the LD_{50} titration of challenge suspension.
- Use at least 3-dilutions of the reference vaccine and similar dilution of the vaccine under examination.
- In each case the dilution are so selection that the dilution protecting 50% of the mice ED_{50} is as near as possible to middle of the dilution range.
- Each dose being contained in a volume, not exceeding 0.5 ml
- For each dilution use 16-24 mice and use i.p. route select a suitable strain of *B. pertussis*, capable of causing the death of mice within 14 days of intracerebral injection.
- Make 2 subcultures after reviving the strain on a suitable medium and suspend the strain on a suitable medium and suspend the harvested growth in a solution containing 1% w/v of Casein Hydrolysate and 0.85% w/v of NaCl having a pH of 7.0-7.2.

- Liquors of challenge suspension frozen in liquid nitrogen with a suitable preservation like 10% DMSO may be used to avoid heterogensity.
- After 14-17 days of immunization, inject intracerebral a dose of 0.02-0.03 ml of the challenge randomly into each immunized mouse.
- In the same inject 4 groups of 10 control mice each for LD_{50} titration of challenge preparation, prepared by a series of dilution from the dilution selected for challenge.
- Exclude any mouse from consideration that dies within 3 days of challenge.
- Count the numbers of mice surviving in each of the group after 14 days.
- On the basis of the numbers of animals surviving in each group of 16-24 mice, calculate the potency of vaccine under examination.
- Agonist the potency of reference preparation.
- Calculate the potency of the vaccine by probity analysis and LD_{50} of challenge suspension by reed and muench method.

Conclusion: Probity-analysis is useful for determination of potency.

Read and muench method is useful for determination of LD_{50} value.

The test is not valid unless

(a) For both the vaccines under examination and the reference preparation, the ED_{50} lies between the largest and the smallest doses given to the mice.

(b) The number of animals, which die to the mice 4 groups of 10 mice injected, with the challenge suspension and its dilution indicate that the challenge contains 100-1000 LD_{50} and LD_{50} not more than 300 colony formation units.

(c) The statistical analysis shows no deviation from linearity i.e., the protective response is graded in relation to the vaccinating dose.

4.1.10 Bioassay of Plague Vaccine

Plague vaccine is a sterile suspension of killed plague bacilli, *Yersinia pestis*. The potency of plague vaccine is estimated by determining the dose necessary to protect mice against a lethal dose of a virulent strain of *Yersinia pestis*.

Test animals

Use white mice, 6 -7 weeks old, each weighing between 20-28 grams and of a strain susceptible to plague infection. The selected strain of mice should be such that an injective dose of 6-12 organisms of virulent strain of not less than 80% of the animals used.

The animals should be healthy and free from intercurrence infection such as salmonella.

Selection of suitable virulent strain:

- A freeze dried virulent culture of *Y. pestis* established to be suitable for challenge is revived by sub culturing 0.5 ml in 9.5 ml of nutrient broth contained in other test tube and incubating at 28 °C for exactly 48 hr.
- Such a culture should contain 300-600 million organisms per ml.
- Make 10-fold dilutions in nutrient broth and test for virulence.
- Use a 10-7 dilution containing 6-12 organisms in 0.2 ml the test infective dose per animals.

Standard challenge dose

Freshly reconstitute the freeze dried culture and dilute with nutrient broth to a strength such that 0.2 ml contains 60 -120 organisms.

Procedure:

Measurement of protective power

- Prepare a series of five graded doses of the preparation under examination arranged in such a manner that the 50% protective dose (ED_{50}) lies about the middle of the selected series. For each dose a batch of 16 mice are used.
- Inject subcutaneously the selected dose in 2 equal parts with an interval of 7 days between them. 7 days after the second half of the dose inject subcutaneously into each group of mice the standard challenge dose. At the same time inject into 10-control mice 8-9 weeks old and weighing between 28-30 gm the standard challenge dose.
- Observe the animals for 15days and record the number of deaths in each group. Carry out a post-mortem on the dead animal and look for signs of plague in them. If plague organisms are not seen, such deaths are excluded from the calculation. The test is not valid unless the number of such death is not more.
- At the end of the period of observation kill all the surviving animals and examine for signs of plague. Calculate the median effective immunizing dose ED_{50} by standard statistical method.
- The vaccine passes the test if it has an ED_{50} of 0.004 [less per mice].

4.1.11 Bioassay of Rabies Vaccine

Rabies vaccine for human use is a freeze dried or liquid preparation of suitable approved, stain of fixed rabies virus grown in an approved cell culture/embryos of duck chicken and inactive by a validated method.

The potency of rabies vaccine is determined by comparing the dose necessary to protect mice against a lethal intracerebral dose of rabies vaccine necessary to provide the same protection.

Test animals

- Use mice of a suitable strain, drawn from a uniform stock 3-4 weeks old, weighing between 11-15 grams.
- Distribute the mice into 6-groups of at least 16 mice each and 4- groups of 10 mice each and must be of the same sex or the sexes must be equally distributed among the groups.
- Throughout the test all mice that die before the 5th day after challenge are excluded from the test and all mice that die with signs of rabies between 5th and 14th day after challenge are counted as failing to resists the challenge.
- The strain of mice suitable for the test is such that when 0.03 ml containing 5-50 LD_{50} of the challenge virus suspension is injected intracerebral per mouse there is 100% mortality.

Standard challenge virus suspension

- A working pool of the challenge virus strains are prepared by injecting intracerebral 0.03 ml of a 10 fold dilution of the CVS strain of rabies virus in 2% v/v sterile inactivated normal horse serum in water for injection into a suitable number of test animals.
- The animals when moribund after showing characteristic signs of rabies are scarified and their brains harvested aseptically.
- They are then washed in chilled saline solution to remove blood clots.
- A 10% suspension of brain is prepared in a suitable dilute and thoroughly homogenized.
- After centrifuging lightly, the supernatant liquid is distributed into sterile vials and freeze dried.
- The sealed and freeze dried supernatant liquid containing vials are stored at –20 °C.
- When stored under prescribed conditions the virus titre of the freeze dried preparation may be expected to be maintained for not less than 3 years.

Virus titer of the challenge virus

- Prepare 10-fold serial dilutions of the standard challenge virus suspension.
- Groups of 10 mice each inject 0.03 ml of the virus suspension intracerebrally into each mouse, using a different group of each suspension.

- Observe the mice for 14 days.
- Calculate the virus titer of the standard challenge virus suspension in LD_{50} per dose of 0.03 ml standard statistical methods.

Determination of potency of the vaccine

- Reconstitute the standard preparation with suitable diluents.
- Prepare at least three 5-fold serial dilutions of the solution of the standard preparation and three 5-fold serial dilutions of the vaccine under examination.
- For both, the standard preparation and the preparation under examination, the serial dilutions should be prepared in such way that the lowest dilution protects more than 50% of the injected mice.
- Allocate one dilution to each of the 6 groups of 16 mice each.
- Inject intraperitonially (I.P.) each mouse in each group with dilution of the vaccine and reference preparation and repeat the injection.
- After seven days, prepare identical dilutions of the vaccine and reference preparation and repeat he injection after a further 7 days, inject each vaccinated mouse intra cerebrally with 0.03 ml of the standard challenge various suspension. Such that on the basis of preliminary titration.
- Observe the mice for 14 days and record the mice surviving the challenge in each group. Calculate potency of the preparation under examination by standard statically methods.

The test is not valid unless

- For both the preparation under examination and the standard preparation, the ED_{50} lies between the largest and smallest doses given to the mice.
- There is no deviation from linearity of the dose response lines.
- The titer of the challenge virus suspension lies between 5-50 LD_{50}.

4.1.12 Bioassay of Hyaluronidase

Hyaluronidase

Hyaluronidase activity may be determined by various biological and physicochemical methods and theoretically any method measuring the depolymerizing activity of hyaluronidase may be considered suitable. The clinical efficacy of hyaluronidase, however, depends mainly on its power to split the highly polymerized mucopolysaccharides in the dermis, thus breaking down the barrier which hinders the inflow or the absorption of injected fluid.

Enzyme preparation

Seven preparations from different sources were used. Five of them were of testicular origin in a more or less purified state. One had been prepared from staphylococci and one from streptococci. Our laboratory standard preparation, with which the other enzymes were compared, consisted of Seitz-filtered bull seminal fluid, distributed in equal amounts into ampoules, and dried from the frozen state. One ampoule contains approximately 50 mg of the dry material. volumes of 0.2 ml were injected with an all-glass tuberculin syringe calibrated to 0.01 ml, through a short 26-gauge needle. Indicator, Horse red cells were washed eight times with 0.9% (w/v) NaCl on the centrifuge in order to remove any serum inhibitor of hyaluronidase, then lacked by the addition of distilled water, and the resulting solution was freeze-dried.

Animals required	:	Albino guinea pigs (300 gm)
Chemicals required	:	0.9% (w/v) NaCl

Procedure:

- Using four two fold dilutions of enzyme, the highest of which produced about 20% increase of the mean area compared with the control, it was ascertained that, within the dose range employed, the departure from linearity of the curves of response (area of spread of indicator) plotted against log dose, was not significant.
- In these assays, however, the site to site variations were excessive and the lesions tended to spread into one another.
- It was therefore decided to use a skin area in which such variations could be reduced to a minimum.
- This area is limited cranially by the interscapular pad of fat, posterior by the pelvis and extends ventrally on both sides to a line parallel to and 1 inch distant from the midline. Within this area two dilutions of the standard preparation (4 and 2, gm/ml) and two appropriate two fold dilutions of the enzyme under test, that is a total of four injections, were distributed at random.
- The dilutions of the test preparation were made as nearly as possible equipotent with the dilutions of the standard. The time elapsing between the animal's deaths, by a blow on the head and bleeding from the neck, and the start of the first injection was usually not more than 1 min; subsequent injections were made at 15 sec intervals.
- After the first injection the skin of the back was flayed, care being taken neither to pull on the skin nor to press on the blebs. The skin, with the inside

- Surface uppermost, was laid beneath a flat glass plate and the outline of each bleb traced on cellophane exactly 12 min after the injection was made. These tracings were copied on parchment paper and the resulting areas determined by cutting out and weighing the pieces of parchment. The time of 12 min. At this time the blebs are still actively diffusing with approximately their initial velocity.

Conclusion: Since two doses of the standard and two of the test enzyme were administered, the assay represents a 4-point design. The estimation of potency and the statistical analysis were performed accordingly, including an analysis of variance and a test for parallelism of the dose-response lines.

4.1.13 Bioassay of Tetanus Antitoxin

Tetanus Antitoxin is a preparation containing the specific antitoxic globulins or their derivatives obtained by the purification of hyper immune serum of horses or other suitable animals and have the specific activity of neutralizing the toxin from by *Clostridium tetani*. Tetanus antitoxin has the potency of not less than 1000 units per ml when intended for prophylactic use and less than 3000 units per ml when intended for therapeutic use.

Biological assay of tetanus antitoxin

Aim: The potency of tetanus antitoxin is determined by comparing the dose necessary to protect mice against the paralytic effects of a fixed dose of a tetanus antitoxin with the dose of standard preparation of tetanus antitoxin necessary to give same protection.

Standard preparation: The standard preparation is the 2nd International standard for Tetanus Antitoxin. It consists of freeze dried hyper immune horse serum or another suitable preparation the potency of which has been determined in relation to International standard.

Method: Test animal: Healthy mice (weight-17-22 gm)

Preparation of test toxin: Prepare tetanus toxin from a sterile filtrate of 8-10 day culture of *Cl. tetani*. Test toxin may be prepared by adding this filtrate to glycerin in the portion of 1 vol. of filtrate to 1 or 2 vol. of glycerin. This solution of test toxin is stored below 0 °C. The toxin may also be prepared in stable form by saturating the filtrate with ammonium sulphate, collecting the resulting precipitate, drying it over P_2O_5 at a pressure of 1.5 to 2.5 kPa and reducing it to fine powder. The powder so obtained is preserved in a dry condition at a low temperature either in sealed ampoules or over P_2O_5 at a pressure of 1.5 to 2.5 kPa.

Determination of test dose of toxin (Lp/10 dose): First determine the limes paralyticum/10 (Lp/10) dose of the test toxin. This is the smallest quantity of toxin which when mixed with 0.1 unit of standard preparation and injection S.C. into mice causes titanic paralysis within 4 days. Prepare the solution of standard preparation in a suitable liquid such that 1 ml contains 0.5 units. Accurately measure or weigh a quantity of test toxin and dilute it with or dissolve it in, a suitable liquid. Prepare mixture such that each contains 2 ml of the solution of standard preparation (1 unit), one of the series of graded volume of solution of the toxin and sufficient of a suitable to give a final volume of 5ml. Allow the mixture to stand at room temperature, protected from light, for 60 min and then inject 0.5 ml of each mixture S.C. into mice, 6 mice being used for each mixture and observe the mice for 4 days. The mixture that contains the largest volume of preparation under examination that fails to protect the mice from paralysis contains 1 unit. The test is not valid unless all the mice injected with the mixture containing 2 ml or less of the solution of standard preparation under examination in units per ml.

Determination of potency of the antitoxin: Prepare a solution of standard preparation in a suitable liquid such that it contain 0.5 units per ml. Accurately measure or weigh a quantity of test toxin and dilute it with or dissolve it in a suitable liquid so that 1 ml contains 5 times the Lp/10 dose as previously determined. Prepare mixtures such that each contain 2 ml of solution of test toxin and 1 of a series of graded volumes of the preparation under examination and sufficient of toxin and 1 of a series of graded volume of 5 ml. Prepare similar mixture containing 2 ml of the test toxin and 1 of series of graded volumes of solution of the standard preparation centered on that volume that contains 1 unit. Allow the mix to standard room temperature protected from light for 60 min and then inoculate 0.5 ml of each mix by s.c. route into each mouse, 6 mice being used for each mix and observe the mice for 4 days. The mix that contains the largest volume of preparation under examination that fails to protect the mice from paralysis contains 1 unit. The test is not valid unless all the mice injected with the mixture containing 2 ml or less of the solution of standard preparation show paralysis and all those injected with more don't calculate the potency of the preparation under examination in units per ml.

4.1.14 Bioassay of Diphtheria Vaccine (ADSORBED)

The potency of diphtheria vaccine (adsorbed) is determined by comparing the dose of the vaccine required to protect guinea-pigs from the effects of either an erythrogenic dose of diphtheria toxin administered intradermally or a lethal dose of diphtheria toxin administered subcutaneously with the dose of a reference preparation, calibrated in International Units, needed to give the same protection. The International Unit is the activity contained in a stated amount of the International Standard which consists of a quantity of diphtheria toxoid adsorbed on aluminum hydroxide. The equivalence in International Units of the International Standard is stated by the World Health Organization.

Diphtheria vaccine (adsorbed) BRP is suitable for use as a reference preparation. The design of the assay described below follows a parallel-line model with 3 dilutions for the test and reference preparations. Once the analyst has sufficient experience with this method for a given vaccine, it is possible to apply a simplified model using a single dilution for both test and reference preparations. Such a model enables the analyst to determine whether the potency of the test preparation is significantly higher than the minimum required but does not give information on linearity, parallelism and the dose-response curve. The simplified model leads to a considerable reduction in the number of experimental animals required and must be considered by each analyst in accordance with the provisions of the European Convention for the Protection of Vertebrate Animals used for Experimental and other Scientific Purposes.

Method of Intradermal Challenge

Selection and distribution of the test animals: Use in the test, healthy, white guinea-pigs from the same stock and of a size suitable for the prescribed number of challenge sites, the difference in body mass between the heaviest and the lightest animal being not greater than 100 gm. Distribute the guinea-pigs in not fewer than 6 equal groups; use groups containing a number of animals sufficient to obtain results that fulfill the requirements for a valid assay prescribed below. If the challenge toxin to be used has not been shown to be stable or has not been adequately standardized, include 5 guinea-pigs as unvaccinated controls. Use guinea-pigs of the same sex or with males and females equally distributed between the groups.

Selection of the challenge toxin: Select a preparation of diphtheria toxin containing 67 to 133 L/100 in 1 Lf (Limes flocculation) and 25,000 to 50,000 minimal reacting doses for guinea-pig skin in 1 Lf. If the challenge toxin preparation has been shown to be stable, it is not necessary to verify the activity for every assay.

Preparation of the challenge toxin solution: Immediately before use, dilute the challenge toxin with a suitable diluents to obtain a challenge toxin solution containing about 0.0512 Lf in 0.2 ml. Prepare from this a further series of 5 four-fold dilutions containing about 0.0128, 0.0032, 0.0008, 0.0002 and 0.00005 Lf in 0.2 ml.

Determination of potency of the vaccine: Using a 9 gm/L solution of sodium chloride, prepare dilutions of the vaccine to be examined and of the reference preparation, such that for each, the dilutions form a series differing by not more than 2.5-fold steps and in which the intermediate dilutions, when injected subcutaneously at a dose of 1.0 ml per guinea-pig, will result in an intradermal score of approximately 3 when the animals are challenged. Allocate the dilutions 1 to each of the groups of guinea-pigs and inject subcutaneously 1.0 ml of each dilution into each guinea-pig in the group to which that dilution is allocated. After 28 days, shave both flanks of each guinea-pig and inject 0.2 ml of each of the 6 toxin dilutions intradermally into 6 separate sites on each of the vaccinated guinea-pigs in such a way as to minimize interference between adjacent sites.

Determination of the activity of the challenge toxin: If necessary, inject the unvaccinated control animals with dilutions containing 80, 40, 20, 10 and 5 millions of an Lf of the challenge toxin.

Reading and interpretation of results: Examine all injection sites 48 hr after injection of the challenge toxin and record the incidence of specific diphtheria erythematic. Record also the number of sites free from such reactions as the intra-dermal challenge score. Tabulate together the intradermal challenge scores for all the animals receiving the same dilution of vaccine and use those data with a suitable transformation, to obtain an estimate of the relative potency for each of the test preparations by parallel-line quantitative analysis.

Requirements for a valid assay: The test is not valid unless or both the vaccine to be examined and the reference preparation, the mean score obtained at the lowest dose level is less than 3 and the mean score at the highest dose level is more than 3, if applicable, the toxin dilution that contains 40 millionths of an Lf gives a positive erythema in at least 80 per cent of the control guinea-pigs and the dilution containing 20 millionths of an Lf gives a positive erythema in less than 80 per cent of the guinea-pigs (if these criteria are not met a different toxin has to be selected), the confidence limits (P = 0.95) are not less than 50 per cent and not more than 200 percent of the estimated potency, the statistical analysis shows no deviation from linearity and parallelism. The test may be repeated but when more than 1 test is performed the results of all valid tests must be combined in the estimate of potency.

4.1.15 Bioassay of Digitalis

Potency of test sample is compared with that of standard preparation by determining the action on the cardiac muscle. Any other equivalent method which gives results similar to those obtained by this method is also valid.

- ***Standard preparation:*** It is a mixture of dried and powdered digitalis (1 unit = 76 mg).
- ***Preparation of extract:*** Exact amount of powder is extracted with dehydrated alcohol in continuous extraction apparatus for 6 hr. The final extract should contain 10 ml (5 ml alcohol + 5 ml water) per 10 grams of digitalis powder. That preparation should be stored in between + 5 °C to –5 °C.

(i) Guinea pig method: (End point method):

Animals required: Guinea pig

Chemical required: Anesthetic agent, Digitalis extract solution

Procedure:

- Standard and test sample extracts are diluted with normal saline in such a way that l gram of digitalis power is diluted to 80 ml.
- A guinea pig anesthetized with suitable anesthetic agent. After giving of anesthesia animal is dissected on operation table.
- Jugular vein is dissected out by removing adhering tissues and connected by means of venous cannula. A pin is inserted in heart such that is gets inserted in area of heart. In this way, we can observe that heart beats by up and down movements of the pin. The injection is continued through venous cannula until the heart arrests systole.
- The amount of extract required to produce this effect is taken as lethal dose of extract.
- Another set of 19 animals of same species are used for this experiment and average lethal dose is determined.
- It is not necessary to determine the lethal dose of standard during each time of experiment but is should be occasionally checked.
- The lethal dose of test sample is determine in a similar way using minimum 6 guinea pigs of some strain.
- The potency of test sample is calculated in relation to that of the standard preparation by dividing the average lethal dose of sample to the test and expressed as units/gram.

(ii) Pigeon method

Animals required: Pigeon

Chemical required: Anesthetic ether, Digitalis solution

Procedure:

- Minimum 6 pigeons are used for testing each sample. They should be free from gross evidence of disease.
- Weight of heaviest pigeon is $\leq 2\times$ lightest pigeon weight.
- Food is withheld l6-28 hr before the experiment.
- Pigeons are divided on basis of their sex, weight and breed into 2 groups.

- Anesthetized with anesthetic ether. After giving of anesthesia one side of wing is dissected and the alar vein is cannulated by means of venous cannula.
- Dilutions are made with normal saline average lethal dose of each sample is determined; results are tabulated and calculated as per guinea pig method.
- Lethal dose/kg of body weight is determined for each pigeon.
- The potency of test sample is determined by dividing the mean lethal dose of standard by mean lethal dose of test sample.
- In pigeons, stoppage of heart is associated with characteristic vomiting response called emesis.
- The milk from the crop sac of pigeons is being ejected out. This may be taken as the point response of digitalis.

4.1.16 Bioassay of HCG

Human Chronic Gonadotropin is a dry, sterile preparation of placental Glycoprotein that has luteinizing activity. It is extracted from urine of pregnant women. That is sterilized by filtration and dried under reduced pressure or freeze dried.

Preparation of standard sample:

- HCG consisting of freeze dried extract of HCG with human albumin.
- Dissolve a sufficient quantity corresponding to the daily doses to be used in sufficient albumin phosphate buffer pH 7.2. So daily dose is about 0.2 ml.
- Add a suitable antimicrobial preservative such as

  0.4% w/v of phenol.

  (or)

  0.002% w/v of thiomersol.
- Store the solution at temperature of 2 °C to 8 °C.

Preparation of Test Sample

= Dissolve the sufficient quantity + Albumin Phosphate Buffer pH 7.2

+ 0.4% w/v of phenol (or) 0.002% w/v of thiomersol

Store solution at a temperature of 2 °C to 8 °C.

Animals required: Female rats

Chemical required: HCG

***Procedure*:**

- Use immature female rats of same strain. Approximately 21 days old and weight approx 25 to 30 gm.
- Assign the rats at random to 4 groups of at least 8 rats. If sets of 4-littermates are available, allot one littermate from each set at random to each group and mark according to the litter.
- Choose 2 doses of standard preparation and test solution. Such that the smaller dose is sufficient to produce a positive response in some of the rats and the large dose does produce a maximum response in all of the rats.
- As an initial approximation, doses of 7.5 and 1.5 units may be tried although the dose will depend on the sensitivity of animals used, which may vary widely.
- Inject s.c. into each rat the daily dose allocated to its group on 4-consecutive days at the same time each day.
- On the 5th day, about 24 hr after last injection kill the rats and remove the seminal vesicles or the prostate glands from each animal.
- Remove any extraneous fluid and tissue from the vesicles or glands and weigh them immediately.

Conclusion: Calculate the result of the assay of standard in statistical methods using the weight of the vesicles or prostate glands as the response. The estimated potency is not less than 80% of the stated potency.

CHAPTER 5

SCREENING METHODS

5.1 INTRODUCTION

Screening techniques of various drugs are used to minimize various toxic effects of newly prepared medications and it is very dangerous to perform studies on human beings. Animal studies are very beneficial to estimate pharmacokinetic parameters (absorption, distribution, metabolism and excretion) of various medications.

Drugs and their uses were well started in pre historical era only. Even beneficial or toxic effects of many plants and animal sources were recognized.

The concept of pharmacology began in 17th century, when observation and experimentation began to replace traditional drug use. Many physicians from Great Britain and of this continent understood the values of experimentation when they applied them to the effects of traditional drugs used in their own practices in the treatment of several diseases. Thus 'Materia Medica' the science of drugs began to develop as the part of pharmacology. But limitation in use was lack of method for purifying active agents from the crude materials and methods for testing hypotheses. Real advances in the basic pharmacology during the time were mainly promoted by the private manufacturers and marketers.

In last two decades many nonomedicines like polymeric nanoparticles, biochips, nanosensors, bioreactors, neural stem cells, immune nanoparticles, nanotubes, micelles, liposomes, quantum dots, dendrimers, fullerenes and hydogels have been developed for the more targeted disease therapy in CVS, CNS, GIT, chemotherapy etc.

So based on previous studies and experience pharmacological products broadly governed by 2 principles:

1. All therapies for healthy should meet the same standards of evidence of efficacy and safety in preclinical and clinical studies

2. Substances used as drugs can be toxic under certain conditions.

PLANEERS OF PHARMAOLOGY:

Father of modern experimental Medicine:	Claude Bemard (1813-1878)
Father of American Pharmacology:	Jhon Jacob Abel (1857-1938)
Father of Indian Pharmacology:	Ramnath Chopra (1882-1973)
Father of Clinical Pharmacology:	Lou Lasagna (1923-2003)
Father of Modern Chemotherapy:	Paul Ehrlich (1854-1915)
Father of Modern Medicine:	Hippocrates (460 BC-370 BC)

Commonly Used Experimental Animals

Selection of an animal model is one of the most important steps in any of the experimental pharmacological study. Animal model preferred for the study must be producing similar disease profile as in the human. Hence suitable animal model should be selected which follows three main objectives:

1. Use of an animal phylogenetically closer to man
2. Use of an animal in which the process under investigation is as close as possible to that in man
3. The anatomy, physiology and biochemistry are considered to be similar.

Experimental Animals

- Rodents (mouse, rat, guinea pig, hamster etc.)
- Nonrodents (rabbit, monkey, dog, cat, pig etc.)
- Miscellaneous (frog, pigeon, zebra-fish, chicken etc.)

(i) ***Mouse (Mus musculus):*** It is smallest laboratory animal.

Its commonest strain is Swiss albino.

Nude mice -hairless genetic mutant which lacks thymus gland.

Beige mice -lack of natural killer cells and are susceptible to cancer.

Mice use their tail to help in thermoregulation.

(ii) ***Rat (Rattus norvegicus):*** Albino (subgroup, Wister and Sprague Dawley)

Wistar rat, wide head and the ear is long where as tail length is less than body length.

Rats, longer and narrow head, tail is longer than the body length.

Do not vomit (due to strong sphincter between the stomach and the esophagus and lack of vomiting center).

Do not have tonsil and gallbladder.

Diffuse pancreas, so not a good model for type 1 diabetes.

Coprophagy (eating their own stools).

Tail of rat helps in thermoregulation of body.

(iii) ***Guinea pig (Cavia porcellus):*** Highly sensitive to histamine (1000 times more sensitive)

Serum containing an enzyme asparaginase, which shows antileukemic action.

Very susceptible to tuberculosis and anaphylactic shock.

Highly sensitive to penicillin (100-1000 times more than rat).

(iv) ***Rabbit (Oryctolagus cuniculus):*** Very sensitive to histamine

Do not vomit (like rat and horse).

Ideal animal for pharmacokinetic studies.

Cytochrome 3A4 is absent which is corresponding to cytochrome 3A6.

Enzyme atropinesterase present in blood which degrade atropine.

Has an ability to taste water, a characteristic absent in humans or rats.

Very important to pyrogen testing in parenteral preparation.

Only unknown mammal from which tubules of the kidney and be dissected with basement membrane intact.

Lacks vasomotor reversal phenomenon (absence of adrenergic vasodilator nerve).

(v) ***Monkey (Macaca mulatta):*** Uterus resembles humans and exhibiting regular menstrual periods

Metabolism is approximately same as human.

Ideal model for pharmacokinetic studies.

Best studying for drugs acting on CNS (memory, anxiety, antidepressant, etc.), CVS (antihypertensive, anti angina etc.) GIT and fertility.

Require regular check up for rabies, tuberculosis and timely immunization.

(vi) ***Dog (Canis familiaris):*** Stomach and Intestinal tract resemble human.

Distinct structure of pancreas allowing it as good model for the research on diabetes.

It may develop spontaneous hypertension resembling human.

Cervical sympathetic and vagal nerves are run together hence stimulating of nictitating membrane through preganglionic sympathetic is complicated by central vagal stimulation causing reflex variations in blood pressure.

(vii) ***Frog (Rana tigrina):*** Oxygen can pass through their highly permeable skin and hence "breath" largely through their skin.

Camouflage is a common defensive mechanism in frogs (hiding or color change).

Very commonly used in the CVS related experiments or bioassay.

Table 5.1 About laboratory animals.

Animal	Weight (gm)	Life span (year)	Food intake (gm/day)	Water intake (ml/day)	Gestation period	Animal house temperature	Humidity
Mouse	18-40	1.5-3	3 to 5	6 to 7	19 to 21	19 to 23 °C	40 to70
Rat	150-400	2 to 4	10 to 100	10 to100	21 to 23	19 to 23 °C	40 to70
Hamster	85-150	1 to 3	5 to 7	10 to100	15.5 to 16	15.5 to 16 °C	40 to 60
Guinea pig	600-1200	4 to 8	6 to 100	10 to100	59 to72	18 to 26 °C	40 to 70
Rabbit	1000-3500	6 to 12	5 to 100	10 to100	31 to 32	16 to 20 °C	40 to 60

In vitro Pharmacology Studies

These studies are conducted with isolated part of any laboratory animals, in cooperation with leading research groups we have established several tests using different tissue culture models to quality control of pharmaceuticals. This offers you the opportunity to investigate a variety of pharmacological aspects at considerably lower costs compared to clinical trials or animal studies. We offer a wide range of services from initial pharmacological screening to functional cellular assays accompanying clinical trials.

In vivo Pharmacology Studies

These studies are conducted with live animals only, parameters also calculated on live animals only. Knowledge of pharmacodynamic and pharmacokinetic parameters is essential for the characterization of active substances. The primary screening of compounds for pharmacological and antimicrobial activities can assist in selecting candidate substances for further development. There is an increasing relevance on generating information on the pharmacokinetic and metabolic behavior early during the developmental process. We provide a wide range of services to accelerate your candidate development from tailor-made proof-of-concept studies and early assessments of drug metabolism and pharmacokinetics to regulatory IND-enabling safety pharmacology studies.

5.2 SCREENING METHODS FOR DRUGS ACTING ON CNS

5.2.1 Screening Methods for Sedatives

Sedatives refers to decreased responsiveness to any level of stimulation, is associated with some decrease in motor activity and ideation. Drugs that are subdues excitement and calms the subject without inducing sleep, though drowsiness may be produced.

Screening methods:

(i) Hole board test in mice
(ii) Chimney test in mice
(iii) Grip strength in mice
(iv) Rotarod test in mice
(v) Test for muscle co-ordination
(vi) Inclined plane test in mice
(vii) Open field test

(i) Hole board test in mice

Aim: In this use an open field with holes on the bottom into which the animals could poke their noses. This phenomenon indicates the curiosity component of the behavior of mice. The whole board test has been widely used and modified by a number of workers.

Animals required	:	Swiss albino mice (20-25 gm)
Chemicals required	:	Benzodiazepines, Test and standard only
Equipments used	:	Whole board (size of 40E 40 cm in which 16 holes of 3 cm diameter) Electronic device

Procedure:

- Albino mice are use and also hole board used. The hole board is elevated so that the mouse poking its nose into the hole does not see the bottom.
- Nose poking is considered as an indication of curiosity/exploratory or by electronic devices in more recent modification.
- Usually 6 animals are used for each dose and as control.
- After 30 min of test drug administration animals are subjected to test for 5 min.

- The average count of nose poking of treated animals is calculated as the percentage of control animals.

Conclusion: Poking of nose into hole is a typical behavior of mice indicating a certain degree of curiosity. Benzodiazepines have been shown to suppress nose poking of relatively low doses.

(ii) Chimney test in mice

Aim: The chimney test is used as an additional test for determining the muscle relaxant activity of test drug.

Animals required	:	Male Swiss albino mice (16-22 gm)
Equipments required diameters	:	Pyrex glass cylinder (30 cm length different from 22-28 cm depending on lot of mice)

Procedure:

- Albino rats are used. Glass cylinders are called chimney are used for this test.
- Initially cylinder is held in a horizontal position. At the end of cylinder near a 2 cm mark from the base, a mouse is introduced with the head forward.
- When the mouse reaches the other end of the cylinder, the tube is moved to a vertical position. Immediately, the mouse tries to climb backwards and performs coordinated movements similar to an alpinist to pass a chimney in the mountains. That is why the name of chimney has been given to this test.
- The time required by the mouse to climb backwards to the top of the cylinder is noted.

Conclusion: The ED_{50} with 95% confidence limits, the dose at which 50% of the animals fail to climb backwards within 30 sec is calculated using log- probity analysis method. The chimney test is used as an additional test for determining the muscle relaxant activity of test drug.

(iii) Grip strength in mice

Aim: In this method disturbance of the grasping reflex can be considered while giving of test drug.

Animals required	: Swiss albino mice (20-30 gm)
Equipments required	: Horizontal thin metallic wire suspended about 30 cm in air,
	Forceps,
	Cages, etc.

Procedure:

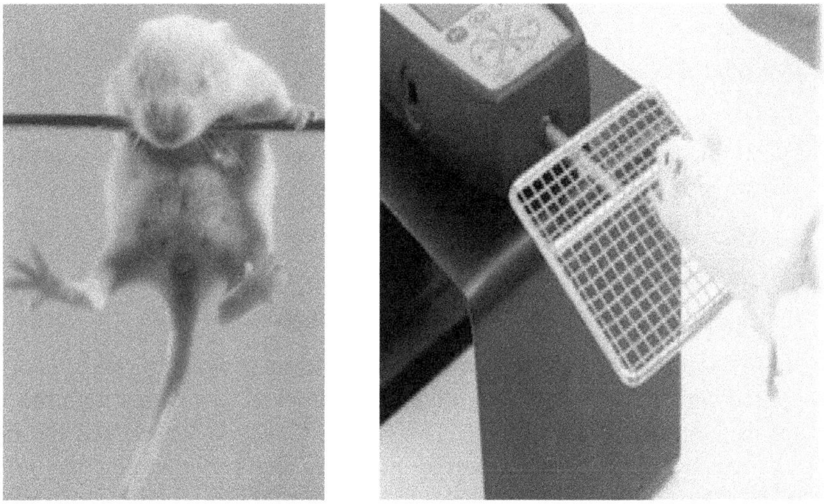

Fig. 5.1 Grip strength apparatus.

- Swiss albino mice are used in this test.
- This test is used to assess muscular strength in rodents which can be influenced by muscle relaxants and sedative drugs.
- In a preliminary experiment the animals are tested for their normal grip strength by exposing them to horizontal thin metallic wire suspended about 30 cm in the air, which they immediately grasp with their forceps. Thc mousc is thcn rclcascd to hang on with its forclimbs.
- Normal animals are able to catch the wire with the hind limbs and climb on to it within 5 seconds.
- Only animals which fulfill this criterion are included in the test.
- Ten mice are used in each group.
- After oral or parental administration of test standard drugs the animals are tested every 15 min for 2 hr.
- Animals which are not able to climb on to the wire with hind limbs with in 5 sec or fall off are considered to be impaired by drug effect.
- After the completion of this test the animals are observed for their behavior in the cages.
- If their behavior and mobility in the cage appears to be normal, the disturbance of the grasping reflex can be considered to be caused by central relaxation.

Conclusion: The percentage of animals loosing the grip strength is recorded using different doses of rest standard drugs and LD_{50} values are calculated.

(iv) Rotarod test in mice

Aim: One of the classical methods introduced by Dunham and Miya in 1957 for the evaluation of drugs interfering with motor coordination activity by testing their ability to remain on a revolving rod.

Animals required	:	Male Swiss mice (20-30 gm)
Chemicals required	:	Test or standard
Equipments required	:	Rotarod apparatus

About apparatus: Rotarod consists of horizontal wooden rod or metal rod coated with rubber with 30 cm diameter attached to a motor with the speed set at 2 rotations per minute. The rod is 75 cm in length and divided in sections by plastic discs, thereby allowing the simultaneous testing of 6 mice .The rod is placed at a height of about 50 cm above the table top in order to discourage the animals from jumping off the roller. Cages kept below the sections save to restrict movements of animals when they fall off from the roller.

Procedure:

- Male Swiss mice undergo as per test on the apparatus.
- Only those mice, which demonstrate their ability to remain on the revolving rod for at least 60 sec are chosen for the test.
- 30 min after i.p. or 60 min after oral administration of test or standard drugs.
- The animals are placed on the rotarod for 1 min.
- The number of animals falling with in 1 min are counted.
- Percentage of animals falling from the rotarod within the test period is calculated for every drug concentration tested.

Conclusion: ED_{50} is defined as the dose of the drug at which 50% animals fall from the rotarod.

5.2.2 Screening Methods for Hypnotics

Hypnotics are the drug that includes and or maintaining sleep, similar to normal arousal sleep. This is not to be confused with hypnosis meaning a Trans like state in which the subject becomes passive and highly suggestible. An ideal hypnotic drug is expected to produce a normal night sleep from which the patient can be aroused without a lingering hangover.

While screening these drugs on experimental animal the parameters usually monitored are indicative of a much deeper stage of central depression as they are associated with lose of muscle tone and righting reflexes. Hence most of pharmacological models are of questionable value with regard to the productivity of the attributes of an ideal hypotonic for human use. Some of the tests are based on potential of sleeping induced by other hypnotic and sedative. Most of sedative in higher doses produce hypnosis.

Screening Methods

(i) Potentiation of hexobarbitone induced sleeping time.

(ii) Recording of EEG in conscious CATS.

(iii) Experimentally induced insomnia in rats.

(i) Potentiation of hexobarbitone induced sleeping time

Aim: This test is indicative of a CNS depressant activity of test compound. Loss of lighting reflex is used as the criterion for the duration of sleep in this model.

Animals required	:	Swiss albino mice (20-25 gm)
Chemicals required	:	Diazepam 3 mg/kg standard,
		Hexobarbitone sodium injection
Equipments required	:	Thermostatically wormed pad (37 °C)

Procedure:

- Groups of 10 male Swiss albino mice weighing between 20-25 gm are used to test orally, s.c or i.p.
- Diazepam in dose of 3 mg/kg orally may be used a reference standard.
- 30 min after parental or 6 min after oral dose of test or standard drugs.
- 60 mg/kg of hexobarbitone sodium injected i.v. through tail vein.
- Then animals placed on their back on thermostatically warmed pad (37 ^{0}C) and the duration of the loss of righting flex, starting from the time of hexobarbitone sodium injection is measured until the animals regain their righting reflexes.
- Hexobarbitone (i.v.) cause anesthesia for 15 min mean values of the duration of anesthesia in min are recorded in control and experimental groups. The percentage change in duration of anesthesia is calculated in the experimental group as compared to those of control.

Conclusion: EP_{50} of test drug is defined as the dose of the drug producing a 100% prolongation in duration of anesthesia in 50% animals. The test is considered non specific as compound which inhibits the metabolism of hexobarbitone in live, the microsomal enzyme inhibitors, may also prolong the hexobarbitone sleeping time and thus give false positive results.

(ii) Recording of EEG in conscious cats

Aim: In this method the effect of hypnotics can be studied on the sleep pattern if EEG on conscious freely moving cats with chronically implanted electrodes.

Animals required	:	Female cats (3 to 4 kg)
Equipments required	:	Bipolar sub cortical electrodes, 2 Teflon coated steel wires, ECG dental acrylic experimental chamber (70 × 80 × 80 cm dimension)

Procedure:

- Cats are anaesthetized and prepared with bipolar sub cortical electrodes in reticular formation, dorsal hippocampus and caudate nucleus.
- Cortical screw electrodes are places over the anterior suprasylvian, lateral and medial suprasylvian and ectasylvian gyro.
- 2 Teflon coated steel wires are placed in the cervical neck muscles. All wires are connected to a subminiature socket and implanted in dental acrylic. Cats of this chronic colony are then intermittently utilized for drug experiments by inter drug intervals of at least 2 weeks.
- On the days of experiments the cats are taken into on experimental chamber 70 × 80 × 80 cm dimensions. The box is lighted and ventilated with room air at 21 °C.
- The cat is then connected to a cable which exists through the top center of the cage into mercury swivel. This prevents the cable from becoming twisted and restricting the cat's movement.
- Recording of the cortical EEG, cervical neck muscle tone and reticular formation multiple unit activity is obtained.
- Continuous recording for up to 96 hr are amplified and stored in a recorder.
- The recordings of cortical EEG, cervical neck muscle tone and reticular formation multiple unit activity are analyzed for REM sleep, slow wave sleep and wakefulness.
- Since a first night was observed, drugs are given on the third or fourth day.

Conclusion: The data so obtained are analyzed by ANOVA with subjects, days and drug as factors.

5.2.3 Screening Methods for Anti Epileptic Activity

Epilepsy is common disorder with an incidence of approximately 0.3-0.5% throughout world. The characteristic event is seizure which is paradoxical event due to abnormal, excessive, hyper synchronous discharges from an aggregate in

CNS. Epilepsy is characterized by recurrent seizures. Pathophysiology of epilepsy involves alternation in voltage dependent ion channels.

(a) Reduction in inhibitors i.e., GABA – mediated

(b) Increase in excitatory i.e., Glutamate – mediated inputs.

Epileptic seizures have been classified into:

- Partial seizures
- Being focally in cortical site and may or may not generalize
- Includes simple partial seizures
- Complex partial seizures
- Generalized seizures

  Involves both the cerebral hemispheres from onset. Includes
  - Absence seizures (petit mal)
  - Generalized tonic – clonic (grand mal)
  - Myoclonic seizures
  - Atonic seizures

Anti epileptic drugs act by modularly GABA or Glutamate transmission or by modularly sodium and calcium ion channels.

A. *In vitro* Methods

(i) Hippocampal slices

(ii) *In vitro* assay for GABAergic compounds

(iii) Excitatory amino acid receptor binding assay

(iv) Electrical recording from isolated brain cells

B. *In vivo* Methods

(i) Electrically induced seizures

(ii) Other methods of kindling

(iii) Chemically induced convulsions

(iv) Seizures induced by focal lesions

(v) Models of status epileptics

(vi) Models of infantile spasm

(vii) Genetic animal models of epilepsy

A. *In vitro* Methods

(i) Hippocampal slices

Aim: *In vitro* brain slice systems are being increasingly used for study of neurophysiologic mechanism of epilepsies. *In vitro* Hippocampal slices have been especially useful due to involvement of hippocampus in generation of complex partial seizures.

Animals required	:	Any rodent (rat, mouse or pig)
Equipments required	:	Micropipettes, holding chamber, perspex chamber (1.5 × 4 cm)
Chemicals required	:	Saline

Procedure:

- Animals decapitated, brain removed hippocampus is dissected out.
- Using a vibratome, slices of about 0.5 mm thickness are made.
- Cutting approximately perpendicular to long axis of hippocampus preserves the three – neuron synaptic circuit and associated recurrent circuitry.
- After cutting the slices are incubated for 2 hr in holding chamber in which they are kept in 28 °C worm saline equilibrated with 95% O_2 and 5% CO_2.
- Slices can be kept healthy for more than 18 hr if handled properly.
- For recording, the slices are transferred to Perspex chamber and attached to its bottom.
- Slices are either kept in 3 mm thick layer of 32 °C warm saline or submerged in liquid artificial CSF.
- Intra cellular recording from the pyramidal neurons in the slice are done by passing micropipettes (tip diameter < 0.5 mm) into the stratum pyramidal under microscopic control.

  Conclusion: Reading is taken by adding drug to the slice medium and recording the spontaneous or shock evokes repetitive fixing of neurons.

(ii) *In vitro* assays for GABAergic compounds

- (^{3}H) GABA – receptor binding assay
- $GABA_a$ – receptor binding assay
- $GABA_b$ – receptor binding assay
- GABA – Uptake in Rat cerebral cortex
- (^{35}S) TBPS – binding assay
- (^{3}H) Muscimol – receptor binding assay
- (^{3}H) SR 95531 – receptor binding assay

Gamma Amino Butyric Acid (GABA) is principle inhibitory neurotransmitter in CNS. It exerts its action by acting on 2 distinct types of receptor. They are

$GABA_a$ which is ligand gated ion channel or inotropic receptor.

$GABA_b$ which is of protein coupled receptor family or metabotropic receptor.

In epilepsy abnormalities in function of GABA will occur. In relations to epilepsy it has been suggested that enhancing GABA mediates synaptic inhibition could reduce neuron excitability and raise the seizure threshold. Benzodiazepines, barbiturates, vigabatrin, tigabine are the more using drugs, which act by enhancing GABAergic inhibition.

[^{3}H] GABA receptor binding assay: It is a simple and sensitive method

Animals required	:	Male Wister rats (100-150 gm)
Chemicals required	:	Sucrose
		Tris maleate buffer
		Triton X-100
		Liquiscint
Equipments required	:	Centrifuge
		Liquid scintillation photometry

Procedure:

- Rats are decapitated and brain removed.
- The brains are homogenized in 15 volumes of ice cold 0.32M sucrose and centrifuged for 10 min at 1000 rpm.
- Supernatant is recentrifuged for 20 min at 20000 rpm.
- After discarding the supernatant, the pallet obtained is homogenized in 15 volumes of distilled water and centrifuged for 20 min at 8000 rpm and then centrifuged for 20 min at 48000 rpm.
- The pallet (Synaptic membrane pellet) so obtained is resuspended in 15 volumes of distilled water and centrifuged for 20 min at 48,000 rpm.
- After discarding the supernatant, the centrifuge tubes, containing the pellets are copped with paraffin and stored at –70 °C.
- Homogenize a frozen membrane pellet in 15 volumes of 0.05M Tris maleate buffer (pH 7.1) at 4 °C.

- Add Triton X-100 to a final concentration of 0.05% and incubate the suspension for 30 min at 37 °C.
- This is now centrifuged for 10 min at 48000 rpm. Discard the supernatant and resuspended the pellet by homogenization in 15 volumes of buffer at 4 °C.
- The assay tubes are prepared in triplicate. The tissue homogenate is incubated with (^{3}H) GABA (15 min) in the Trismaleate buffer (0.05M) alone or along with either the test drug or with isoguvacine (0.1mM) or muscimol (0.1 mm) at 4 °C for 5 minutes and then centrifuge for 15 min at 500 rpm. After washing the pellet with buffer twice, radio activity is quantified with liquiscint using liquid scintillation photometry.

Conclusion: Specific [^{3}H] GABA binding, radioactivity that can be displaced by a high concentration of unlabelled GABA is calculated difference between total bound radioactivity and radioactivity bound in the presence of 0.1mM of isoguvacine i.e., non specific binding gives the specific binding. % of specifically bound [^{3}H] GABA displaced by a given concentration of test compound is calculated and its IC_{50} value with 95% confidence limits obtained using computer derived linear regressive analysis.

GABA$_a$ receptor binding assay

- GABA$_a$ receptor mediates the bulk of postsynaptic inhibitory action of GABA. It is a ligand gated channel. It exits as pentamer, composed of 3 different submits (α, β, γ). The receptor submits each exist in several subtypes giving heterogeneity to GABA$_a$ receptors.
- Muscimol is a powerful GABA against biculline whereas picrotoxin and SR 95531 are antagonists various centrally acting drugs like benzodiazepines, barbiturates, and neurosteroids also modulate GABA$_a$ receptor function.
- To examine the GABA$_a$ binding sites, [^{3}H] Muscimol agonist and [^{3}H] SR 95531 (antagonist) are used as radioligands.

GABA$_b$ receptor binding assay: GABA$_b$ is metabotropic receptor which acts by inhibiting adenylyl cycles K^+ channel opening or Ca^{2+} channel blockade. It mediates both presynaptic and postsynaptic inhibition in CNS. Baclofen is an agonist at GABA$_b$ receptor. GABA$_b$ receptor binding assay, using [^{3}H] Baclofen, allows the screening of drug with affinity for GABA$_b$ receptor.

Procedure: The tissue homogenate is incubated in buffer along with [^{3}H] Baclofen (1.8-2×10^{-8} M) and either Baclofen (0-1.2×10^{-6} M) or GABA or test drug for 60 min at 4 ^{0}C. The binding is terminated by rapid vacuum filtration over glass fiber filters. Filters are washed with ice cold buffer and radioactivity counted after addition of ethylene glycol monomethyl either and liquiscint.

Evaluation: Difference of binding of [^{3}H] Baclofen in presence or absence of Baclofen gives the specific binding dissociation constant (K_1) of the test drug i.e., the concentration of test drug at which 50% of receptor are occupied is calculated.

(iii) Excitatory amino acid receptor binding assay

[^{3}H] CPP – binding assay

[^{3}H] TCP – binding assay

[^{3}H] Glycine – binding assay

Disadvantages of in vitro models: Provide insight into the mechanism of action of putative antiepileptic drugs and serve initial screen for drug discovery but they are not give any indication of Pharmacokinetic, Pharmacodynamic or Pharmacokinetic - Pharmacodynamic interactions of compound when introduced into living animal or human being. Further it is not possible to study the compensatory changes that occur in body when a drug is given.

B. *In vivo* Methods

(i) Electrically induced seizures

(a) Threshold models
(b) Maximal electroshock seizures
(c) Focal electrical stimulation such as kindling
(d) Other models of kindling-PTZ test

(a) *Threshold models*

Aim: Used to screen drugs with efficacy against generalized tonic clonic and focal seizures.

Procedure:

Animals required : Mice (18-30 gm)

Equipments required : Electrical stimulator

- Group of 8-10 male mice (18-30 gm) used for dosing.
- Corneal or ear electrodes are used to provide electrical stimulation from stimulator (at constant frequency of 50-60/sec for 0.2 sec duration).

- Threshold is usually determined current or voltage inducing hind limb extension in 50% of animals i.e., CC_{50} and CV_{50} or EV_{50} respectively.
- Control thresholds in mice are about 6-9 mA (CC_{50}) or 90-140 with (CV_{50} or EV_{50}) depending on stain age and method of stimulation.

Evaluation: Evaluation of test drug is taken as measure of its efficacy. Comparison of drug effects required calculation of dose that elevates the threshold by 20%.

Control threshold determination should be undertaken on each day parallel to threshold determinations in drug treated animals. Use of an animal more than once a day is not recommended as post octal rise in seizure threshold has been noted.

(b) ***Maximal Electroshock Seizure (MES) Test***

Aim: Merritt and Putain (1938) develop this anticonvulsive effect of diphenyl hydantoin using this test. Useful to primary and secondary generalized tonic – clonic seizures.

Procedure:

- Group of 8-10 animals used per dose of drug (rats or mice).
- Electrical stimulation applied with corneal or electrodes with stimulator constant voltage at frequency of 50-60/sec. Electrodes are moistened with saline solution before application.
- Usually 2-5 times current strength.
- 50 mA in mice and 150 mA in rats.

Evaluation: Potency is determined by calculation of ED_{50} for suppression of tonic hind limb extension.

(c) ***Corneal electroshock kindling:*** Kindling can be done in rats and mice by giving electroshocks *via* corneal electrodes.

Mice kindled by daily of 3 mA current 60 Hz frequency.

Rat kindled by daily of 8 mA current60 Hz frequency.

Occurrence of Racine stage 5 seizures indicates that the animal is kindled.

Evaluation: Putative anti epileptic drugs can be tested after animals have had 5 seizures for 10 consecutive times.

Class 1 – Immobility, eye closure, twitching of vibrissae stereotypic sniffing.

Class 2 – Facial clonus and head nodding

Class 3 – Facial clonus (contra lateral to focus)

Class 4 – Rearing, often accompanied by bilateral forelimb clonus

Class 5 – Rearing with loss of balance and falling accompanied by generalized clonic seizures

In kindled animals

1. Seizure latency: Time from stimulation to 1st sign of seizure activity.
2. Seizure severity
3. Seizure duration
4. After discharge duration

(d) Pentylenetetrazole (*PTZ*) *Test:* PTZ is tetrazole derivative with consistent convulsive effect in mice, rat, cats, primates etc. Used for screening the drugs effective in petit mal or absence seizures. Threshold for clonic seizures after i.v.

Infusion of PTZ

- 8-10 mice are taken. 1% solution PTZ i.v. infusion at the rate of 0.3 ml per min is given.
- Animals develop seizures as one or more isolated jerks followed by generalized clonic seizures with loss of righting reflexes followed by maximal tonic clonic seizures.
- Dose for the production of generalized clonic seizures with loss of righting reflex is preferably taken as an end point.
- Threshold is calculated as the mean dose of PTZ that induces seizures in the group tested and is about 50 mg/kg for clonic seizures and 90 mg/kg for maximal tonic – clonic seizures in mice.

(ii) Other models of kindling

Kindling by stimulation of other brain areas are done by chemicals.

(iii) Chemically induced convulsions

Numerous chemical compounds produce seizures.

1. Chemoconvulsants including generalized seizures after systemic administration.

   Examples: Pentylenetetrazol, Bicucullin, Picrotoxin, Penicillin, Isoniazid, Thiosemicarbazide, allylglycine, DMCM, B-CCM,

Strychnine, Pilocarpine, NMDA, Kainic acid, GABA, DDT and Methionine sulfoxinine.

2. Chemoconvulsants including focal seizures after central administration.

   Examples: Penicillin, Kainic acid, Quinolinic acid, Pentylenetetrazol.

5.2.4 Screening Methods for Anxiolytic Activity

Anxiety is a subjective human phenomenon and except for some of the associated somatic and autonomic changes, it has no obvious part in experimental animals. In biological terms anxiety may be regarded as a particular farm of behavioral inhibition that occurs in response to environmental events that are novel, non-rewarding or punishing. In animals this behavioral inhibition may take pressing to obtain food. To develop new and more effective to have animal tests that give a good prediction at activity in man and considerable effort has one into developing and validating such tests. These models are divided into following broad categories:

Models which use changes in ongoing, non-evoked behavior

Models which set up an artificial in which animal's behavior changes

Models which use anticonvulsant activity as a measure of anxiolytic drug potential

Models which use anti-aggressive activity as a measure of anxiolytic activity

Some of the more commonly used models of anxiety from these categories are being described in this chapter.

Screening Methods

(i) Yohimbine induced convulsions

(ii) Maternal aggression in Rats

(iii) Anti-Anxiety test (Light –Dark model) in mice and Rats

(iv) mCPP induced anxiety in Rats

(i) Yohimbine induced convulsions

Aim: Potential anxiolytic and GABA – mimetic drugs have shown antagonism of Yohimbine – induced seizures in mice. This model is considered to have predictive value for identifying potential anxiolytic and GABA-mimetic agents.

Animals required : Swiss albino mice (20-30 gm)

Chemicals required : Yohimbine hydrochloride (s.c) 45 mg/Kg

Equipments required : Trasparent Propylene cages

Procedure: Male Swiss mice (20-30 gm) are individually placed in transparent propylene cages and test and reference drugs are administered i.p. 30 min prior to the s.c. injection Yohimbine hydrochloride in a dose of 45 mg/kg. The animals are then observed for the onset and number of clonic seizures for 60 minutes.

ED_{50} values with 95% confidence limits are calculated for the antagonism of Yohimbine induced clonic seizure by means of Light field – Wilcoxon procedure and compared with the reference standard.

(ii) Anti-aggressive activity

Maternal aggression in rats

Aim: Oliver et al., (1985) described this model of maternal aggression in rats. Entry of intruder (male or female) in the cage of a parturient female rat, induces high levels of aggression against such intruders. Maternal aggression in such a case is characterized by short latency attacks of high intensity, mostly directed toward the head or neck of the intruder and is particularly pronounced during the part of the locating period.

Animals required	:	Female rats weighing 250-350 gm
Chemicals required	:	Pentobarbitone
Equipments used	:	Home cages with iron gauge, ejaculation plugs, video tape

Procedure:

- Female rats weighing 250-350 gm are placed with a breeding male in their home cages. An iron gauge is placed on the bottom of each cage which enables collection of ejaculation plugs.
- After detecting an ejaculation plug, the male is left for another week with the female after which female is placed in the observation cage provided with nesting material. These cages are kept in an observation room under reversed day/night rhythm.
- The day of birth is marked as day 0. Every parturient female is tested each day against a male intruder, having about 25 gm less body weight than the female. Tests are performed during first part of dark period under red light conditions.
- One male intruder is placed in the female's home cage for 5 min. The ongoing behavior is videotaped and analyzed later.
- Each intruder is used only one and sacrificed immediately afterwards with an i.p. overdose of pentobarbitione followed by shaving and

describing the wound on wound charts. The aggressive behavior of the female is the scored with the help of the video-tape recording and autopsy reports.

- Drug experiments are performed on post partum days 3, 5, 7 and 9. Preceding days (day 1 and 2), intervening (4, 6 and 8) and following (10, 11, 12 and 13) days are used to establish an aggression base line and as wash out days. Drugs are administered orally 60 min before testing.

  ANOVA is employed to detect overall significance, followed by Wilcoxon matched pairs comparison between dosages, Kruskal – Wallis analysis is used to test the differences in the bite areas after drug treatment.

(iii) Anti-anxiety test (Light-Dark Model) in mice and rats

Aim: Crawley and Godwin (1980) have described this simple behavior model to detect compounds with anxiolytic effects. Mice and rats tend to explore a novel environment, but they retreat from the observe sight of a brightly light open field. Animals are placed in a two chambered system, where they can freely move between a brightly – light open field and a dark corner. After the treatment with an anxiolytic they show more crossings between the two chambers and more locomotor activity. The number of crossings between the light and dark sites is recorded.

Animals required	:	Native mice or rats
Equipments required	:	Dark and light chamber

Procedure:

- The apparatus consists of a dark and a light chamber which are divided by a photocell equipped zone.
- A polypropylene animal cage of 44×21×21 cm dimensions is darkened with black spray over one-third of its surface.
- A partition containing a 13 cm long × 5 cm high opening is used for separating the dark one-third from the bright two-thirds of the cage. This cage shows an activity monitor which counts total locomotor activity.
- Another electronic system consisting of four sets of photocells across the partition automatically counts movements through the partition and records the time spent in the light and dark compartments.
- Experiments are conducted on native mice or rats. They are treated 30 min before the experiments with test drugs or vehicle given i.p. placed in the cage and observed for 10 min. Groups of 6-8 animals should be used for each dose.

- Finally, the dose response curves are plotted and number of crossings through the partition between the light and the dark chamber are compared with total activity counts during the 10 min.
- It has been reported that anxiolytics like diazepam and meprobamate produce a dose dependent facilitatory effect whereas the non anxiolytics are not effective in this model.
- The relative potency of anxiolytics in increasing the exploratory behavior agress well with their potency observed in lineal trials.

(iv) mCPP induced anxiety in rats

Aim: mCPP is a metabolite (1-(3-chlorphenyl) piperazine) of antidepressant drug trazodone, which has been classified as 5 HT_{2C} against. It has been shown to anxiogenic in man and in rats. mCPP includes induces hypophagia and hypolocomotion, inhibits social interaction in rats, diminished exploratory activity of rats in the open field test and in the light-dark box test, induces hyperthermia and reduces ultrasound induced defensive behavior in rats. Antagonism of these symptoms has been used for the screening of anxiolytic drugs.

Animals required	:	Male Sprague Dawley rats (200-250 gm)
Chemicals required	:	mCPP 7 mg/kg (i.p)
Equipments required	:	Locomotion activity cages

Procedure:

- Male Sprague Dawley rats (200-250 gm) are housed in groups of six exposed to 12 hr light/dark cycle with free access to food and water.
- Locomotion study – Test compound or vehicle are administered orally 1 hr or i.p. 30 min before the locomotion test. mCPP is injected i.p. in a dose of 7 mg/kg 20 min before the test.
- Thereafter the animals are placed individually in an automated locomotor activity cages and locomotion is recorded for 10 min.
- Hypophagia study – Rats are individually placed in cages on day 1. After getting acclimatized to their home cages, they are deprived of food on day 3 for 24 hr.
- They are then treated with the test drug or vehicle orally and returned with 5 mg/kg mCPP or saline i.p. After a further 20 min weighed quantity of their normal food pellets are placed in their food hampers and the amount remaining after 1 hr is measured.
- The quantity of food consumed by each animal during this period is calculated.

Conclusion: The effects of test compound of mCPP induced hypolocomotion is determined by one-way ANOVA and Newman-Keuls test and the effect on hypophagia is determined by one-way ANOVA and Dunnett's test. The dose producing 50% disinhibition of locomotion is also calculated for comparison with a standard drug.

5.2.5 Screening Methods for Neuroleptics and Anti Psychotic Activity

"Phyche" means mind and "osis" means diseased or abnormal condition. It has been used as an alternative to insanity and mania. The etiopathology of psychosis is complex and genetic basis has been understood to play a definite role in its genesis.

Risk of developing schizophrenia	**(%)**
General population	1
Fraternal twins	10
Sibling of schizophrenic	10
Child of one parent schizophrenic	10-15
Child of both parents schizophrenic	30-40
Identical twins	40-50

- Antipsychotic or neuroleptic drugs are those agents used to treat hallucination, psychosis and mania.
- Symptoms of psychosis – hallucinations, delusions, thought disorders.
- *Rauwolfia serpentina*, Chinese herb-ma-hung and ergot are antipsychotic drugs used to modify behavior, mood and emotions.
- Antipsychotic agents also include tricyclics, phenothiazines, thioxanthenes, dibenzazepines, and butyrophenones. But they also produce some neurological effects like sedation, hypotension and autonomic side effects. They block D_2 dopamine receptor in forebrain and also in D_1 dopaminergic, 5-HT_2 serotonergic and adrenergic receptor.
- Number of antipsychotic drugs were developed but has extra pyramidal side effects, so there is a need of creating newer agents with less side effects.
- Animal models can be divided into 3 sets namely with predictive validity, face validity and construct validity.
- Animals models with face validity are based on symptom similarity and exhibit behavioral, impaired performance and social withdrawal. These models are few difficult to design, interpret and replicate. Models that mimic the psychopathologic disturbances underlying the disease are constructs validity genetic model.

A. *In vitro* and *ex vivo* models

(i) ^{3}H – Prazosin competition binding for 1 adrenoreceptors.

B. *In vivo* models

(i) Inhibition of amphetamine – induced stereotypy in rats.

(ii) Genetic models.

(iii) Single unit recording of A_9 and A_{10} midbrain dopaminergic neurons.

(iv) Phencyclidine induced social withdrawal measured in social interaction test.

(v) Conditioned avoidance reflex in rats.

(vi) Neuro developmental models are
- Gestational malnutrition model
- Viral infection
- Obstetrical and birth complications
- Early stressful experience

(vii) Extra pyramidal side effects prime monkey model.

(viii) Catalepsy in rodents.

(ix) Phencyclidine induced bizarre pattern of locomotors activity and stereotypy.

A. *In vitro* Models

(i) ^{3}H- Prazosin competition binding for adrenoreceptors

Aim: Direct intern between compound and α_1 adrenergic receptor is determined by measuring the inhibition of binding of radioactive ligand (^{3}H-prazosin) to receptor.

Animals required :	Male Wistar Rats (200-250 gm)
Chemicals required :	50 mm Tris-HCL buffer pH 7.6
Equipments required:	Homogenizer
	Centrifuge
	Whatman filters

Procedure:

- Rats (Male Wistar 200-250 gm) are housed 12 hr day and night cycle free access food and water animals sacrificed their brains quickly removed cerebral cortex is taken out and frozen is stored at –70 °C.

- Membrane prepare of rat frontal cortex is prepared and protein content is measured accordingly to method of Lowry et al., tissue is homogenized in 20 vol. of 50 mm Tris-HCl buffer, pH 7.6.
- Supernatant recentrifuged at 25000 rpm for 30 min stored at -20 °C until incubation.
- Pellet reconstituted in 50 mm Tris–HCl buffer pH 7.6.
- Final incubation contains 450 ml membrane suspension.
- 50 ml of radio ligand and 50 ml of Tris–HCl buffer or of solution of displacer. Nine concentrations of test drug are incubated in presence of concern (0.146 mnM) of [^{3}H] prazosin standard – phentolamine or prazosin – filter with what man filters.

- Filters washed with ice cold Tris – HCl buffer and placed in scintillation cocktail.
- Radio activity is measured in liquid scintillation counter and binding is corrected for protein content.

K_i value is calculated from formula

$$K_i = IC_{50}/ (1+L/K_d)$$

where L = Concentration of radio ligand.

K_d = Dissociation constant

K_i = Value for each comp studied is mean + SEM

Conclusion: From at least 3 independent competitions – binding studies of radioactive binding sites to receptors represents ^{3}H- Prazosin competition binding for adrenoreceptors shows the antipsychotic activity of sample drug.

B. *In vivo* models

(i) Inhibition of amphetamine induced stereotypy in rats

Aim: Amphetamine is an indirect sympathomimetic agent. It includes characteristic stereotypic behavior (lip smoking, grooming, catalepsy, gnawing) in rats, which can be successfully prevented by classical neuroleptic agents. It binds With D_2 receptor and shows antagonism effect.

Animals required	:	Wistar rats (180-200gm)
Chemicals required	:	d-amphetamine (5 mg/kg. i.p.)
Equipments required:		Wire cages (21cm × 21cm × 23 cm)

Procedure:

2 groups adult Wistar rats (180-200 gm)

- Treated with either test or standard drug and then placed in individual wire cages (21 cm × 21 cm × 23 cm)
- They are injected with d-amphetamine (5 mg/kg. i.p.) after 30 min intervals for 3 hr.
- Animals are protected if behavior is reduced or abolished.
- The intensity of stereotype activity is assessing on an arbitrary rating scale from 0-4 for normal, periodic sniffing, licking, gnawing and biting behaviors respectively.

Conclusion: A reduction in mean stereotypy score is indicative for antipsychotic effect.

(ii) Genetic models

Schizophrenia is a hereditary disorder targeted gene deletions or gene transfer techniques been used to set up the animal models of schizophrenia. These models show construct validity. However, the behavior exhibited in these models does not mimic disease.

(iii) Single unit recording of A_9 and A_{10} midbrain dopaminergic neurons

Aim: Dopamine D_3 receptor are richly located in limbic areas.

D_3 receptor involved in pathogenesis of schizophrenia target of Antipsychotic drugs electro physiological recordings.

Animals required	:	Albino Sprague Dawley rats (200-225 gm)
Chemicals required	:	Anesthesia (chloral hydrate 400 mg/kg,) i.p.
Equipments required:		Stereotoxic instrument.

Briefly number of spontaneously active midbrain dopamine neurons are recorded and studied in anesthetized rats increases in number of spontaneously active Ventral Tegmental Area (VTA) (A_{10}) and Substantia Nigra Compacta (SNC) (A_9) DA neurons produced by repeated administration of compound may be correlated with their therapeutic and neurological side effects respectively.

Alternatively, extra cellular single unit activity is also recorded to assess the clinical antipsychotic efficacy and side effects of Dopamine receptor blockers on A_9 and A_{10} Dopamine neurons.

[Male albino Sprague Dawley rats (200-225 gm) anaesthetized (chloral hydrate 400 mg/kg, i.p.) mounted in stereotoxic instrument].

5.2.6 Screening Methods for Anti Depressants

Depression is a major affective disorder it belongs to heterogeneous group of mental disorders characterized by extreme aggregations and disturbances of mood which adversely affect cognition and psychomotor functions. It is a psychobiologic phenomena resulting from abnormal brain mechanism. An imbalance in central cholinergic and adrenergic tone is the critical pathophysiology mechanism in affective disorders.

The biogenic amine hypothesis proposes

An increase in	NE (Nor epinephrine)
Reduction in level of	5HT (Serotonin)
	DA (Dopamine)
	GABA (γ–amino butyric acid)

As the etiologic mechanism for genesis of depression, the current therapy includes- MAO inhibitors (Tranylcypromine, clorgilene, moclobemide).

Tricycles and related campounds (Imipramine, amitriptyline, desipramine, fluoxetine, fluvoxamine).

However, the typical antidepressants are some of the most toxic psychopharmacological agents and include sedation, hypotension and arrhythmias along with anti cholinergic symptoms. These factors limit their use.

- Major problems in search for new antidepressant drug are lack of animal models that resemble depressant treatments.
- Most of available screening methods are based mainly on empirically established relationships between clinical efficacy of known antidepressants and their effects on various pharmacological test models.
- In combination with study of motor activity these tests allow assessment of specificity of anti depressant activity by establishing ratio between "Anti depressant" dose and "Stimulant" or "Sedative" dose. Same dose if ratio is close to 1.

***In vivo* Methods**

(i) Water wheel model.
(ii) Tail suspension test.
(iii) Reserpine induced hypothermia.
(iv) Isolation induced hyperactivity.
(v) Learned helplessness test.
(vi) Amphetamine potentiating.
(vii) Apomorphine antagonism.

(viii) Resident intruder paradigm in rats.

(ix) Muricidal behaviour in rats.

(i) Water wheel model

Aim: This model is based on behavioral despair activity of test drug by animals are allowed to forced swim

Animals required	:	Albino mice (20-25 gm)
Chemicals required	:	Imipramine
Equipments required	:	Plexiglass water tank (40 cm × 18 cm × 18 cm)
		Plexiglass shaft (diameter 3 cm, length 6 cm)

Procedure:

- The animal is forced to swim without any escape in a water tank.
- A rotating wheel in water tank poses as an option for escape but adds on to the despair as it turns under the weight of animal and the animal has to keep rotating the wheel in order to stay afloat.
- Keep its head above water.
- The apparatus consists of a Plexiglass water tank (20 cm × 18 cm × 18 cm) with a water wheel in its centre.

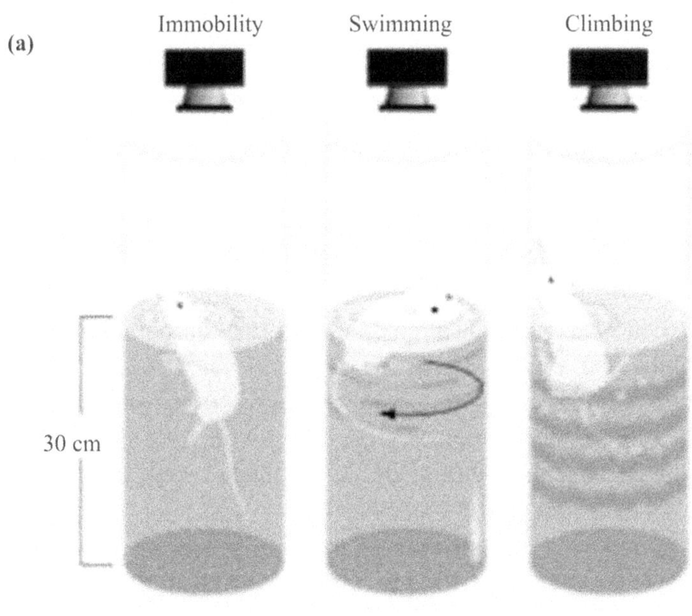

Fig. 5.2 Water wheel apparatus.

- Water wheel is made of Plexiglass shaft (diameter 3 cm, length 6 cm) on which 6 paddles (0.5 cm width) move when loads of more than 5 gm are attached and number of rotations of water wheel are counted.
- Tank is filled up to height of 30 cm, 25 °C.
- That paddles just touch the surface of water.
- On discovering the water wheel, they climb onto it and begin turning it due to their weight. After a few minutes of attempted escape, they climb to wheel and just float in water showing complete immobility.
- For this method, mice (20-25 gm) randomly received control, standard and test group. 1st count number of rotations after that vehicle, Imipramine, test drug and rechallenged water wheel.

Conclusion: Potential antidepressant will increases the number of counts of water wheel turns, indicating increase effort at escape behavior. The classical tricycle antidepressants reduce immobility time in this model. But opiates and antihistaminic gives false positive results.

(ii) Tail suspension test

Aim: This model is a modification of behavior despair test.

Animal required	:	Mice (25-30 grams)
Equipment required	:	Hanging wire
		Water container

Procedure:

Mice are resoled immobile by suspending from tail to induce behavioral despair. An animal in that situation alternates between 2 kinds of behavior agitation (mobility) and immobility.

- The cumulative immobility time is a measure of animal's degree of helplessness depression.
- Treatment with antidepressant drugs reduces immobility time. It has been observed that mice exhibit better reproducibility of results than rats.
- In a typical experiment the mouse (20-30 gm), either sex housed under standard laboratory condition with food and water ad libitum is hang on wire in an upside down posture such that its nostril touches the water surface in a container.
- Initially the animal tries to escape by making vigorous movements, but is unable to escape and becomes immobile. The period of immobility during 5 min observation period is noted.

This test used for serotonergic pathway.

Conclusion: Computerized system with 16 channels is available as a single channel basic configuration for measuring time of activity, time of immobility of the animal in real time. The tail suspension monitor is a device for screening antidepressants in mice.

(iii) Reserpine induces hypothermia

Aim: In this method depression is produced by inducing reserpine.

Animals required	:	Swiss albino mice (25-30 grams)
Chemicals required	:	Reserpine 2.5-mg/kg s.c
Equipment required	:	Temperature detector

Procedure:

- The test measures ability of compounds to inhibit Reserpine induced hypothermia in mice.
- Used to screen potential antidepressants mice (male albino Swiss 25-30 gm) 12 hr day-night cycle and free access to food and water. Reserpine in dose 2.5-5.0 mg/kg, s.c. induces ptosis, hyperthermia, and catalepsy.
- Reserpine given 2 hr before to test drug.
- Rectal body temperature is measured every 30 min for 3 hr after drug injection.
- Measure initial temperature.

Conclusion: By measuring of temperature, according to intensity of temperature anti depressant activity of test drug is estimated.

(iv) Isolation induced hyperactivity

- It is observed that rats when socially deprived for period of 15 days, exhibit depressive behavior. There is a reduction in spontaneous locomotors activity, exploratory behavior rearing, and stereotypy.
- Adult Wistar rats of either sex (200-250 gm) housed singly in cages (30 cm × 26 cm × 20 cm) any visual or auditory their normally housed counter parts for 10-15 days.
- Animals are subjected to behavior testing on an arbitrary scale for sleep, reduced response to external stimuli, ambulatory behavior, and stereotype posture.
- Both classical and newer antidepressants reduce isolation induced depressive behavior.

5.2.7 Screening Methods for Anti Parkinsonism Activity

- More than 2.1 million people worldwide suffer from Parkinson's disease (PD)
- A neurological syndrome characterized by bradykinesia, postural instability, rigidity and involuntary tremors. Extensive loss of dopaminergic neurons of substantia nigra.
- Biochemically there is depletion of dopamine increases of Acetycholine (Ach).
- Neurotoxicity in CNS and basal ganglia and produces neurological symptoms.
- Belladonna alkaloids, antispasmodics and antihistamics, are traditionally used for management of Parkinsonism. Current drug therapy with levodopa which is decorboxylated to dopamine in dopaminergic neurons which helps to maintain adequate motor functions.

Screening Methods

I. *In vitro* and *Ex vivo* models

(i) Experiments using Rat striatal slices.

(ii) Dopamine stimulated adenylyl cyclase activity.

(iii) Radioligand studies for D_1 and D_2 dopamine receptors.

(iv) Dopamine release from synaptosomes.

II. *In vitro* models

(i) Neuroprotective efficacy.

III. Behavioral models of parkinson's disease

(i) Reserpine induced Parkinsonism

(ii) Neuroleptics induced Parkinsonism

(iii) Cholinomimetics induced Parkinsonism

(iv) Surgical induction

(v) Monitoring dopamine concentration using micro dialysis

(vi) Effect of dopamine receptor stimulation.

(vii) Electrophysiological output from rat basal ganglia.

I. *In vitro* and *Ex vivo* models

(i) Experiments using rat striatal slices

Aim: Striatus is the brain region, which is primarily affected in Parkinsonism. The release of neurotransmitters like dopamine and Ach in response to test agent services as good *in vitro* marker of its activity

Animals required	:	Male Sprague Dawley rats (150-250 gm)
Chemicals required	:	Ice cold Kreb's solution,
		Dopamine, Choline, Nomifensine
		Pargyline chloride, Hemicholinium,
		0.1 mm ascorbic acid
Equipments required	:	Tissue chopper
		Incubator
		Super fusion chamber

Procedure: Male Sprague – Dawley rats (150-250 gm) are decapitated, the skull is opened and the right and left striata are removed and placed in ice – cold kreb's solution.

- The striata is cut into 0.4 mm thick slices using tissue chopper. The slices are kept floating for 30 min in kreb's solution continuously aerated with 95% O_2 and 5% CO_2 at room temperature.

  [Krebs's solution (in mM) concentration]

NaCl	118
NaOH CO_3	25
KCl	4.85
$C_6 H_2 O_4$	11
$CaCl_2$	1.3
KH_2PO_4	1.15

- The slices are labeled by incubating for 30 min at 37 °C with {^{3}H} dopamine (5 µl/ml).
- The slices are labeled by incubating for 30 min at 37 °C {^{3}H} dopamine (5 µl/ml) and Choline (2 µl/ml).
- In presence of 0.15 mm Pargyline, chloride and 0.1 mm ascorbic acid.
- Labeled slices are transferred to super fusion chambers and per fused with Kreb's solution at 37 °C.
- After washing and stabilization 5 min fractions of superfast are collected.
- The perfusion buffer contains 1 mm nomifensine to inhibit dopamine reuptake 10 mm hemicholinium to inhibit Choline. The slices are subjected to field stimulation with rectangular pulses of alternating polarity with a current strength of 10-15 mA/cm^2 and pulse duration of 2 msec at a stimulating frequency of 3HZ for 5 min.

- Drugs to be tested are present in the super fusion fluid. The radioactivity is the superfustate samples and in the tissue is determined by liquid scintillation counting.
- The standard drug action compared with test drug (radio labeled actions)

II. *In vitro* models

(ii) *In vitro* neuroprotective efficacy

Aim: To measure the efficacy of test drug as neuroprotective agent against a stress of H_2O_2.

Requirements	:	Human neuroblastoma cells
Chemicals required	:	Dulbecco's culture
		Eagle's medium
		Fetal calf serum
		Penicillin/streptomycin
		H_2O_2, HCl
		Isopropanol
Equipment required	:	Micro plate reader.

Procedure:

- Human neuroblastoma cells, SH – SY5Y are cultured and maintained in Dulbecco's modified eagles medium supplemented with 10% (V/V) fetal calf serum and 1% (V/V) penicillin/streptomycin antibiotic mixture.
- SH – SY5Y cells are seeded at a density of 4×10^4 cells/well in 96 well culture plates and allowed to attach overnight.
- The cells are subjected to stress by incubating with hydrogen peroxide (100 or 300 μm) for 6 hr.
- Appropriate concentration of test drug is added to culture plate 0.5 hr before H_2O_2. So as to evaluate its efficacy as neuroprotective agent.
- The cell survival is evaluated, by performing MTT. Briefly, MTT is added to the cultures at a final concentration of 0.2 mg/ml and after incubation at 37 °C for 2 hr, the media is removed carefully and the reaction is stopped by addition of isopropanol containing 0.04N HCl. The absorbance of each well is measured at 590 nm by using a micro plate reader.

Conclusion: Increase in viability of the cells in test wells may indicate the efficacy of test drug as neuroprotective agent against a stress of H_2O_2. Less than of test drug

III. Behavioral model of parkinsonism

(i) Reserpine induced parkinsonism

Aim: Quantitative effect of test drug

Animals required	:	Male Sprague Dawley rats (150-250 grams)
Chemicals required	:	Reserpine
Equipments required	:	Metal rod, Woolen box

Procedure:

- Reserpine is an alkaloid extracted from dried roots of rauwolfia serpentine belonging to the family, Apocynaceae.
- Used for hypertension and psychosis
- Interfering with vesicular uptake and storage of NE, DA and 5HT (Centrally and peripherally)
- Depletion of biogenic amines – impair sympathetic activity, which takes at weeks to restore after discontinuation of drug.
- i.v. (5 mg/kg) and i.p. (2.5 mg/kg) injection of reserpine in rats. Produce signs and symptom of Parkinson's disease.
- After 20-30 min of drug administration, motor disorders are apparent. Animals are sedated and markedly hypnotic with poor movement coordination.
- Hind limb rigidity, arched body position fixed facial expression and ptosis are other typical effects of reserpine
- Effects peak at 1-2 hr post administration and subside with in 24 hr.
- The animals are divided into 3 groups, test, standard and vehicle control given to them for each group.
- About 30 min after reserpine administration the test standards drug may be administration % inhibition of peak reserpine effect evaluated.

Conclusion: Inhibition of reserpine effects are evaluated and test drug % inhibition and compared with standard drug is compared and drug potency is measured.

5.2.8 Screening Methods for Drugs Influencing Learning and Memory (NOOTROPICS)

- Nootropics are also referred as smart drugs, memory enhancers, and cognitive enhancers. They are reported to improve mental function such as cognition, memory, intelligence, motivation, attention and concentration.
- They are thought to be work by altering the availability of brains supply of neurochemicals, by improving the brains oxygen supply or by stimulating nerve growth. Nootropics are also referred as smart drugs, memory enhancers, and cognitive enhancers.
- They are reported to improve mental function such as cognition, memory, intelligence, motivation, attention and concentration.
- They are thought to be work by altering the availability of brains supply of neurochemicals, by improving the brains oxygen supply or by stimulating nerve growth.
- The main features of nootropic drugs are, the enhancement, at least under same conditions of learning acquisition as well as resistance of learned behaviors to agents that tend to impair them, the facilitation of inter hemispheric flow of information, partial enhancement of the general resistance of the brain and particularly its resistance to physical and chemical injuries and increase in the efficacy of the tonic cortical sub cortical control mechanisms.

Screening methods for drugs used to enhancing memory and intelligence

***In vivo* models:**

(a) Morris water maze test
(b) Assessment of learning memory using Y maze apparatus
(c) Passive shock avoidance paradigm
(d) Assessment of learning and memory using Hebb's William Maze (rectangular maze)
(e) Scopolamine induced amnesia (Interceptive Behavior model)
(f) Elevated plus maze (Exteroceptive behavior model)
(g) Shuttle box avoidance (Two way shuttle box)
(h) Passive avoidance paradigm (Exteroceptive behavior model)

***In vitro* models:**

(a) *In vitro* inhibition of acetylcholine-esterase activity in rat striatum
(b) *Ex vivo* cholinesterase inhibition
(c) [H]-N-methyl scopolamine binding in the presence and absence of GPP(NH)p

(d) [^{3}H]N-methylcarbamylcholine binding to nicotinic cholinergic receptors in rat frontal cortex.

(e) Cultured neurons/astroglial cells

***In vivo* models:**

(i) Morris water maze test

The modified procedure from morris method. The Morris water maze is a circular pool (90 cm in diameter and 45 cm in height) with featureless inner surface. The circular pool was filled to a height of 30 cm with water (18 ± 1°C), in which 500 ml of milk was mixed. A white platform (6 cm in diameter and 29 cm in height) was centered in one of four quadrants of the pool (Southest area) and submerged 1 cm below the water surface so that it was invisible at water level. In the water maze experiments the first week of the experiment was dedicated to swimming training for 60 sec. All animals were four groups we investigated the 3 weeks for treatment. In these days the mice were given one session of two trails each day for

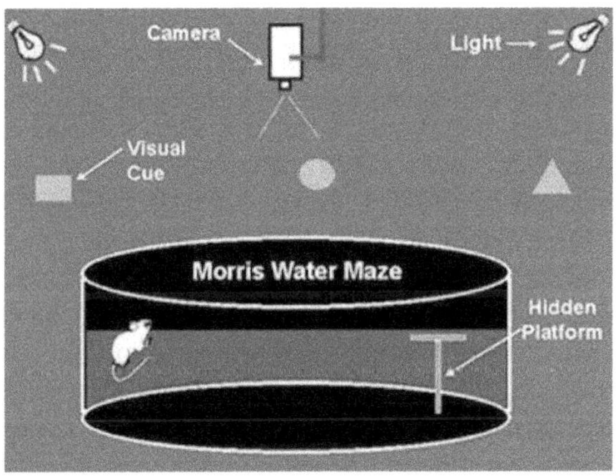

21 days. During each trial, the mouse's escape latency, measured with a stop watch, were recorded. The parameter was averaged for each session of trials and for each mouse. Once the mouse located the platform; it was permitted to remain on it for 10 sec. If the mouse did not locate the platform within 120 sec, it was placed on the platform for 10 sec. During this period, the platform was located in a fixed position. In the last day of training, mice were given a probe trial which considered of removing the plat form from the pool and allowing the mice to swim for 60 sec in search of it. A record was kept of the swimming time in the pool quadrant where the platform had previously been placed. Solutions of test sample were given orally 30 min prior to the consecutive training. After that swimming time in the pool was compared.

(ii) Assessment of learning and memory using Y Maze Apparatus

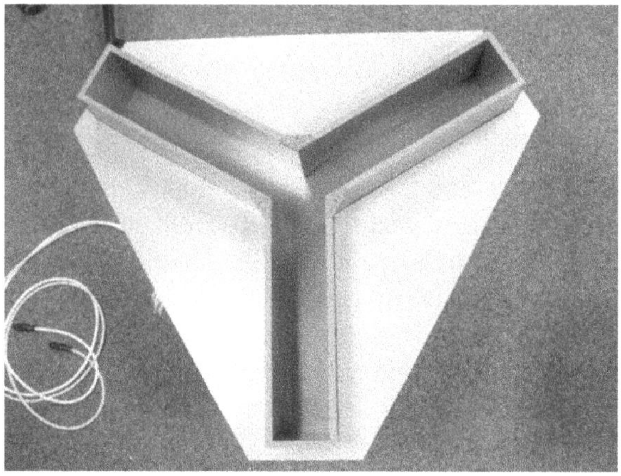

The Y-maze is a simple two-trial recognition test for measuring spatial recognition memory, it does not require learning of a rule, and thus is useful for studying memory in rodents, and in particular for the study of genetic influences on the response to novelty and recognition processes. Y-maze made of wood, consists of three arms with an angle of 120° between each of the two arms. The arm dimensions are 8 cm × 30 cm × 15 cm (width × length × height). The three identical arms were randomly designated: start arm, in which the mice started to explore (A), novel arm (B, with food stimuli), and the other arm (C). Mice tend to explore the maze systematically, entering each arm in turn. The ability to alternate requires that the mice know, which arm they have already visited. On the first day, all the mice were allowed to explore the Y maze apparatus for a period of ten minutes each. From the 2nd to 5th day the mice received four consecutive trials of training per day in the maze of 8 min duration. In each trial the mice were placed in the entry chamber (A) and the series of arm entries in all the three arms, including possible return into the same arm was recorded visually. Alteration is defined as the number of successive entries into the three arms on overlapping triplet sets. The percentage of alteration is calculated as the total number of arm entries minus two, and multiplied by 100. Pretreatment with amnestic agent 30 min prior to trials induces a marked decrease in spontaneous alteration performance with a concomitant increase in the total number of arm entries. Administration of agents that possesses memory enhancing effects is expected to reverse the changes. During learning assessment the animals were exposed to food and water add libitum only for 1 hour after the maze exposure for the day was completed to ensure motivation towards reward area (B).

***In vitro* methods**

(i) *In vitro* inhibition of acetylcholine-esterase activity in rat striatum

Aim: The purpose of this assay is to screen drugs for inhibition of acetylcholine-esterase activity.

Animals required	:	Male Wistar rats
Chemicals required	:	NaH_2PO_4
Equipments required	:	Potter-Elvehjem homogenizer, Beckman DU-50 Spectrophotometer

Procedure:

Tissue preparation: Male Wistar rats are decapitated, brain rapidly removed, corpora striata dissected free, weighed and homogenized in 19 volumes (approximately 7 mg protein/ml) of 0.05M NaH_2PO_4, pH 7.2 using a Potter-Elvehjem homogenizer. A 25 μl aliquot of this suspension is added to 1 ml of the vehicle or various concentrations of the test drug and reincubated for 10 min at 37 °C.

Assay: Enzyme activity is measured with the Beckman DU-50 spectrophotometer. This method can be used for IC_{50} determinations and for measuring kinetic constants. Reagents are added to the blank and sample cuvettes as follows:

Blank	:	0.8 ml PO_4 buffer/DTNB
		0.8 ml buffer/Substrate
Control	:	0.8 ml PO_4 buffer/DTNB/Enzyme from control animals
		0.8 ml PO_4 buffer/Substrate
Drug	:	0.8 ml PO_4 buffer/DTNB/Drug/Enzyme From treated animals
		0.8 ml PO_4 buffer/Substrate

Blank values are determined for each run to control for non-enzymatic hydrolysis of substrate and these values are automatically subtracted by the kindata program available on kinetics soft-Pac module. This program (Beckman DU-50 series spectrophotometer, kinetics) Soft-Pac TM module operation instructions: 1–7 also calculates the rate of absorbance change for each cuvette.

Evaluation: For IC_{50} determinations: Substrate concentration is 10mM diluted 1:2 in an assay yielding a final concentration of 5mM. DTNB concentration is 0.5mM yielding 0.25mM final concentration.

$$\% \text{ Inhibition} = (\text{slope control} - \text{slope drug/slope control}) \times 100$$

IC_{50} values are calculated from log probity analysis.

5.2.9 Screening Methods for CNS Stimulants

These are the drugs used to stimulate the central nervous system.

Examples

(a) ***Cerebral or psychomotor stimulants:*** Xanthine (caffeine), Ephedrine, Amphetamine, Methyl phenidate, Atropine, Pemoline.

(b) ***Brainstem stimulants or analeptics:*** Pentylenetetrazole (Metrazol), Picrotoxin, Doxapram.

(c) ***Spinal convulsants:*** Strychnine.

Preclinical Screening for Central Nervous System Stimulants

Some screening methods for CNS stimulant drugs are described as follows:

***In vivo* methods**

(i) Sandauswurf'' (displacement of sand) method
(ii) Runway test
(iii) Ptosis test
(iv) Registration of motor activity
(v) Open field test
(vi) Hole-board test
(vii) Combined open field test

***In vivo* methods**

(i) Sandauswurf'' (Displacement of Sand) method

Aim: This method is useful for detecting stimulant of all types. Amount displaced sand in graduated cylinder is measuring parameter of this method.

Procedure:

- A cylinder diameter 10 cm height 12 cm. The cylinder cages have a rubber torus around its lowest part to prevent motion of cages.
- Then the cage is placed in glass funnel so that on rubber torus touches the funnel.

- The cage is loaded with 50 ml dry sand contains 10 ml blue gel for absorption for moisture.
- Beneath the glass funnel, graduated glass cylinder having volume (10 ml), capable of being read to 0.1 ml. Quantity of sand is recorded every 15 minutes.

Conclusion: Amount of sand displaced by control group is compare to the test group.

(ii) Runway test

Aim: To study the effect of a drug on spontaneous activity and motor coordination.

Animals required	:	Wistar rats
Equipments required	:	Symmetrical Y shaped runway

Procedure:

- Age of 115-140 days Wistar rats are used for the experiment. 8-19 rats are used for each dose the apparatus is symmetrical Y shaped runway made of wood and 13 inches high.
- Each arm is 15 inches long and 5 inches wide. A trial consists of placing a rat in the center of the Y and leaving it in the apparatus for 5 minutes. The number of times it enter the arms of the apparatus, so that all of its feet are arm, is recorded as a measure of activity.
- In order to estimates the degree of ataxia, the rat is then placed on a runway covered with paper, so that footprint record of control rat shows that the regularity of spacing, is a measure of ataxia.
- The group of control rats had as the mean of spontaneous activity. Amphetamine at a dose of 0.19 mg/kg caused this number to increase to 20 times entries. Amylobarbitone sodium at a dose of 15 mg/kg caused it to increase to 22 times entries. But at high doses; decreases in the number of entries were found.

Conclusion: There were increase in the mean value of various CNS stimulants at specific dose than the control animal group.

(iii) Ptosis test

Aim: Reserpine causes the complete ptosis (depletion of neurotransmitter leads to depression like state) owing to central depression & this state is useful in evaluating CNS stimulant.

Animals required	:	Male albino mice
Chemicals required	:	Reserpine, deoxyephedrine 5 mg/kg Lysergic acid diethylamide 2 mg/kg Cocaine 40 mg/kg, 5% ascorbic acid

Procedure:

- Reserpine in 5% ascorbic acid and test compounds in aqueous solution, are administered i.p. to male albino mice. With about 4 mg/kg Reserpine, complete ptosis is reached at about 3 hr. 2-3 quarters hours after the reserpine injection, the test compound is administered.
- The ptotic rating is made 15 min later: 4 for complete ptosis; 3 for ¾ complete; 2 for ½ complete; and 1 for ¼ complete. Two reading on each mouse are taken, are averaged.
- Compound which antagonized the ptosis cause by reserpine, and which served as guides were: deoxyephedrine, 5 mg/kg; cocaine, 40 mg/kg and lysergic acid diethylamide, 2 mg/kg. Some compounds were effective only when given 2 hr before reserpine administration.

Conclusion: There are two unique neuropharmacological effects of reserpine in mice: ptosis and facilitation of extensor seizures. Reserpine induce Ptosis is generally considered to be owing to central depression. Thus central stimulants overcome the effect.

(iv) Registration of motor activity

Aim: This method may be used to detect increase motor activity.

Animals required	:	Mice
Chemicals required	:	0.9% sodium chloride
Equipments required	:	Rectangular cage, Photo electric cell, Digital counter, Light beam

Procedure:

- The rectangular cage is constructed with floor and ends of wood, and with plastic sides. A beam of light is passed through a plastic side to a photo electric cell, so adjusted that, when a mouse breaks the beam of light, the cell activates a digital counter.
- The drug is dissolved in a 0.9% sodium chloride and injected intraperitonially the number of counts or interruption of the light beam from the time of injection until 15minutes later is noted.

Conclusion: The ratio of this count to the count for control mice is measure of activity. For screening, a drug is tested initially at dose level of 50% and 10% of its LD_{50} for comparison, amphetamine, 5 mg/kg or more is used.

(v) Open field test

Aim: Interruption of light beams as a measure of movements of rats or mice in a cage. General motor activity also locomotion, rearing and the speed of locomotion can be determined.

Animals required : Adult male Sprague-Dawley rats (wt. 280-350 gm)

Equipments required: Open field area 8 photo cells micro computer

Procedure:

- The rats are observed in a square open field area (68 × 68 × 45 cm) equipped with 2 rows of 8 photocells, sensitive to infrared light, placed 40 and 125 mm above the floor, respectively.
- The photocells are spaced 90 mm apart and the last photocell in a row is spaced 25 mm from the wall.
- Measurements are made in the dark in a ventilated, sound-attenuating box.
- Interruptions of photocell beams can be collected by a micro computer and the following variables can be evaluated.
- Motor activity: All interruptions of photo beams in the lower rows. Peripheral motor activity: Activation of photo beams in the lower rows, provided that the photo beams spaced 25 mm from the wall were also activated.
- Rearing: All interruption of the photo beams in the upper rows. Peripheral rearing: Interruption of beams in the upper rows, provided that the photo beams spaced 25 mm from the wall were also activated.
- Locomotion: Successive interruptions of photo cells in the lower rows when the animal is moving in the same direction.
- Speed: The time between successive photo beam interruptions during locomotion collected in 0.1 categories. Adult male Sprague-Dawley rats with a weight between 280 and 320 gm are used. Drugs are injected subcutaneously 10 to 40 min before test. The rats are observed for 15 min whereby counts per min are averaged for 3 min intervals.

Conclusion: Dose-response curves can be obtained for sedative and stimulant drugs, whereby the various parameters show different results. The effects of various doses are compared statistically with the values of controls and among themselves.

(vi) Hole-board test

Aim: Evaluation of certain components of behavior of mice such as curiosity.

Animals required : Mice of either sex

Equipments required : Hole board with sixteen holes, light beams

Procedure:

- Mice of either sex (NMRI strain) with a weight between 18 and 22 gm are used. The hole board has a size of 40 × 40 cm sixteen holes with a diameter of 3 cm each are distributed evenly on the floor.
- The board is elevated so that the mouse poking its nose into the hole does not see the bottom.
- Nose-poking is thought to indicate curiosity and is measured by visual observation in the earliest description and counted by electronic devices in more recent modifications.
- Moreover, in the newer modifications motility is measured in addition by counting interruption of light beams.
- Usually, 6 animals are used for each dose and for controls.
- Thirty minutes after administration of the test. Compound the first animal is placed on the hole-board and tested for 5 min.

Conclusion: The number of counts for nose-poking of treated animals is calculated as percentage of control animals.

(vii) Combined open field test

Aim: The simultaneous determination of locomotion and curiosity by using a modification of the hole-board test and a photo-beam system has been proposed as a relatively simple test several types of such equipment are commercially available.

Animals required	: Male mice
Equipments required	: Open-field box with black plexi glass cage, photo cell beams

Procedure:

- Male mice (NMRI-strain) with an average weight of 30 gm are used. Each animal is tested individually in an automated open-field box which consists of a black plexiglass cage (35 × 35 × 20 cm^3) with a post (8 × 8 × 20 cm^3) in the center of the cage.
- Two evenly spaced photo cell beams perpendicular to the wall and 2 cm above the floor divide the box into 4 compartments.
- Every photo cell beam interruption is registered automatically as an activity count. Each wall of the cage contains 4 evenly spaced 2 cm diameter holes in a horizontal array 7 cm above the floor.
- A row of 4 photocell beams is mounted 1 cm outside of the holes and automatically records. Every exploratory nose-poke. Thirty min after intraperitoneal and 60 min after oral administration of the test

compound the animal is placed into the cage and the behavior recorded for a period of 5 min. Ten mice are used for each dose as well as for controls.

Conclusion: Counts for motility (interruption of photo cell beams inside the cage) and for curiosity (interruption of photocell beams outside the cage due to nose-poking) are recorded individually. The mean values of the treated groups are expressed as percentage of the control group. Using different doses, dose-response curves can be obtained.

5.3 SCREENING METHODS OF DRUGS ACTING ON AUTONOMIC NERVOUS SYSTEM

5.3.1 Screening Methods for Sympathomimetics

Autonomic nervous system is largely involuntary and is responsible for maintaining the internal homeostasis. Two subdivisions of autonomic nervous system include the sympathetic nervous system and parasympathetic nervous system. Neurotransmitter released at post ganglion sympathetic neuron is noradrenalin. Adrenaline secreted by adrenal medulla provides generalized sympathetic stimulation.

Adrenergic Receptors α, β.

Sub types - α1, α2, β1, β2, β3.

Which are present in heart, bronchi, blood vessels, uterus G.I.T, eyes etc.

Pharmacological actions of sympathomimetics

- Increased heart rate.
- Increased B.P.
- Dilution of pupils.
- Dilution trachea and bronchi.
- Stimulation of conversion of liver glycogen into glucose.
- Shunting of blood away from the skin and viscera to the skeletal muscles, brain, and heart.
- Inhibits peristalsis in G.I.T.
- Inhibition of contraction of bladder and rectum stimulation of uterus and contraction of spleen capsule.
- Sympathomimetic drugs are agents with activity that mimics the responses of adrenaline or stimulation of sympathetic nervous system.

Screening methods used

***In vivo* methods**

(i) The rat blood pressure non invasive model.
(ii) Cat spleen model.
(iii) The rat blood pressure invasive model.
(iv) Cat model of nictitating membrane prolapse.
(v) Mouse eye model.
(vi) Pithead rat model.
(vii) Rat heart and uterus model.

***In vitro* methods**

(i) Cat splenic strip model.
(ii) Rabbit pulmonary artery model.
(iii) Cat spleen model.
(iv) Rat vas deferens model.
(v) Rat seminal vesicle model.
(vi) Guinea pig tracheal chain model.
(vii) Guinea pig isolated heart model.
(viii) Rat sub maxillary tissue model.
(ix) Mice metabolic stimulation model.
(x) Marine macrophage model.

***In vivo* methods**

(i) Rat blood pressure non-invasive model

Aim: Sympathomimetic drug induced changes in (increased) blood pressure and heart rate can also record in a non invasive model.

Animals require	:	Adult male Wistar rats (250-300 grams)
Equipments required	:	Cannula
		Heating pads
		Tail cuffs
Chemicals required	:	Anesthesia, Cannula
		Polyethylene catheters
		Vinyl tubing
		Heparin (100 units)

Procedure:

- Adult male Wistar rats (250-300 gm) are used.

- The Jugular Vein is cannulated in anaesthetized rats using a curved polyethylene catheter.
- The vinyl tubing is under the skin of neck and exposed on the surface if back to allow for infusion of drugs.
- The catheter is flushed with heparin (100 units) to prevent clotting.
- Rats are allowed to recover for at least 24 hours before starting the experiment.
- On the day of experiment rats are first placed on heating pads (35-37 °C) for 20-30 mints. The tail cuff and pulse sensor is placed at proximal end of tail and is inflated. The heart rate is determined by manually counting the number of beats per unit. The value for each parameter is taken as average of at least 4 measurements.
- The measurements are done on three successive days to determine the baseline values.
- After baseline measurements the drug vehicle standard drug are injected through the catheter jugular vein and changes in heart rate and blood pressure are measured to evaluate sympathomimetic activity in invasive model.

Conclusion: If the sample drug increases the heart rate and blood pressure, then the drug has sympathomimetic activity. And when comparing with standard drug test drug baseline is more than standard means its potency is more than standard vice versa.

(ii) Cat spleen model

Aim: After the injection of sympathomimetic amines or electrical stimulation of pre and post ganglionic sympathetic nerves, spleen contracts.

Animal required	:	Cats
Chemicals required	:	Chloroform
		Heparin
		Warm paraffin
Equipment used	:	Cannula
		Centrifuge
		Electrical stimulator
		Scintillation counter

Procedure:

- Cat is anesthetized by using chloroform.

- Abdomen is cut and opened by giving a midline incision and the intestine is removed from the mid-duodenum to the terminal colon.
- The vascular connection between spleen and omentum are being cut. The splenic nerves are also cut to avoid liberation of catecholamine from other sites. The adrenal glands are also removed which is helpful to avoid the artifacts due to the release of pressure amines.
- A ligature is placed around the portal vein just beyond the junction of splenic and superior mesenteric veins and close to the adjoining gastric vein.
- Heparin is injected (i.v.) to prevent clotting of blood.
- The abdominal cavity is filled with warm paraffin and aerated with a mixture of 95% O_2 and 5% CO_2.
- Blood is collected by cannulated and placed in chilled silicon coated, calibrated centrifuge tubes during the period of stimulation together with a subsequent 20 sec period immediately after cessation of the stimulus.
- This is enough to capture more than 80% of NA released into the blood during electrical stimulation at the same time avoids the excessive loss and unwanted dilution of activity in the plasma.

Conclusion: The amount of the noradrenaline present in the blood is estimated by scintillation counter for radio activity measurement.

In vitro **methods**

(i) Cat splenic strip model

Aim: The splenic tissue contracts in response to sympathomimetic agents and therefore can be used for screening of drugs with potential sympathomimetic activity.

Animals required : Cats (1.0 - 2.8 kg)

Chemicals required : Anaesthetized spleen strips (25-30 mm long, 2-3 mm wide)
Kreb's Solution, Sodium pentobarbitone
Phentolamine (standard drug)

Equipments required : Organ bath, Kymograph

Procedure:

- Cats of either sex weighing around 1.0 - 2.8 kg were anaesthetized by i.p. of 4.5 mg/kg sodium Pentobarbitone.

- Then the spleen is removed and spleen strip are placed in organ bath filled with of Kreb's – ringer solution, at 38 °C aerated with 95% oxygen and 5% carbondioxide.
- Isotonic contractions are recorded on kymograph at 0.5 gm tension with magnification 5 to 6 times.
- To induce contractions NE {10^6g/ml} (Nor epinephrine), E {10^{-6}g/ml} (Epinephrine) is administered after 30 min.
- Test drug is then added into organ bath followed by administration of α agonists after 3 min.

Conclusion: Comparison of test drug potency with standard (α agonist).

(ii) Rabbit Pulmonary Artery Model

Aim: Pulmonary artery is very sensitive to sympathomimetic agents.

Animals required	:	Rabbits (1-2 kg)
Chemicals required	:	Kreb's bicarbonate solution
Equipments required	:	Ventricle strip [4 mm by 30 mm of length]
		Organ bath
		Isometric strain gauge, Transducer, Spectrophotometer
		Electrical stimulator [Bipolar platinum electrodes]

Procedure:

- The rabbit is sacrificed by exsanguinations and removal of main pulmonary artery.
- The artery is cut transversely and spirally into vertical strip. That strip suspended vertically in organ both connected by thread to an isometric strain aerated transducer.
- The resting tension 2 gm and artery is superfused in Krebs's bicarbonate solution, flow down the connector thread and tissue rate at 6 ml/min at 37 °C and aerated with 95% O_2 and 5% CO_2.
- Following incubation of 60 min. Artery strip is super fused with kreb's solution 37 °C for 30 min wash out external ^{3}{H} noradrenalin.
- During the experiment, superfusates are collected in vials every 2 min.
- Aliquots of collected samples are then assayed for noradrenalin using scintillation spectrophotometer to count the radio activity after adding scintillation fluid.

- The electrical stimulation given to that either side of strip of 0.3 milli sec duration. Responses to successive 2 min period observed at 16 min intervals.
- Tension produced by tissue increases rapidly after commencement of stimulation and decrease back to original basal value after stimulation has ceased.
- The response produced is accompanied by increased release of tritium onto the superfusate.
- The further reduction in basal radioactivity in the superfusion fluid occurs after each stimulus period as the tissue gradually loses its stored radio activity.
- The total tritium detected in collected superfusates unchanged noradrenaline comprised of approximately 30% during rest period and at least 50% during stimulation.

Conclusion: Stimulation of pulmonary artery with test drug is compared with stimulation percentage given by noradrenalin. Then the potency of test drug is estimated.

5.3.2 Screening Methods for Parasympathomimetics

Parasympathetic nervous system performs maintenance activities and conserves body energy.

- Acetylcholine (Ach) is both preganglionic and postganglionic neurotransmitter of parasympathetic system.
- Ach releases at cholinergic synapse and neuron effectors junction and shows its pharmacological actions through cholinergic receptors (Muscarinic and Nicotinic).
- Nicotinic receptor present at autonomic ganglion and neuromuscular junction.
- Muscarinic receptor present on autonomic effector cells and post ganglionic cholinergic nerves.
- Present in heart, eyes, glands, smooth muscles and blood vessels.
- Muscarinic receptor is 5 types – M_1, M_2, M_3, M_4 and M_5.

Screening Methods

***In vivo* methods**

(i) Cat model for anti cholinesterase activity.

(ii) Rat blood pressure model.

(iii) Mydriasis test.

(iv) Intestinal spasmolytic activity in mice.
(v) Continuous cystometry in rats.
(vi) Guinea pig bronchospasm model.

***In vitro* models**

(i) *In vitro* assay for anti cholinesterase activity.
(ii) Guinea pig trachea model.
(iii) Isolated eye of rodents.
(iv) Isolated frog rectus muscle.
(v) Rat isolated aorta model.
(vi) Guinea pig ileum.
(vii) Guinea pig isolated heart model.

***In vivo* methods**

(i) Cat model for anti cholinesterase activity

Aim: Sample drug contain Anti cholinesterase activity shows sympathomimetic activity.

Animals required	:	Cats
Chemicals required	:	Anaesthesia (Chloralose or Phenobarbitone sodium)
Equipments required	:	Cannula, B.P, Respiration recorders

Procedure:

- Cat is anaesthetized using chloralose or phenobarbitone sodium.
- The common carotid artery is cannulated for recording the blood pressure and the substance to be tested is injected (i.v.).
- The B.P and respiration are recorded in anaesthetized animal at different doses of an anti cholinesterase agent. For instance, at some dose (x) not detectable effect observed.
- At dose 2x - slight bradycardia followed by fall in B.P. by 100-120 mm of Hg developed over period of 5 min.
- At dose 4x – B.P reduces 50-100 mm of Hg with pronounced bradycardia.
- Salivary and bronchioles secretion are seen with fasciculation of skeletal muscles.
- Initially respiration is increased but later on it is depressed.
- Defection and urination are also observed.

- At dose 8x, all effects mentioned are much more prominent as compared to dose 4x.

Conclusion: Presence of all these effects indicates that test drug anti cholinesterase activity.

(ii) Rat blood pressure model

Aim: Administration of cholinergic drugs produces fall in blood pressure

Animals required	:	Sprague Dawley rats (200-350 grams)
Chemicals required	:	Anaesthesia
		Heparin (600 μl/kg)
		Normal saline
Equipments required	:	Tracheostomy tube, Cannula
		Polythene catheters

Procedure:

- Rats are anaesthetized by using a 50:50 mixture of 25% urethane and 1% alpha chloralose at a dose 5 ml/kg body weight.
- A tracheostomy tube is placed to support respiration femoral artery and vein cannulated using polythene catheters.
- The catheters placed in femoral artery are connected to pressure transducer for recording blood pressure and femoral vein catheter is used for administration of drug.
- Immediately after cannulation the animals are injected with heparin 600 μl/kg to avoid clotting.
- After 30 mins of equilibrium period rats are injected with normal saline/ test drug.
- A change of blood pressure is required.

Conclusion: Blood pressure is allowed to return to normal between injections. Evaluate cholinergic activity the injected after administration of muscarinic blocker atropine (1-6 mg/kg).

***In vitro* methods**

(i) *In vitro* assay for anticholinesterase activity

Acetylcholinestrase activity is detected by assay described by Ellman *et al*. This assay is based on measurement of change in absorbance at 412 nm. In this assay thiol ester, acetylcholine was used as substrate. To detect inhibition of enzyme activity, 289 ml phosphate buffer,

0.1 ml DTNB and 10 ml of sample (serum, plasma, blood or brain homogenate) are mixed and incubated for 10 min.

- After addition of substrate, absorbance is recorded using spectrophotometer.
- The rate of change of absorbance is determined and enzyme activity is calculated.
- Different concentration of inhibitors of enzymes is used and again rate of reaction is recorded.
- The percent inhibition as compared to standard activity is calculated.

(ii) Guinea pig trachea model

Aim: Tracheal smooth muscles contracts in response to parasympathomimetic drug like acetylcholine. The evaluation of test drugs can be done in guinea pig tracheal smooth muscle preparation.

Animal required	:	Guinea pig (300-350 gm)
Chemicals required	:	Kreb's solution
		Carbachol
Equipments required	:	Organ bath

Procedure:

- Guinea pig is used and sacrificed by stunning and exsanguinations.
- The trachea is dissected out and transferred to dish containing Kreb's solution.
- The trachea is cut to 2-3 mm wide rings and 6 such rings are connected to each other with the help of a silk thread.
- Then it is placed in organ bath- under 1 gm tension.

  In 10 ml organ bath at 37 °C temperature.

  Aerated with $O_2 + CO_2$ (95:05).
- Carbachol used as standard. Dose response curve for cumulative concentration is measured after wash out same process continued with test drug.

Conclusion: The shift of dose response curve of Carbachol

Right indicates - parasympatholytic activity

Left indicates - parasympathomimetic activity.

5.3.3 Screening Methods of Local Anaesthetic Activity

Local anesthetics have been defined as drugs which reversibly block nerve conduction beyond the point of application when applied locally in an appropriate concentration. This local anesthesia is drug induced reversible blockade of nerve impulses in a restricted region of the body. According to their clinical usage the local anesthetics have been classified as

- Topical anesthetics
- Infiltration and block anesthetics
- Spinal anesthetics
- Epidural and caudal anesthetics

The methods for pharmacological evaluation have also been directed towards these sites and classified similarly with a slight difference in the terminology used for their actions.

Conduction anesthesia

- Conduction anesthesia in the sciatic nerve of frog
- Conduction anesthesia in the sciatic nerve of the rat
- Conduction anesthesia on the mouse tail

Infiltration anesthesia

- Infiltration anesthesia in guinea pigs

Surface anesthesia

- Corneal anesthesia in rabbits
- Inhibition of sneezing reflex in rabbits

Epidural anesthesia

- Epidermal anesthesia in guinea pigs

Intrathecal (Spinal) anesthesia

- Spinal anesthesia in rats

(i) Conduction anesthesia in sciatic nerve of frog:

Aim: The time of onset and duration of anesthesia is measured by this method.

Animals required	:	Frogs
Chemicals required	:	0.65% NaCl
		Anesthesia
Equipments required	:	Bath, Small forceps

- Frogs were decapitated and upper part of spinal cord was destroyed down to level of 3rd vertebra.

- The viscera are removed exposing the lumbar plexus damaging it.
- The frog is then suspended on vertical board.
- Small pieces of white cotton are soaked with different concentration of test preparation (0.05-1%) or the standard and placed gently around the sciatic nerve for 1 min. The cotton swab is removed and frog is placed with it extremities into a bath with 0.65% NaCl solution.
- One side is used for test preparation and other side for standard.
- Every 3 min the frog removed from the bath and toes of legs or ankle joint are pinched 3 times with small forceps. The reflex contraction is abolished when conduction anesthesia is effective.
- The stimuli are repeated every 3 min until anesthesia vanishes.
- 5 frogs are used for every concentration of test.
- The time of onset and duration of anesthesia are recorded for each concentration.

Conclusion: Results can be presented as time responses and dose response curves.

(ii) Infiltration anesthesia

Aim: This is the method of intracutaneous wheals in guinea pigs for assessment of local anesthetic activity of novel compound has become standard proceeding.

Animal required	:	Guinea pigs
Chemicals required	:	Pin prick
		Anesthesia
		0.1 ml saline

Procedure:

- Guinea pigs of either sex at 300-400 gm are taken.
- A day before experiments 2 areas of 4-5 cm diameter are shaved in skin at back of animals.
- Sensitivity of skin is more in middling and slight more in front than back areas.
- So test drug tested in both areas, 6 tests using 3 guinea pigs performed simultaneously.

- The test and standard compound injection in 0.1 ml saline 1 dose from front and 1 dose back.
- The size of wheal is marked with ink, one side use for test and 1 side for standard.
- The reaction to pin prick is tested 5 min after injection 1st normal reaction of animal pin prick is noted outside the wheal. 6 pricks are then applied inside the wheal and number of pricks to which animal fails to react is counted.
- Six pricks are applied every 5 min for 30 min.

Conclusion: After completing the testing guinea pigs, the same solutions are injected in another 3 guinea pigs but solution used for front is now used for back area vice versa. The number of times the prick fails to elicit response during 30 min period is added up and the sum of possible 36, gives own indication of degree of anesthesia.

Using various doses: Dose response curves can be established. Similarly the time response curves can be drawn and duration of action can be found out. This test has been used for studying the influences of vasoconstrictors like adrenaline on intensity and duration of action of local anesthetics.

(iii) Surface anesthesia

Aim: Stimulation of Nasal Mucosa

Animals required	:	New Zealand albino rabbits (either sex (3 kg))
Equipments required	:	Cotton swab

Procedure:

- New Zealand albino rabbits either sex (3 kg).
- Test solution is applied to mucous membrane of nostrils with help of cotton swab.
- Standard drug solution similarly applied after 2-5 min stimulated by fine tip.
- Loss of sneezing refuse is considered as sign of complete.
- Stimulation repeated 3, 5, 10 and 15 min continued every 5 min until sneezing refuse appears.
- Time required for onset of action and duration of anesthetic effect is noted using various concentrations of test comp and standard.

Conclusion: Dose response curve and relative potencies can be established as described under the corneal anesthesia in rabbits.

(iv) Intrathecal (Spinal) anesthesia

Aim: Spinal anesthesia in rat model has been routinely used for screening of local anesthetics.

Animal required : Male Sprague Dawley or Wistar rats (75-100 gm)
Chemicals required : Saline
Equipment required : Needle
Tail flick
25 ml Hamilton syringe
Analgesiometer

Procedure:

- The rat is held firmly by pelvic girdle.
- A 30 gauge needle is attached to a 25 ml Hamilton syringe.
- It is inserted into the tissue on one side of the L5 or L6 portion of spine. This process maintaining on angle of about 200.
- The needle is further advanced to the groove between the spinal and transverse processes and then move forward the intervertebral space at an angle of about 100. At this stage about 0.5 cm of needle is secured in vertebral column.
- Arching of tail following this procedure indicated the correct insertion of needle in the vertebral column of rat.
- Test compound dissolved in saline or water and administered volume of 5 ml.
- Anti nociception is determined by tail flick assay in rats.
- The tail is placed on an analgesiometer providing exposure to a source of focused radiant heat.

Conclusion: The reaction time is noted in each case. The degree of anti nociception is calculated as the % of more possible effect. Using different doses the ED_{50} values of test comp and standard L.A. are worked out for comparison of potency.

5.3.4 Screening Methods for Muscle Relaxants

(i) Rotarod test in mice
(ii) Chimney test in mice
(iii) Grip strength in mice
(iv) Test for muscle co-ordination
(v) Inclined plane test in mice

(i) Rotarod test in mice

Aim: One of the classical methods introduced by Dunham and Miya in 1957 for the evaluation of drugs interfering with motor coordination activity by testing their ability to remain on a revolving rod.

Animal required	:	Male Swiss mice (20-30 gm)
Chemicals required	:	Test and standard
Equipments required	:	Rotarod apparatus

About apparatus: It consists of horizontal wooden rod or metal rod coated with rubber with 30 cm diameter attached to a motor with the speed set at 2 rotations per minute .The rod is 75 cm in length and divided in sections by plastic discs, thereby allowing the simultaneous testing of 6 mice. The rod is placed at a height of about 50 cm above the table top in order to discourage the animals from jumping off the roller. Cages kept below the sections save to restrict movements of animals when they fall off from the roller.

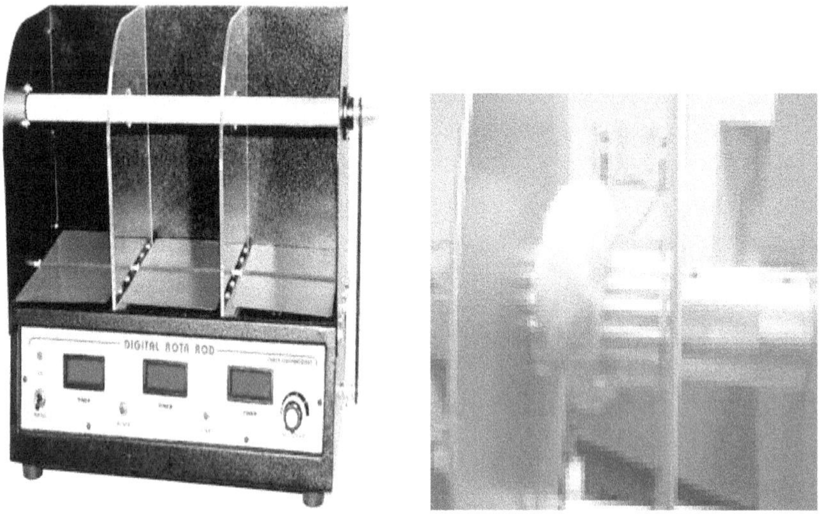

Fig. 5.3 Rotarod apparatus.

Procedure:

- Male Swiss mice undergo as per test on the apparatus.
- Only those mice, which demonstrate their ability to remain on the revolving rod for at least 60 sec are chosen for the test.
- 30 min after i.p. or 60 min after oral administration of test or standard drugs the animals are placed on the rotarod for 1 min.
- The number of animals falling with in 1 mins are counted.

- Percentage of animals falling from the rotarod within the test period is calculated for every drug concentration tested.

Conclusion: ED_{50} is defined as the dose of the drug at which 50% animals fall from the rotarod.

(ii) Chimney test in mice

Aim: The chimney test is used as an additional test for determining the muscle relaxant activity of test drug.

Animal required	:	Male Swiss albino mice (16-22 gm)
Equipment required	:	Pyrex glass cylinder (30 cm length different diameters from 22-28 cm)

Procedure:

- Albino mice are used. Glass cylinders are called chimney are used for this test.
- Initially cylinder is held in a horizontal position. At the end of cylinder near a 2 cm mark from the base, a mouse is introduced with the head forward.
- When the mouse reaches the other end of the cylinder, the tube is moved to a vertical position. Immediately, the mouse tries to climb backwards and performs coordinated movements similar to an alpinist to pass a chimney in the mountains. Because of this reason the name of chimney has been given to this test.
- The time required by the mouse to climb backwards to the top of the cylinder is noted.

Conclusion: The ED_{50} with 95% confidence limits, the dose at which 50% of the animals fail to climb backwards within 30 sec is calculated using log- probity analysis method. The chimney test is used as an additional test for determining the muscle relaxant activity of test drug.

(iii) Grip strength in mice

Aim: In this method disturbance of the grasping reflex can be considered while giving of test drug.

Animal required	:	Swiss Albino mice (20-30 gm)
Equipments required	:	Horizontal thin metallic wire suspended about 30 cm in air
		Forceps
		Cages

Procedure:

- Swiss albino mice are used in this test.
- This test is used to assess muscular strength in rodents which can be influenced by muscle relaxants and sedative drugs.
- In a preliminary experiment the animals are tested for their normal grip strength by exposing them to horizontal thin metallic wire suspended about 30 cm in the air, which they immediately grasp with their forceps. The mouse is then released to hang on with its forelimbs.
- Normal animals are able to catch the wire with the hind limbs and climb on to it within 5 seconds.
- Only animals which fulfill this criterion are included in the test.
- Ten mice are used in each group.
- After oral or parental administration of test standard drugs the animals are tested every 15 min for 2 hr.
- Animals which are not able to climb on to the wire with hind limbs with in 5 sec or fall off are considered to be impaired by drug effect.
- After the completion of this test the animals are observed for their behavior in the cages.
- If their behavior and mobility in the cage appears to be normal, the disturbance of the grasping reflex can be considered to be caused by central relaxation.

Conclusion: The percentage of animals loosing the grip strength is recorded using different doses of test and standard drugs and LD_{50} values are calculated.

5.4 SCREENING OF DRUGS ACTING ON CARDIOVASCULAR SYSTEM

5.4.1 Screening Methods for Anti Hypertensive Agents

Introduction

Hypertension is the most common cardiovascular disease and is a major public health issue in developed as well as developing countries. Although it is common and readily detectable, but if left untreated it can often lead to lethal complications. Because of its high incidence and morbidity, various classes of drugs and regimens have been proposed for the control of hypertension. Despite the large armamentaria of drugs being available for the treatment of hypertension, the last two decades have witnessed the introduction of a number of new antihypertensive drugs. Recent research during this period has also added considerably to our knowledge of the mechanisms involved in the pathogenesis of hypertension.

The animal models of hypertension share many features which are common to human hypertension. Many of these models have been developed by utilizing the etiological factors that are presumed to be responsible for human hypertension such as excessive salt intake, hyperactivity of Renin Angiotensin-Aldosterone System (RAAS) and genetic factors. These models are also used in the pharmacological screening of potential antihypertensive agents. In the past, hypertensive animal models have been used infrequently for testing antihypertensive potential of drugs. As new molecules are being synthesized in a large number, the use of animal models is increasing for testing these molecules. New animal models of hypertension are being developed as new insights in to the pathogenesis of hypertension are revealed.

***Different models of inducing hypertension in rodents*:** The various types of animal models of hypertension are:

1. Renovascular hypertension
   (i) Goldblatt method
      - Two kidney one clip (2K1C) hypertension
      - One kidney one clip (1K1C) hypertension
      - Two kidney two clip (2K2C) hypertension

   (ii) Hypertension induced by external compression of renal parenchyma
      - Page hypertension

   (iii) Grollman hypertension
      - Two kidney one ligature (2K1L)
      - One kidney one ligature (1K1L)
      - Coarctation of aorta
      - Reduced renal mass
2. Dietary hypertension
   - Increased salt intake
3. Endocrine hypertension
   - Mineralocorticoid induced hypertension
   - Adrenal regeneration hypertension
4. Neurogenic hypertension
   - Denervation of sinoaortic baroreceptors

5. Psychogenic hypertension
6. Genetic hypertension
7. Other models
   - Obesity related hypertension
   - Hypertension induced by cholinomimetic agents
   - Angiotensin-II induced hypertension
   - Hypertension induced by cadmium

1. Renovascular hypertension

(i) Goldblatt method

Aim: It was reported that a partial constriction of renal arteries in dogs produced hypertension. U-shaped silver ribbon clip is used to constrict the renal arteries in rabbits and rats.

Three types of hypertension are produced by goldblatt method

- ***Two Kidney One Clip (2K1C) hypertension:*** The renal artery is constricted on only one side with the other artery (or kidney) left untouched which causes sustained increase in BP due to increased Plasma Renin Activity (PRA), which in turn increases circulating angiotensin-II, a potent vasoconstrictor. However, there is no salt and water retention because of the other normal kidney being intact. Therefore, the resultant hypertension at this stage is renin-angiotensin dependent. After about 6 weeks, the increased angiotensin-II releases aldosterone from adrenal cortex leading to a gradual retention of salt and water. Decreased renin production is because of the retention of salt and water. From this stage onwards, hypertension is volume dependent. This clearly shows that salt and water balance is critically involved in the pathogenesis of renovascular hypertension. Increased BP and increased renin activity returns to normal by unclipping or removal of the affected kidney.
- ***One Kidney One Clip (1K1C) hypertension:*** Constriction of renal artery is done on one side and the contralateral kidney is removed. BP rises within few hours. As there is no other kidney, there is no pressure diuresis and natriuresis, so rapid salt and water retention is there. Plasma renin activity is usually normal. Hypertension soon becomes volume dependent
- ***Two Kidney Two Clip (2K2C) hypertension:*** Constriction of aorta or both renal arteries is done. There is a patchy

ischemic kidney tissue, which secretes renin causing increased BP. The remaining kidney tissue retains salt and water. In fact, one of the most common causes of renal hypertension in human beings is such a patchy ischemic kidney disease.

(ii) **Hypertension induced by external compression of renal parenchyma:** This type of hypertension is produced in dogs, rabbits and rats. The following methods are used to produce this type of hypertension:

- ***Page hypertension:*** A sheet of cellophane is covered around the kidney and held in place by silk sutures tied loosely around the renal hilus. Both kidneys are wrapped or one kidney is wrapped and other is removed. A fibrocollagenous shell is formed around the kidney in 3-5 days because of reaction of the tissue to the foreign material. Renal vascular pressure is decreased due to the shell compressing renal parenchyma. This expands the extracellular volume leading to increased peripheral resistance and hence increased BP.

(iii) **Grollman hypertension:** In this method, kidney tissue is compressed by securing a ligature around the kidney. The ligature around the kidney forms a figure resembling number 8. This type of hypertension can be produced in dogs, rabbits and rats.

It is of two types:

1. Two kidney one ligature (2K1L)
2. One kidney one ligature (1K1L)

Coarctation of aorta: Renal blood flow can be decreased by compressing the aorta. Coarctation can be done just above the renal arteries, between renal arteries and superior mesenteric arteries or between two renal arteries with the right artery above and the left artery below the site of coarctation. An increase in BP similar to 2K1C model can be produced by applying a rubber band to abdominal aorta along with constriction of right renal artery for 8 weeks. Coarctation can be followed by unilateral nephrectomy to produce this type of hypertension.

Reduced renal mass: Reducing renal tissue to five-sixth ($5/6^{th}$) by renal mass ablation produces hypertension. The right kidney is removed and 2 or 3 branches of left renal artery are ligated to produce infarction of approximately $2/3^{rd}$ of the left kidney in this method.

2. **Dietary hypertension**

   Increased salt intake: Physiologically, normal kidney has the ability to excrete easily the daily salt load without allowing a marked rise in extracellular volume. Excess salt intake produces hypertension in rats, which mimics human hypertension. High salt intake hypertension has been produced in rats, rabbits and chicks by replacing drinking water with 1-2% sodium chloride for 9-12 months.

3. **Endocrine hypertension**

   1. ***Mineralocorticoid induced hypertension:*** It was first demonstrated that deoxycorticosterone acetate (DOCA) produces hypertension in rats. Increased blood volume and hence increased BP is due to increased DOCA-induced reabsorption of salt and water. Vasopressin secretion is increased leading to water retention and vasoconstriction. Additionally, altered activity of RAAS leads to increased sympathetic activity. Rats are prone to DOCA-salt induced hypertension. This type of hypertension can also be produced in dogs and pigs. Other mineralocorticoids (e.g., aldosterone) and glucocorticoids can also produce this type of hypertension.
   2. ***Adrenal regeneration hypertension:*** Hypertension is produced in rats by unilateral nephrectomy followed by removal of right adrenal gland and enucleation of left adrenal gland. Enucleation is carried out by making a small incision in the capsule of adrenal gland through which the bulk of glandular tissue is extruded by gentle application of pressure with curved forceps. Drinking water is replaced with 1% saline. Hypertension develops during regeneration of adrenal glands in about 2 weeks.

4. **Neurogenic hypertension**

   1. ***Denervation of sinoaortic baroreceptors:*** This is the most often used neurogenic model of hypertension. In dogs, cardioaortic nerve is located at the junction of superior laryngeal and vagus nerve and runs in the form of several fine strands. These strands unite and may be traced back as a white band lying within the vagal sheath alongside the cervical sympathetic nerve. Following bilateral vagotomy and carotid sinus denervation, the region is painted with 5% phenol and then alcohol to ensure complete denervation of the carotid sinus. There is sudden increase in BP. The dog is allowed to equilibrate for approximately 30 min and a bolus of the test compound can be given by intravenous administration. BP returns to normal within about 2 days because the response of vasomotor center to the absent baroreceptors signals fades away, which is called "resetting of baroreceptors". Thus, this is only an acute type of hypertension.

5. **Psychogenic hypertension:** Reports depict that elevation of BP resulting from repeated exposure to stressful situation may lead to a state of persistent hypertension. Borderline Hypertensive Rats (BHR) are useful for psychogenic hypertension. BHRs that were exposed to daily sessions of either short (20 min) or long (120 min) duration air-jet stimulation developed hypertension within 2 weeks in comparison to home cage controls. Animals exposed to 120 min stress sessions had significantly higher systolic BP relative to the 20 minute group.

6. **Genetic hypertension:** Aoki introduced a new model of experimental hypertension that required no physiological, pharmacological or surgical intervention. The so called 'Spontaneous Hypertensive Rat (SHR)' was developed by meticulous genetic inbreeding that uniformly resulted in 100% of the progeny having naturally occurring hypertension.

7. **Other models**

    1. ***Obesity related hypertension:*** Wistar fatty rats (WFR) derived from cross between obese Zucker and Wistar Kyoto rats show persistent hyperinsulinemia and hypertension after 16 weeks of age and may be a good model to elucidate the relationship between hyperinsulinemia and hypertension.

    2. ***Hypertension induced by cholinomimetic agents:*** Physostigmine (10-80 μg/kg, *i.v.*), a cholinesterase inhibitor, and oxotremorine(20-40 μg/kg, *i.v.*), a direct muscarinic cholinergic agonist; cause a dose-dependent increase in BP. The cholinomimetic-induced hypertension has been shown to be elicited through activation of central cholinergic mechanism and mediated peripherally through sympathetic nervous system

    3. ***Angiotensin-II induced hypertension:*** Subcutaneous infusion of angiotensin-II (0.7 mg/kg/day) using mini pump elicits hypertension in 4-8 weeks.

    4. ***Hypertension induced by cadmium:*** Hypertension is produced by the chronic administration of $CdCl_2$ (1 mg/kg/day, i.p. for 2 wk). $CdCl_2$-induced hypertension might be due to the fact that the metal ion might mimic Ca^{2+} ion as a partial agonist and produce a direct contractile effect on vascular smooth muscle.

5.4.2 Screening Methods of Anti Arrhythmic Activity

An arrhythmia is any deviation from or disturbance of normal heart rhythm. The basic rhythm of the heart is a tightly regulated phenomenon designed to insure maximal efficiency and optimal performance. The cardiac rhythm involves several different microscopic and microscopic structures within the normal heart.

- An arrhythmia may occur when any portion of this sequence is interrupted or disturbed.
- Arrhythmia may be begin, symptomatic life threatening or even fatal. Cardiac arrhythmias are required problem in clinical practice, occurring in up to 25% of patients treated with digitals, 80% of patients with acute myocardial infarction.

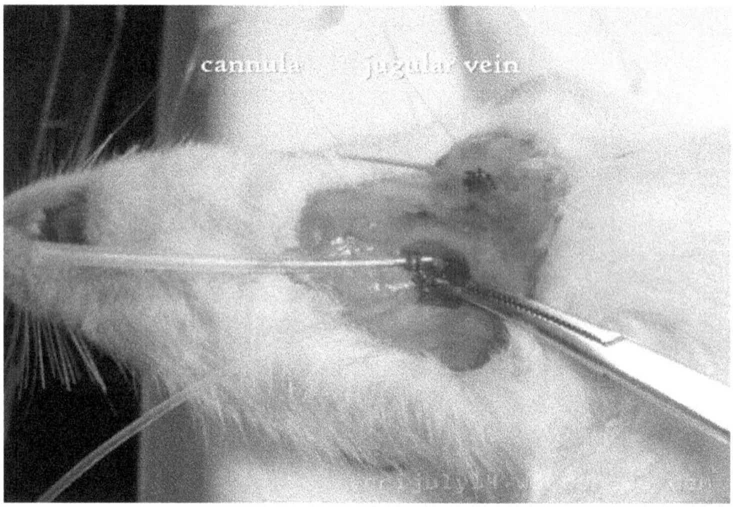

Fig. 5.4 Cardiac puncture.

Arrhythmia is manifested as either as ventricular extra systole. Impulse originates from the site other than SA node. Early QRS complex with wide abnormal morphology is observed, ventricular tachycardia.

- Rapid series of regular ventricular contraction at the rate of 140-170 beats per min is observed.
- QRS complex is widened or ventricular fibrillation. Disorganized very rapid rhythm of ventricle is observed. Rate is about 100 beats per min.

The anti arrhythmic agents have traditionally divided into 4 distinct classes on basis of their mechanism of action.

- Class I: Drugs act by blocking the sodium channel, subdivided into 3 groups.

  IA, IB and IC based effects on phase depolarization and repolarization.

  IA-drugs has moderate potency to block sodium channels has prolonged repolarization (increased QRS).

IB-drugs has lowest potency to block sod channels shorten repolarization.

IC-drugs most potent sodium channel blockers have little effect on repolarization.

- Class II: Drugs act indirectly on electrophysiological parameters by blocking beta – adrenergic receptors.
- Class III: Drugs act by mechanisms that are not well understood (interference with potassium conductance is one possible mechanism) but act to prolong repolarization with little effect on the rate of depolarization.
- Class IV: Drugs are relatively selective AV nodal calcium channel blockers, primarily L type channels.

Annulations in rat jugular vein.

Screening methods:

Cell culture techniques

(i) Studies on Isolated ventricular myocytes.

***In vitro* methods**

(i) Langendorff technique.
(ii) Acetylcholine or potassium induced arrhythmia.
(iii) Isolated guinea pig papillary muscle.
(iv) Action potential and refractory period in isolated pig papillary muscle.

***In vivo* methods**

Chemically induced arrhythmia

(i) Aconitine antagonism in rats
(ii) Digoxin induced arrhythmia in guinea pigs
(iii) Strophanthin or Waban induced arrhythmia
(iv) Adrenaline induced arrhythmia
(v) Calcium induced arrhythmia

Electrically induced arrhythmia

(i) Ventricular fibrillation electrical threshold
(ii) Programmed electrical stimulation induced arrhythmia
(iii) Sudden coronary death model in dogs

Exercise induced ventricular fibrillation

Mechanically induced arrhythmia

(i) Reperfusion arrhythmia in dogs
(ii) Two stage coronary ligation in dogs

Genetically induced arrhythmia

Genetic arrhythmia

***In vitro* methods**

(i) Langendorff technique

Aim: The basic principle involved in this technique is that heart is perfused in a retrograde direction from the aorta either at constant pressure or constant flow with oxygenated saline selection.

Animals required	:	Guinea pigs (30-500 gm)
Chemicals required	:	Ringers solution
Equipments required	:	Cannula, Plexiglass perfusion apparatus.
		Chronometer
		Poly graph

Procedure:

- Guinea pigs of either sex weighing 300-500 gm are sacrificed by stunning.
- The heart is removed as quickly as possible and placed in a dish containing ringers solution at 37 °C associated pericardial and lung tissues are removed.
- The aorta is located and cut below the point of division. The cannula is inserted into the aorta and tied and the heart is perfused with oxygenated ringers solution.
- The heart is transferred to a double wall Plexiglas perfusion apparatus maintained at 37 °C oxygenated ringer solution is perfused at constant pressure of 40 mm Hg at temperature of 37 °C.
- Ligature is placed around the LAD coronary artery and occlusion is maintained for 10 min followed by reperfusion.
- Test compound is administered through perfusion medium either before or after occlusion.
- An epicardial ECG electrode is used for pulsatile stimulation and induction of arrhythmias (rectangular pulses of 0.75 msec duration, usually of 10 V frequency 400-1800 shocks per min).
- A small steel hook with a string is attached to the apex of the heart.
- Contractile force is measured isometrically by a force transducer and recorded on a polygraph.

Conclusion: Heart rate is measured through a chronometer coupled to the polygraph. Drugs are injected into the perfusion medium. Incidence and duration of ventricular fibrillation or ventricular tachycardia is recorded in the control as well as test group.

(ii) Acetylcholine or potassium induced arrhythmia

Aim: Test drug fibrillation is measured by this method.

Animals required	:	New Zealand white rabbits (0.5-3 kg)
Chemicals required	:	Ringer solution, Potassium chloride (0.10 gm)
Equipments required	:	Kymograph, bath

Procedure:

- New Zealand white rabbits of weight range 0.5-3 kg are used for the study.
- The animals are sacrificed and heart removed immediately. Atria dissected from other tissue and placed in ringers solution.
- The atria are attached to an electrode in lower part of bath and are suspended.
- Fibrillation is produced when the atria are exposed to acetylcholine (3×10^{-4} gm/ml) or (0.10 gm) potassium chloride.
- After 5 min of exposure to acetylcholine or potassium the atria are stimulated with rectangular pulses of 0.75 min duration, usually of 10 V (frequency 400-1800 shocks per min).
- A mechanical record is taken on kymograph control arrhythmias are produced and allowed to continue for up to 6-10 min.
- After 30 min rest period, fibrillation is again induced and after allowing the arrhythmia to produce for 30 min a test compound is added to the bath.
- If the atria do not cease to fibrillate within 8-10 min following the addition of the test compound, the preparation is washed and allowed to return to normal contraction.

Conclusion: Test compound is found to be effective if fibrillation disappears immediately or within 5 min following test drug supplementation to the organ bath.

***In vivo* methods**

Chemically induced arrhythmia

A large number of agents alone or in combination are capable of inducing arrhythmias. Administration of anesthesia like chloroform, ether, halothane followed by a precipitating stimulus such as i.v. adrenaline, ovalbumin, alkaloids causes arrhythmia. The sensitivity of these arrhythmogenic substances differ among various species.

(i) Aconitine antagonism in rats

Aim: Aconitine a plant alkaloid from aconite root acts persistently on sodium channels and activates it resulting in ventricular arrhythmias. Drugs considered to have anti arrhythmic properties can be tested in aconite intoxicated rats.

Animals required	:	Male Ivanovo rats (300-400 kg)
Chemicals required	:	Urethane, Aconitine (5 μg/kg)
		HNO_3 0.1N
Equipments required	:	Lead II ECG

Procedure:

- Males Ivanovo rats (300-400 gm) are anesthetized i.p. with urethane (125 gm/kg).
- Aconitine (5 μg/kg) is dissolved in 0.1N HNO_3 and continuously infused into the rats saphenous vein at a rate of 0.1 ml/min.
- Lead II ECG is recorded every 30 sec test compound is injected orally or i.v. 5 min before the aconite infusion.
- A higher dose of aconitine in the test group compared to untreated group gives an anti arrhythmic activity.

Conclusion: Anti arrhythmic effect of test compound is measured by amount of aconite 100 gm animal (infusion duration) and includes ventricular extra systoles, tachycardia, fibrillation and death.

Mechanically induced arrhythmia

(i) Reperfusion arrhythmia in dogs

Aim: Coronary artery ligation in dogs may result in increased heart rate, heart contractility, left ventricular end diastolic pressure, blood pressure and ventricular arrhythmias especially in the reperfusion duration.

Animals required	:	Dogs (20-25 kg)
Chemicals required	:	Thio-butobarbital sodium (30 mg/kg),
		chlorasole (20 mg/kg), urethane (250 mg/kg)
		Morphine (2 mg/kg)
Equipments required	:	Artificial respiration,
		Cannula, Lead II ECG recorder

Procedure:

- Dogs are anaesthetized with thio-butobarbital sodium (30 mg/kg) i.p. and maintained on intravenous chloralose (20 mg/kg) and 250 mg/kg urethane i.v. followed by SC administration of 2 mg/kg morphine.
- Animal is subsequently maintained on artificial respiration.
- A peripheral vein (saphenous vein) is cannulated for the administration of test compound.
- ECG is recorded continuously in lead II.
- Femoral artery is cannulated to measure blood pressure and connected to a pressure transducer.
- Left ventricular and diastolic pressure and heart rate are determined from the left ventricular pressure curves.
- Myocardial contractility is measured as a rise of left ventricular pressure.
- The experimental procedure followed is similar to that in rats. Coronary artery is ligated for 90 min and 20 min prior to ligation the test compound is administered.
- Animals are reperfused for 30 min.

Conclusion: All parameters are recorded during whole experiment changes in parameters (mortality, hemodynamic and arrhythmia) in drug treated animals are compared to vehicle controls.

5.4.3 Screening Methods for Cardiac Stimulants

- Congestive Heart Failure (CHF) or heart failure is a condition in which the heart is unable to pump enough blood to body's other organs. This can result from narrowed arteries that supply blood to heart muscle, part heart attack, myocardial infarction either scar tissue that interferes with heart muscles normal work, high blood pressure, heart value disease due to part rheumatic fever, cardiopathy, congenital heart defects, endocarditis and/or myocarditis. An early symptom of congestive heart is fatigue. As CHF program swelling (edema) of the ankles and legs or abdomen may be noticed.
- In addition fluid may accumulated in the lungs, causing, shortness of breath particularly during exercise and when lying flat. Accumulation of fluid in the liver and intestine may cause nausea, abdominal pain and decreased appetite. This CHF normally occurs in middle age and older age people. Although it is believed that the primary defect in early heart failure resides in excitation contraction coupling machinery of the heart the clinical condition also involves may other process reflexes the sympathetic

nervous system kidney rennin angiotensin-aldosterone system, vasopressin and death of cardiac cells.

- Traditional therapy includes of CHF includes cardiac glycosides (digitalis) that increase cardiac output and alter the electrical function of the heart.
- They increase cardiac contractility that correct the imbalance associated with failure clinical research has show that therapy directed at non cardiac target may be more valuable in long term treatment of cardiac failure than positive inotropic agents, cardiac glycosides. Thus drugs acting on kidneys (diuretics) have been considered at least as valuable as digitalis for this condition. During the last decades, ACE inhibitors and vasodilators have come into common use β-adrenoceptor blocking drugs are also used as treatment for CHF.

Screening methods used

***In vitro* methods**

(i) Isolated hamster cardiomyopathic heart
(ii) Isolated cat papillary muscle
(iii) Ouabain binding

***In vivo* models**

1. Rat models of heart failure
   (a) Rat coronary ligation model
   (b) Rat aortic binding
   (c) Dahl salt sensitive rats
   (d) Spontaneous hypertensive rat
   (e) Spontaneous hypertensive heart failure rats
2. Dog models of heart failure
   (a) Chronic rapid pacing
   (b) Volume overload
   (c) Coronary artery ligation and microembolization
3. Rabbits models of heart failure
   (a) Volume and pressure overload
   (b) Tachycardia pacing
   (c) Doxorubicin cardiomyopathic
4. Guinea pig model
   (a) Aortic bonding
   (b) Syrian hamster model
   (c) Cardiomyopathic hamster
   (d) Transgenic mice model

***In vitro* methods**

(i) Isolated hamster cardiomyopathic heart:

Animals required	:	Syrian hamster
Chemicals required	:	Heparin (5 mg/kg) Langendorff ringer solution
Equipments required	:	Polygraph, Cannula Chronometer Electro flow meter

Procedure:

- Isolated Syrian hamster hearts can be used for evaluation of cardio tonic drugs.
- Hamsters with cardiomyopathic of the age group (50 weeks) are used for the study.
- Normally Syrian hamsters if same age is used as controls.
- The animals are pretreated with heparin (5 mg/kg) i.p. and after 20 min heart is isolated and placed in Langendorff and perused with ringer solution at 60 min at 32 °C.
  - The force of contraction is recorded somatically by force transducer connected to a polygraph.
  - The heart rate is measured using a chronometer.
  - The coronary flow is measured using an electro flow meter.
  - Test compounds are injected *via* the aortic cannula into the inflowing heart ringer solution.
  - The contractive force and coronary flow in heart of the treated and the shown control group are compared using students test.

Conclusion: % improvement is calculation and the efficacy of the drug evaluated in increasing flow and contractile force.

(ii) Isolation cat papillary muscle:

Aim: In this method prolonged electrical stimulation of isolated cardiac tissue results in decrease in performance cardiac glycosides restores the force of contraction.

Animals Required	:	Cats (2.5-3 kg)
Chemicals Required	:	Anesthetics (ether) Ringer solution Ouabain (standard)
Equipments Required	:	Organ bath Electrical stimulator, Polygraph

Procedure:

- Cats of either sex are anesthetized with ether thought a left thoracotomy heart is exposed papillary muscle from right ventricle is isolated and fixed in an organ both containing ringer solution (at 37 °C).
- One end of papillary muscle is tied to other end to the muscle.
- Electrical stimuli of 4-6 V is applied to the stimulation for 1 hr the muscle contraction start diminishing.
- The cardiac glycosides are added to the bath at this point to restore the contractile force.
- Ouabain is the standard glycoside that is added at a dose of 300 mg/ml.

Conclusion: Evaluation is based on increase in contractile force on adding the glycoside. Contractile fore is calculated as percentage of the predose level and comparisons between different groups are made.

***In vivo* models**

(i) **Rat models:** Rat models are in expensive so used for long-term pharmacological inter venations. But some limitations also there for M.I. Rat myocardium exhibits a very short action potential which normally lacks a plateau phase. Calcium removal from cytosol is predominated by activity of sarcoplasmic reticulum calcium pump where as Na^+/Ca^+ exchanger activity is less relevant.

In normal rat myocardium, myosin heavy chain isoform predominates and a shift toward the β-myosin isoform occurs and a hemodynamic bad or hormonal change take place. Resting heart rate is five times that of humans and the force-frequency relative is inverse.

(ii) **Dahl salt sensitive rats:**

Aim: This model is well studied to study the transition from compensated hypertrophy to failure. This strain of rats develops systemic hypertension after receiving a high-salt diet.

Animals Required	:	Sprague Dawley rats
Chemicals Required	:	Saliva solution
		High salt diet
		NaCl solution.

Procedure:

- Sprague Dawley rats are selected for this study.

- Drinking water replaced with 1% NaCl (saline) solution high Dahl salt diet is prepared in laboratory by mixing salt with regular diet.
- Animals and fed the prepared diet and 1% NaCl solution ad libitum.
- The treatment group rats are administered the drug orally for 1 month. After the completion of experimental duration the animals of both groups are sacrificed.
- Their hearts are removed and cardiac mass, weight of left and right ventricle are weighed and compared.
- It is observed that the animals in the sham control group develop concentric left ventricular hypertrophy at 8 weeks followed by market left ventricular dilation and over clinical heart failure at 15-20 weeks failing heart dies within a short period of time.

  Conclusion: The ability of the test drug to reverse this change is studded. The test drug potency is compared with sham control compound.

(iii) Dog model

Dog as an animal model of heart failure allow the study of left ventricular function and volume more study of left ventricular function and volume more accurately than rodent models. Particular they allow better chronic instrumentation and also similar to human myocardium. However dog models are costly and require substantial resource with respect with to housing and care.

(iv) Coronaries artery ligation and micro remobilization

Aim: Coronary artery ligation and micro remobilization have been used to produce myocardial infarction and CHF in dogs.

Animals required	:	Dogs (30 kg) either sex
Chemical required	:	Anesthesia [pentobarbitone] Microsphere
Equipments required	:	Transducer, Cannula Microtip catheter Cardiac index computer Angiogram catheter Artificial respiration

Procedure:

- Dogs of either sex are anaesthetized with i.v. injection of 35 to 40 mg/kg pentobarbitone.

- Animals are maintained on artificial respiration.
- The femoral and carotid arteries are cannulated.
- Transducer is connected to right femoral artery for recording peripheral systolic, diastolic and mean blood pressure.
- A microtip catheter is inserted *via* the left carotid artery for determination of left ventricular pressure systolic, diastolic and mean pulmonary capillary pressure and cardiac output are measured by term dilution technique using a cardiac index computer.
- Heart is exposed though a left thoracotomy between 4th and 5th intercostals space and pericardium is opened. Microsphere is injected through the angiogram catheter into the left atrium.
- Initially a 10 ml (1 mg/ml) microsphere is injected and later a 5 ml bolus about 5 min apart.
- The Microsphere injection produces stepwise elevation of left ventricular end diastolic pressure (LVEDP) embolism is terminated when LVEDP has increased to 16-18 mm Hg or heart rate reaches 200 beats/min.

Conclusion: Intravenous bolus injection or continuous infusion administers the test substance. Recording is obtained before and Remobilization and administration of test compared at various time intervals.

(v) **Transgenic mice model:** Recent Development of techniques to alter specifically the expression of genes has greatly improved the understanding of pathophysiology of heart failure. Moreover, several genetic models of heart failure by addition or deletion of genes in mice have been developed and miniaturized physiology techniques to evaluate the resulting cardiac phenotypes have been established.

These models allow the identification of genes that are causative for heart failure and to evaluate the molecular mechanism responsible for the development and progression of the disease. Gene targeted description of the muscle LIM protein (MLP) in mice is a new model of heart failure.

MLP is a regulator of gynogenic differentiation. Mice that were homogenous for the MLP knockout develop dilated cardiac Myopathy associated with myocardial hypertrophy. Adult mice show clinical and hemodynamic signs of heart failure similar to those in humans. Development of cardiomyopathy was also observed in mice with knockout of gynogenic factor.

Transgenic mice over express either β-adrenergic receptor kinase of G-Protein Coupled receptor kinase resulting in uncoupling of β-adrenergic receptor also exhibit reduced contractility but without clinical signs of over CHF.

A recent model of transgenic over expression of tropomodulin exhibited dilated cardiomyopathy 2-4 weeks after birth with reduced contractile function and heart failure. This was associated with loss of myofibrillar organization.

5.4.4 Screening Methods for Atherosclerosis

Angina is a symptom of Coronary Artery Disease (CAD) the most common type of heart disease. CAD occurs when plaque builds up in the coronary arteries. Thus build up of plague is called atherosclerosis. A plaque buildup the coronary arteries become narrow and stiff. Blood flow to the heart is reduced. This decreases the oxygen supply to the heart muscle. Angina pectoris is severe, sudden, substernal chest pain due to ischemia (lack of blood and hence oxygen supply of the heart muscle).

The pain may also radiate to the shoulders, arm, neck jaw or back. This pain usually occurs during the excretion severe emotional stress or after heavy meal. During these periods, the heart muscle demands more blood oxygen than the narrowed coronary arteries can deliver. Atherosclerosis also can occur in people with valvular heart disease, hypertrophic, cardiomyopathy (this is an enlarged heart due to disease) or uncontrolled high blood pressure.

Screening method for atherosclerosis

***In vitro* methods**

(i) Langendorff heart preparation
(ii) Calcium antagonism in pitched rat
(iii) Isolated heart lung preparation
(iv) Isolated rabbit aorta preparation
(v) Relaxation of bovine coronary artery
(vi) Coronary artery ligation in isolated rat heart
(vii) Plastic costs technique in dogs

***In vivo* methods**

(i) Occlusion of coronary artery
(ii) Microspheres – included acute ischemia
(iii) Isoproterenol – induced myocardial necrosis

(iv) Stenosis – induced coronary thrombosis model

(v) Electrical stimulation induced coronary thrombosis

(vi) Myocardial ischemic preconditioning model

(vii) Models of coronary flow measurement

(viii) Coronary inflow measurement in anesthetized dogs

(ix) Coronary outflow measurement in anesthetized dogs

(x) Electromagnetic flow meter

***In vitro* methods**

(i) Langendorff heart preparation: Langendorff is a highly reproducible preparation which can be studied quickly in large number at relatively low cost. It allows measurement of broad spectrum of biochemical, physiological and morphological indices. Measurements are made in absence of the confounding effects of other organs, both global and regional ischemia can be studied using this model.

The basic principle involved is that heart is per fused in a retrograde direction from the aorta either at constant pressure or constant flow with oxygenated saline solution. Retrograde perfusion closes the aortic valves, just as in the *in site* heart during diastole. The perfuse is displaced through coronary arteries flowing off the coronary sinus and opened right atrium. Parameters usually measured are contractile force, Coronary flow and cardiac rhythm.

Animals Required	:	Guinea pigs (300 – 500 gm)
Chemicals Required	:	Cold perfusion solution (4 °C)
		Oxygenated ringer Solution
Equipments Required	:	Thoracic cage
		Chronometer
		Cannula
		Double wall plexiglass perfusion apparatus
		Small steel hook
		Force transducer
		Polygraph

Procedure:

- Guinea Pigs of either sex weighing 300 to 500 gm used for study and they are sacrificed by stunning.
- Diaphragm is assessed by transabdominal incision and cut carefully to expose, the thoracic cavity. Thoracic is opened by bilateral incision

along the lower margins of last to first ribs. Thoracic cage is reflected over the animals head exposing the heart.

- The heart is cradled between fingers and lifted before incising the aorta, enclave pulmonary veins.
- Immediately after excision, heart is dipped in cold perfusion solution (4 °C to limit ischemic injury during period between excision and restoration of vascular perfusion). The Aorta is located and cut below the point of division.
- Cannula is inserted into the aorta and tied and the heart is per fused with oxygenated ringer's solution.
- Then heart is transferred to a double wall plexiglass perfusion apparatus maintained at 37 °C, 40 mm Hg pressure, small steel hook with a string is attached to apex of the heart. Contractile force is measured isometrically by a force transducer and recorded on a polygraph.
- Heart rate is measured through a chronometer coupled to the polygraph.
- Then drugs (standard, test) are injected into the perfusion medium.
- The atherosclerosis effect of test drug is indicated by an increase in coronary blood flow.

Conclusion: The incidence and duration of ventricular fibrillation, Coronary flow, in atrophic state and K^+ levels after treatment with drug are compared with control.

(ii) Calcium antagonism in pitched rat

Aim: This model can differentiate calcium entry blockers from other agents that do not directly block entry of calcium.

Animals Required	:	Sprague Dawley Rats (250 to 350 gm)
Chemicals Required	:	Anesthesia by methohexital sodium (50 mg/kg)
Equipments Required	:	Cannula
		Artificial respiration
		Electrical stimulator
		Transducer

Procedure:

- Rats are anesthetized with methohexital sodium (50 mg/kg i.p.).
- Trachea is cannulated. There after the rats are pitched through the one orbit and immediately maintained an artificial respiration. The pitting

rod is used as a stimulating electrode and continuous electrical stimulation of the thoracic spinal cord with square wave pulses at supramaximal voltage (frequency 0.5 Hz and duration 0.5 min) produces a cardio-acceleration responses.

- Only rats with a resulting tachycardia (100 beats/min) are induced for the study.
- The jugular vein is cannulated for administration of drugs and blood pressure is recorded *via* carotid artery using a pressure transducer.
- In the femoral region, an indifferent electrode is inserted subcutaneously.
- When cardio acceleration response is established for 3-5 min, calcium channel blockers and β blockers are administered.
- The test compound dose dependently blocks tachycardia.

Conclusion: The level of tachycardia immediately prior to drug administration is taken as 100% and response to drugs is expressed as % of pre dose tachycardia. ID_{50} is calculated and compared.

(iii) Isolated heart – lung Preparation:

Aim: The isolated heart lung preparation is used to study various physiological and pharmacological processes.

Animals Required	:	Wistar Rats [300 – 500 gm]
Chemicals Required	:	Pentobarbitone sodium
		Ice – cold saline
		Krebs ringer, bicarbonate buffer
Equipments Required	:	Cannula
		Artificial respiration
		Electrical amplifier

Procedure:

- Wister rat is anaesthetized with pentobarbitone sodium (50 mg/kg).
- The trachea is cannulated animal is maintained on artificial respiration.
- The chest cavity is opened and ice – cold saline is injected to arrest the heart.
- The aorta, superior and inferior vena cave are cannulated.
- The heart lung preparation is per fused with Krebs-Ringer bicarbonate buffer [pH -7.4] containing rat RBC (hematocrit 25 %).

- The perforate is pumped from the aorta and is passed through the pneumatic resistance and collected in a reservoir maintained at 37 °C.
- It is then returned to inferior vena cava thus perfusing only the heart and the lung.
- Test drug is administered into the perforate 5 min after start of experiment.
- Cardiac output is recorded with an electromagnetic blood flow meter and mean arterial pressure from the pneumatic resistance.
- With the help of a bio electrical amplifier heart rate is recorded.

Conclusion: Hemodynamic data and recovery time of the test drug group and control group (without any treatment) is compared using ANOVA and Kruskal – Wallis test respectively.

***In vivo* models**

(i) Occlusion of coronary artery

Compounds that reduce size are studied using this model.

Animals Required	:	Dogs either sex (30 kg)
Chemicals Required	:	Anesthesia (Pentobarbitone sodium 35 mg/kg i.p.)
Equipments Required	:	Cannula Artificial Respiration Electromagnetic flow meter

Procedure:

- Dogs are anesthetized by pentobarbitone sodium.
- Trachea is cannulated and animals are maintained on artificial respiration using a positive respirator.
- Through the left thoracotomy, heart is exposed at 4th and 5th inter costal space and the pericardium is removed.
- Two poles of electromagnet are placed in opposite sides of coronary vessel. Two chromium-vanadium electrodes are placed adhering to the coronary artery.
- A magnetic field perpendicular to blood flow generates voltage in the conductor (blood stream)
- It then picked up by electrodes, amplified and recorded.
- This method mostly records phasic flow.
- Mean flow is recorded by electrical damping.

- Jugular vein is cannulated for administration of test compared and carotid artery for measurement of blood pressure.
- Changes in coronary outflow and homodynamic parameters before and test drug administration are compared.

Conclusion: To avoid polarization at pickup electrodes, magnetic current is reversed either of square waves or since wave type. Initially probes were big but with advanced technology now-a-day, small sized probes are available. They are used mainly in chromic anesthetized whole animal experiment by running lead wire through the skin.

5.5 SCREENING FOR DRUG ACTING ON RESPIRATORY SYSTEM

5.5.1 Screening Methods for Anti Asthmatics and Bronchodilators

Asthma is a chronic disease in this airway occasionally constricts, becomes inflamed and lined with excessive amount of mucus, often in response to one or more triggers.

Environmental stimulant are (or allergen) cold air, warm air, exercise or exertion or emotional stress.

In children the most common triggers are viral illnesses such as those that cause the common cold. Airway narrowing causes symptoms such as wheezing shortness of breath, chest tightness and coughing. Symptoms, which can range from mild to life threatening, can usually, controlled combination of drugs and environmental changes. Patients usually have reduced forced expiratory volume in one sec (FEV_1) as well reduced airflow.

Short term relief is most effectively achieved with bronchodilator, agents that positive airway caliber relaxing air way smooth muscle α–adrenoreceptor stimulant (α_2–agonists) most widely used. Theophylline, Methyl Xanthenes drugs, Anti muscarinic agents (Ipratropium bromide) are also used for reversal of airway constriction.

- Long term anti inflammatory inhaled corticosteroids (budesonide).
- Inhibitors of mast cell degranulation, Example: Cromolyn or nedocromil sodium.
- Of the several drugs currently available neither clinicians nor patients are completely satisfied with their effects.

There is no doubt that there is an urgent need of new and effective drugs, which are able to treat or even possibly cure the allergic inflammation, Wide variety of animal models have been developed use of an appropriate model could help us to develop new chemical entities for treatment of human allergic disorders in a more predictable way.

I. *In vitro* methods

(i) Binding assays

(a) Histamine receptor assay

(ii) Cell culture method

(a) Culture technique

(b) WST assay

(iii) Test in isolated organs

(a) Spasmolytic activity in guinea pig

(b) Vascular and airway responses lungs to the isolated lung

(c) Relativity of isolated perfused guinea pig trachea

II. *In vivo* methods

(i) Air way inflammation in mice

(ii) Bronchial hyper activity in guinea pigs

(iii) Bronchospasmolytic activity in anesthetized guinea pigs

(iv) Arachidonic acid or PAF–induced respiratory and vascular dysfunction in guinea pigs

(v) Anaphylactic micro shock in guinea pigs

(vi) Sedation aerosol induced asphyxia in guinea pig

(vii) Histamine induced bronchoconstriction in anesthetized guinea pigs

(viii) Pneumotachograph in guinea pigs

(ix) Micro shock in rabbits

(x) Airway micro vascular leakage in guinea pigs

I. *In vitro* methods

(i) Binding assay: (Histamine receptor assay)

Aim: This method evaluates affinity of test compare to histamine – H_1 receptor to measure their inhibitory activity on binding of pyrilamine (H_1 antagonist) to guinea pig brain plasma membrane preparation.

Animals required	:	Male guinea pig (300 – 600 gm)
Chemicals required	:	Ice – cold Tris buffer, aliquots 1 ml, ^{3}H pyrilamine mepyramine (10^{-5} m)
Equipment required	:	Centrifuge, liquid scintillation counter

Procedure: Male guinea pig (wt 300 – 600 gm) is sacrificed by CO_2 necrosis.

- Brain is homogenized in ice – cold Tris buffer (pH 7.5, in 30 ml buffer) and homogenate is centrifuged for 10 minute at 4 °C at 50,000 rpm.
- Supernatant is discarded and pellet is resuspended in buffer– centrifuge again
- The pellet obtained after centrifugation is re-suspended in this buffer (1 gm/5 ml) and aliquots of 1 ml are frozen at 70 °C.
- In a shaking bath maintained at 25 °C. 50 ml ^{3}H pyrilamine (2 × 10^{-9}mM), 50 ml test compound (10^{-5}-10^{-10}mM), and 100 ml membrane suspension from guinea pig whole brain (10 mg/ml) per sample age incubated for 30 min incubation buffer used is Tris HCl buffer (50mM, pH 7.5) with 11 concentration of ^{3}H pyrilamine (0.1–50 × 10^{-9} m) saturation experiments are performed.
- Total binding is determined in presence of incubation buffer non-specific binding in presence of mepyramine (10^{-5}m).
- By rapid vacuum filtration through glass fiber filters reaction is stopped.
- Subsequently the membrane bond is separated from the radio activity. The retained membrane bound reactivity on filter is measured after addition of 3 ml, scintillation cocktail/sample in liquid scintillation counter.
  - ➢ The parameter calculated are total binding of ^{3}H pyrilamine, non-specific binding and specific binding (total binding – non-specific binding) and % of inhibition of ^{3}H pyrilamine binding (10 – specific binding as % of control value).
  - ➢ The dissociation constant (K_i) and IC_{50} value of test compound are determined from experiment of ^{3}H pyrilamine with non-labeled drug by computer supported analysis of binding data.
- Incubation buffer used in Tris HCL buffer (50mM, pH 7.5) with 11 concentrations of ^{3}H pyrilamine (0.1 – 50 × 10^{-9}mM) saturation experiments are performed.
- Total binding is determined in presence of incubation buffer, non specific binding in presence of mepyramine (10^{-5}m).

- By rapid vacuum filtration through glass fiber filters reaction is stopped.
- Subsequently the membrane bound is separated from the radio activity. The retained membrane bound reactivity on filter is measured after addition of 3 ml scintillation cocktail/sample in liquid scintillation counter.

Conclusion: The parameter calculated are total binding of ^{3}H pyrilamine, non specific binding and specific binding (total binding – non specific binding) and % inhibition of ^{3}H pyrilamine binding (100 – specific binding as % of control value). The dissociation constant (K_i) and IC_{50} value of test compound are determined from experiment of ^{3}H pyrilamine Vs non labeled drug by computer supported analysis of binding data.

(ii) Cell culture method:

WST Assay:

Requirements: 96 well micro plate, micro plate reader
RPMI medium
Trypsin
9.9 ml Casytons
Electronic cell counter

- Cells are transferred from cell exposure vessels to conventional RPMI medium per well.
- 500 micro liters of medium with 100 ml of WST-1 dye is layered on attached cells and removed after 1 hr of incubation.
- Aliquots of 100 ml are transferred into 96 well micro plate for measuring their absorbance at 450 nm/630 nm using a micro plate reader.
- Additional cells from same membrane are trypsinized by adding at 37 °C, the enzymatic activity is stopped after adding 25 ml of Trypsin inhibitor (10,000 BAEE units/mg protein).
- The cells are gently suspended and 100 μl so suspension diluted in 9.9 ml Casytons.
- Aliquots are analyzed with an electronic cell counter.
- Thus CULTEX technique enables treatment of bronchial epithelial cells with sample atmospheres for subsequent *in vitro* assays.

Conclusion: The introduction of these cultivation and exposure techniques offers new testing strategies for toxicological evaluation of a broad range of airborne and inhaled compounds.

***In vivo* methods**

(i) Airway inflammation in mice:

Animals required	:	Balb/c mice
Chemicals required	:	Ovalbumin
		Coagulated egg white
		BAL fluid

Procedure:

- Balb/c mice sensitized with ovalbumin and challenged by repeated exposure to ovalbumin yields marked eosinophilia in influx varies dramatically in mice of the different stains.
- Stains such as 129/sv, CBA belong to none or low responder.
- Straining such as SWR, FVB, C57BL/6 respond to antigen challenge with marked increased of eosinophils both in BAL and in lung tissue.
- Bulb/c mice used for study s.c. implanted with heat coagulated egg white.
- 14 days later the mice are challenged intratracheally with heat aggregated ovalbumin.
- Drug administered s.c., i.p or orally.
- 48 hr after Ag challenge, bronchial alveoli lavage fluid is collected from animals of both groups. Total number of eosinophils, neutrophils and eosinophils peroxides activity are assessed.

Conclusion: The animals are then sacrificed and histopathological evaluation is carried out based on results if histopathological study and BAL fluid examination, protection that is offered by the test drug is evaluated.

(ii) Bronchial hyperactivity in Guinea pigs

Aim: Inhalation of histamine or other spasmogens can induce symptoms like asphyxia convulsions resembling bronchial asthma in guinea pigs.

Animals required	:	Guinea pigs (300-400 grams)
Chemicals required	:	0.1% solution of histamine hydrochloride
Equipments required	:	Aerosols
		Ultrasound nebulizer
		Inhalation cages
		Infusion pump

Procedure:

- The challenging agents are applied as aerosols produced by an ultrasound nebulizer.
- Early symptoms breathing frequency, forced inspiration and final anaphylactic convulsion.
- Antagonist drugs can delay the occurrence of these symptoms. Preconvulsion time can be measured.
- Male albino guinea pigs (300-400 gm) are used. The inhalation cages consist of three boxes each ventilated with air flow of 1.5 l/min.
- The animal is placed into box A to which the test drug or standard is applied using an ultra sound nebulizer which provides an aerosol of 0.2 ml solution of the test drug injected in an infusion pump with in 1 min.
- Alternately, the animal is treated orally or s.c. with test drug or standard.
- Box B serves as sluice through which the animal is passed into box C.
- There aerosol of 0.1% solution of histamine hydrochloride provided by an ultrasound nebulizer.

Conclusion: Time until appearance of asphyctic convulsions is measured. Then the animal is immediately removed from inhalation box. % increase of Prcconvulsion timc is calculatcd versus controls.

- ED_{50} (50% increase in preconvulsion time) is also calculated. By comprising with standard drug the test drug potency is measured and compared.

5.5.2 Screening Methods for Antitussives and Expectorants

Protocol for irritant aerosol induced antitussive evaluation

Male guinea pigs, five in each group were used in the study (body weight 500-600 gm). Unanaesthetized unrestrained animals were placed individually in a transparent test chamber, dimensions 30 cm × 20 cm × 20 cm and exposed to a nebulized aqueous solution of i.e., 0.1 gm/ml of citric acid for 7 min. The output of nebulizer was 0.65 ± 0.04 ml solution per minute and continued for 7 min. The same nebulizer was used throughout the experiment. During the last 5 min of the exposure, the animals were watched continuously by a trained observer, and the numbers of coughs were determined. Coughs could easily be distinguished from sneeze since there is a clear difference in sound as well as in behaviour of the animals.

The above protocol was performed 10 min after exposing animals to aerosols of the following solutions for a period of 7 min:

(i) Codeine solution (0.03 gm/ml, positive standard drug)

(ii) Test drug

Conclusion: All the experiments were performed randomly with 2 hr resting period between each two experiments. Coughs and sneeze are compared between control group and test group.

(i) ***SO_2 induce antitussive evaluation:*** Antitussive effect against SO_2 induced cough the experimental model is shown in where V_1 is 500 ml. Three-necked flask containing aqueous saturated solution of sodium hydrogen sulphite.

By opening the stopcock of a burette V_2, the concentrated sulphuric acid was introduced to generate SO_2 gas. The chemical reaction that occurred in the flask A is

$2NaHSO_3 + H_2SO_4 = 2SO_2 \uparrow + Na_2SO_4 + 2H_2O$

Previously, SO_2 gas was filled in V_1 and V_3 gas reservoirs, and then by opening the cocks 3 and 2, pressure in the gas reservoir V_3 was elevated which was recorded by the water manometer V_4. Then the stopcock 2 was closed and stopcock 4 was opened slightly till the pressure in V_4 (11 mm i.d.) reached 75 mm water, when the stopcock was closed. The procedure was operated in a draught.

- The mice were divided into 3 groups, each containing 10 mice. One group served as a control group receiving only 2% v/v aqueous Tween 80 solution (10 ml/kg^{-1}, p.o.).
- One group was used for methanol extract of *C. cretica* (100 mg kg^{-1} p.o.) and the remaining group was used for standard drug codeine phosphate (10 mg kg^{-1} p.o.).
- Both the extract and codeine phosphate were suspended separately in 2% v/v aqueous Tween 80 solution. Initially, the cough responses of all groups of animals were observed (0 min) by placing the animals individually in a desiccator V_5. The cocks 3, 6 and 5 were opened in order and when the pressure in V_4 became 0 mm of water, all the cocks were closed immediately.
- A certain amount of SO_2 gas (5 ml which was kept constant throughout the experiment) was introduced in the desiccator in this way.

- After 1 min of introduction of the gas, the mice were taken out of the desiccator and the frequency of cough was observed for 5 min in an open-ended filter funnel with a stethoscope at the tip in which the mice were confined in this way the frequency of cough was observed for all animal groups at 0 min (before the drug administration)
- After drug treatment also cough was observed test group is compared with control group.

5.6 SCREENING METHODS FOR ANALGESICS, ATIPYRETICS AND ANTI INFLAMMATORY AGENTS

5.6.1 Screening Methods for Analgesics and Antipyretics

Pain is an unpleasant sensory and emotional experience associated with actual and potential tissue damage. Various types of pains are seen in humans are there. Such as

- Somatic pain (arising from skin, muscles, joints, ligaments and bones)
- Visceral pain
- Referred pain
- Neuropathic pain
- Cancer pain etc.

Chemical mediators of pain are numerous. These mediators come from sources intrinsic to neuron. Including various neurotransmitters such as 5-HT and substance P and intrinsic to Nervous system. Including to substances from inflammatory or immune cells and red blood cells such as prostaglandins, kinins, cytokines, chemokines and ATP that are released following injury to tissue. Pain is produced by excitation of particular receptor, the nociceptors or of their afferent fibers and also physical (heat, cold and pressure) and chemical stimuli.

Pain can be classified as acute or chronic, that is based on nature of pain itself.

***Acute pain*:** It is of soft tissue damage, infection or inflammation will be short of duration.

***Chronic pain*:** It is lasts of 6 months or larger than that period.

Example: Cancer pain, neuropathic pain and arthritic pain.

Screening methods

***In vivo* methods**

I Models using thermal stimulus

- Hot plate method
- Tail flick method
- Tail flick test using radiant heat
- Tail flick test using Immersion of tail

Modifications:

- Cold tail flick test
- Cold ethanol tail flick test

II Models using electrical stimulus

- Tooth pulp test
- Monkey shock titration test

III Models using chemical stimulus

- Formalin test
- Writhing test
- Distension of hollow organs using chemical stimulus
- Rat sigmoid colon model
- Inflammatory uterine pain model

IV Model using mechanical stimulus

- Haffner's tail clip method
- Randall selitto test

V Animal models of chronic pain

- Neuropathic pain models
- Vincristine induced neuropathy model
- Diabetic neuropathy model
- Persistent post thoracotomy pain
- Cat model of incisional pain

VI Models of cancer pain

- Rat model of bone cancer pain

***In vitro* methods**

(i) μ- opiate receptor binding assay

(ii) ^{3}H- naloxone binding assay

(iii) Assay to study cannabinoid activity

***In vivo* methods**

(i) Hot plate method

Aim: Hot plate method has been widely used to evaluate opioid analgesics

Animals required	:	Albino mice
Chemicals required	:	Test compound
Equipment required	:	Hot plate at 55-56 °C (electrically heated plate)

Procedure:

- Animals are placed on the hot plate, which consists of electrically heated surface. Temperature on the hot plate is maintained at 55-56 °C.
- Responses such as jumping, withdrawal of the paws and licking of the paws are seen.
- The time period (latency period), when animals are placed and until responses occur, is recorded by a stopwatch.

Conclusion: Test compounds are administered orally or subcutaneously and latency or latency period is recorded after 20, 60, 90 min. These values are compared with the values before administration of the drug by using t-test.

(ii) The tail flick method

Aim: The tail flick test is a widely and reliably used test for revealing the potency of opioid analgesics.

This test is normally conducted by radiant heat method or immersion of the tail method.

Animals required	:	Albino mice (18-22 gm)
Chemicals required	:	Exerting radiant heat
Equipments required	:	Cages leaving tail exposed out

Procedure:

- Animals are placed in small cages leaving the tail exposed out. Mice tail is held gently by the observer.
- A light beam is focused (exerting radiant heat) to the proximal third of the tail. The mouse tries to pull the tail away and rotates the head this reaction is known as escape reaction.
- The reaction time movement is recorded. The reaction time varies with the surface area stimulated.
- The test drug and standard are administered either orally or s.c.

- Same procedure is repeated and reaction time is noted after 30, 60,120 min.
- A lengthening of the reaction time is interpreted as an analgesic action of test drug.

Conclusion: At each time interval those animals that show higher reaction time than the time before drug administration are regarded as positive. Percentage of positive animals are counted for each time interval and each dose and ED_{50} values of test compounds can be calculated according to Litchfield and Wilcoxon method. Codeine, pethidine and morphine are used as standard.

(iii) Tooth pulp test:

Aim: In the electrical stimulus is given in rabbits tooth pulp.

Animals required	:	Rabbits weighing 2-3 kg each
Chemicals required	:	Thiopental 15 mg/kg
Equipment required	:	Dental drill tooth pulp
		Clamping electrodes

Procedure:

- Animals are anaesthetized with thiopental in the doses of 15 mg/kg i.v.
- Using dental drill, tooth pulp chambers are exposed close to the two front upper incisors.
- Clamping electrodes are placed into the drilled holes.
- After 30 min electrical stimulus is applied by rectangular shape current (frequency 50 Hz) upto 1 sec.
- Current is started with 0.2 mA and increased until animals starts licking.
- After that, a threshold is determined at least 3 times in each animal.
- Animal serves as its own control.

***Conclusion*:** Test compound is administered orally or i.v. After 15, 30, 60 and 120 min threshold current is measured and compared with the threshold current prior to drug administration.

***In vitro* method**

(i) μ opiate receptor binding assay:

Aim: Opioid drugs exert their analgesic action mainly through μ opioid receptors only. The compounds that inhibit binding of ^{3}H-Dihydromorphine in a synaptic membrane preparation from rat brain can be identified by this assay.

Animals required	:	Male Wistar rats
Chemicals required	:	20nM stock solution of ^{3}H-Dihydromorphine
		0.1mM stock solution of levallorphan tartrate
		1mM of test stock solution
		Ice cold 0.05M Tris buffer
Equipments required	:	Homogenizer
		Scintillation vials
		Whatman GF/B filters

Procedure:

All compounds are taken in 3 test tubes. 50 μg of ^{3}H-Dihydromorphine and 20 μg of levallorphan tartrate are added to each tube. In the assay final concentration of ^{3}H-Dihydromorphine and levallorphan tartrate are 0.5nM and 0.1μM respectively and concentration of test compounds range from 10^{-6}-10^{-9}M. Total volume of assay mixture is 2 ml.

- Male Wistar rats are used. Animals are sacrificed by decapitation.
- Whole brains without cerebella are removed, weighed and homogenate in 30 volumes of ice cold 0.05M Tris buffer, pH 7.7. Centrifuge of homogenate is performed at 48000 rpm for 15 min and pellet is resuspended in the same volume of buffer.
- This homogenate is incubated to remove the endogenous opiate peptides and centrifuged again. The final pellet is resuspended in 50 volumes of 0.05M Tris buffer.
- In test tubes a mixture consisting of 50 μl tissue suspension, 80 μl distilled water, 20 μl vehicle or levallorphan tartrate or appropriate concentration of drug and 50 μl ^{3}H-Dihydromorphine is prepared.
- Then incubation is performed for 30 min at 25 °C. The assay is stopped by vacuum filtration through Whatman GF/B filters, which are washed twice with 5 ml of 0.05M Tris buffer.
- The filters are placed into scintillation vials with 10 ml liquiscient scintillation cocktail and counted. Specific binding is the difference between total binding and binding in the presence of 0.1mM levallorphan.

Conclusion: At each drug concentration IC_{50} values are calculated from the percent specific binding.

5.6.2 Screening Methods for Inflammatory Drugs

Inflammation is a universal host defensive process involving a complex network of cell-cell, cell-mediator and tissue interaction. Inflammation is response to variety of harmful stimuli physical, chemical, traumatic antigen challenge, infectious agents and ionizing radiations.

Exogenous factors (physical, chemical, mechanical, nutritional and biological etc.)

Endogenous factors (immunological reactions, neurological and genetical disorders) are contributed to inflammation. Inflammation most commonly occurs when microbial invasion or tissue injury overcomes the body's non specific defence mechanism.

The inflammation could be acute, sub acute or chronic in nature.

Acute inflammation	-	short lasting
Chronic	-	May persist for weeks, months or years

There are three principle components of inflammatory responses

- Increased blood flow
- Increased capillary permeability
- Increased migration of leucocytes into effected area

Active hyperemia, exudative and accumulation of neutrophils & macrophages is observed at inflammatory site in an inflammatory response.

Erythema, swelling, heat, pain, loss of function are features in inflammatory condition. Inflammatory diseases cover a broad spectrum of conditions including auto immune diseases.

Example: Rheumatoid arthritis, osteoarthritis, inflammatory bowel disease multiple sclerosis, asthma, chronic obstructive pulmonary disease, allergic rhinitis, infectious diseases various types of cancers and cardiovascular diseases.

Research in last few decades has shown that inflammation is regulated by a large number of pro & anti inflammatory medication such as histamine, PG (PGT2 & Prostacyclins), leukotrienes (LTB4) serotonin, bradykinin, cytokines (IL-1, IL-6, IL-8, IL-n, TNF - α) reactive oxygen species, growth factory, lysosomal, contents of neutrophils, adipokines (leptin, adiponectins, resistin) etc.

Many genes for pro-inflammatory enzymes, (e.g.: COX2, NOS-2) and acute phase proteins and cytokines (TNF–α) contain binding sites for multiple transcription factory in their regulatory elements. Which are activated by variety of inducing agents like bacterial lip polysaccharide (LPS), tumor promoter's cytokines (IFN – G, IL-6) and growth factor.

***In vitro* methods**

- Cox assays
- Mast cell degranulation
- Inhibition of number of production induced by TNF – α in mouse macrophages
- Measurement of number of productions in mouse macrophages
- Adhesion assays
- Platelet – neutrophils adhesion
- Neutrophils adhesion to hypoxia – stimulated porcine aorta
- LPS induced expression of INOS protein, no production, TNF – α expression and P38 MAP kinase in mouse, macrophages
- FMLP – induced O_2 generation by polymorphonuclear cells (PMNs)
- FMLP – induced adhesion of PMN of HUVEC
- Cell based reporter gene assay

***In vivo* methods**

- UV – B induced erythema in guinea pigs
- Carrageen induced paw edema model
- Plural exudation method
- Cotton pellet induced granuloma
- Adjuvant arthritis
- Papaya latex induced arthritis
- *Candida albicans* induced septic arthritis in mice
- Induction of accelerated arthritis by collagen/LPS
- Experimental osteoarthritis in rabbits
- Air pouch mode
- Croton oil induced ear edema in mice
- Arachidonic acid induced ear edema in mice
- Dextran sulphate sod induced colitis in mice

(i) COX Assay

- COX catalyses conversion arachidonic acid

  COX 1

  COX 2 – 2 isoforms, Major ride in inflammations.

COX – 1 Assay

10 ml of sample solution added to 19 ml of 0.1M of L- adrenaline, Dihydrogen tartrate and 10 μM if hematin. After adding 0-2 units of COX 1 it is pre incubated for 5 minutes by adding 10 μl of 10% formic acid. The PGE_2 concentration is measured with a PGE_2 enzyme immune assay.

COX – 2 Assay

- Drugs can be tested for COX 2 inhibitory activity spectrophotometrically by measuring in velocity of oxidation of N, N, N^1, N^1 Tetramethyl-P-phenylenediamine dichloride (TMPD). TMPD is oxidized during the reduction PGG_2 TO PGH_2.
- The assay mixture consists of 100 mm rod phosphate, 1 μm of hematin gelation, 2.5 μl of test compound in DMSO.
- The total volume of assay mixture is 180 μl. This is pre incubated for 15 minutes at 22 °C and the 20 μl of solution of 1mM arachidonic acid and 1mM TMPD in the assay buffer is added.
- The assay buffer contains the assay solution except hematin and enzyme. The absorbance at 400 nm is measured over the fast 36 sec and % inhibition calculated.
- The enzymatic oxidation of TM PD in the absence of COX-2 is also observed and subtracted from activity in presence of COX-2.

(ii) Mast cell degranulation

- Peritoneal mast cells are isolated heparinized Tyrode's solution is injected into the peritoneal cavity of exsanguinated rat (Sprague Dawley).
- After abdominal message, the cells in the peritoneal fluid are harvested and the separated through 38% bovine serum albumin (BSA). Cells are washed and suspended in Tyrode's solution with 0.1% BSA at (1 – 15) × 106 cells/ml.
- The cell suspension is pre incubated with test drugs at 37 °C for 3 min. After 15 min dilution of compound 48/80 (standard compound for mast cell degranulations) glucuronidase (1mM phenolphthalein-D-glucuronidase in 0.1M acetic acid buffer pH – 4) is used as substrate, absorbance monitored at 550 nm after alkalization. And histamine (0.2% O–phthaladehyde condensation in pH 12.5 fluorescence is monitored at 350/450 nm after acidification) in supernatant are determined.

- The total content is measured after treatment of ell suspension Triton x-100.
- The % release determined is index of anti – inflammatory activity.

(iii) UV-B induced erythema in guinea pigs

- Erythema (Redness) is earliest sign of inflammation, not yet accompanied by plasma exudation and edema.
- Usually guinea pigs are used pure erythema reaction appears 21 hours after exposure of depilated skin to ultraviolet irradiation.
- Guinea pigs are pretreated with the test drugs half an hour, before UV – exposure from a UV lamp that emits radiation in the wavelength of 200-400 nm.
- This model can be used as a pure measure of vasodilatory phase in the inflammatory reaction.
- However the test suffers from the drawback that shaving of skin in required before application of irritant.
- The test also depends on skin thickness and intensity of erythema. It is difficult to quantify also the required a skilled investigation.

(iv) Arachidonic Acid (A.A) Induced Ear-Edema In Mice

- A.A. is generated from membrane phospholipids by enzymatic process. To test anti-inflammatory activity A.A. has been successfully used as a topical inflammation to induce ear edema in mice.
- A.A. is freshly prepared in vehicle consistence of acetone: pyridoxine: water (97: 2:1 v/v/v) after 15 minutes test compound is administered via the tail vein, A.A. is applied (0.5 mg in 20 μl of vehicle).
- Inner side of both ears of mice allowed to dry. Animals are sacrified by cervical dislocation 1 hour after topical application of A.A.
- 7 mm diameter ear section is removed from ear by means of a metal punch and weighed to assess the anti-inflammatory activity.
- A.A. has been dissolved just in acetone also and applied topically to ears of mice. These investigators have recorded the weight (mg) as well as thickness (mm) of each ear of mice to assess the anti inflammatory activity.
- A.A. induced ear edema model is suitable for screening lipoxygenase inhibitory.

5.7 SCREENING METHODS FOR DRUGS ACTING ON URINARY SYSTEM

5.7.1 Diuretic Activity

Diuretic agents are very useful for several critical conditions like hypertension, heart failure, renal failure, nephrotic syndrome, and cirrhosis. The various methods for screening of diuretic agents provides useful tool to evaluate the safety and effectiveness of the drugs. It is also useful for determining the dose level of particular class of diuretic agents.

These are the drugs which cause net loss of sodium and water in urine. Diuretics are among most widely prescribed drugs. Application of diuretics to management of hypertension has outstripped their use in edema. Availability of diuretics has also had a major impact on understanding of renal physiology. Various applications of diuretics:

- Used in congestive heart failure
- Essential hypertension
- Acute and chronic renal failure.
- Nephritic syndrome
- Oedema of varied origin & glaucoma

Currently used screening methods are based on effect of drug on water and electrolyte metabolism in rats.

Various methods used:

***In vivo* methods**

(i) Diuretic activity in rats (LIPSCHITZ TEST)
(ii) Saluretic and diuretic activity in dogs
(iii) Saluretic activity in rats
(iv) Stop flow technique
(v) Micro puncture technique in rat.

***In vitro* methods**

(i) Carbonic anhydrase inhibition *in vitro*
(ii) Patch clamp technique in kidney cells
(iii) Isolated perfused kidney

In vivo methods

(i) Diuretic activity in rats (Lipschitz test)

Aim: In 1943diuretic activity in rats (Lipschitz test) purpose to determine diuretic activity of test drug by lipschitz method by comparing water and sodium excretion in test animals.

Requirements

Animals	:	Male Wistar rats (150 - 200 gm)
Equipments	:	Metabolic cages – wire mesh at bottom and funnel for collection of urine Stainless steel sieves, Flame photometer.
Chemicals	:	Test drug, normal saline, urea

Procedure:

- Rats divided into 4 groups of 3, each placed in metabolic cages, provided with wire mesh at bottom and funnel for collecting urine.
- Stainless steel sieves placed in funnel retain feces and allow only urine for measurement.
- The rats fed with standard diet and water ad libitum.
- 15 hr prior to test stop food and water.
- 3 animals are placed in one metabolic cage.
- 2 groups (6 rats) used for 1 dose of test drug. Test drug is given by orally to these 6 rats.
- To other 2 groups (6 rats)

  For one group 1gm/kg of urea was administered.

  To another group 5 ml of normal saline solution per 100 gm by oral route is given.

Evaluation: Urine excretion is recorded after 5 hr upto 24 hr. Sodium content of urine is estimated by flame photometer depending upon response doses of test compound, adjusted for graded response, determined by ED_{50}.

Results for calculation

$$\frac{\text{Urine volume excreted}}{100} \times \text{body wt.}$$

Urine volume excreted/100 gm body weight is worked out expressed as "lipschitz value".

$$\text{Ratio} = \frac{T}{U}$$

T – Response of test compound

U – Response of urea treatment

- If ratio is 1 and more indicates the positive diuretic effect (Calculated for 5 hr upto 24 hr).
- Similar quotients can be calculated for sodium excretion.

(ii) Saluretic and diuretic activity in dogs

Aim: Dogs are most dependable animals for screening diuretic to study renal physiology and action of diuretics.

Because of renal physiology of dog is similar to human than that of rat.

Requirements:

Animals required	:	Beagle dogs (either sex)
Chemicals required	:	Urea
Equipments required	:	Metabolic cages, plastic catheter, gavage, Osmometer

Procedure:

- Dogs are subjected to intensive training for accepting feeding through gavage and hourly catheterization without any resistance. Then placed in metabolic cages.
- Minimum 4 dogs used as control group receiving water only, 1 gm/kg urea p.o. or 5 mg/kg furosemide orally is given to test group.
- 24 hr prior to experiment, food is withdrawn, and water is withdrawn on morning of that day urinary bladder is emptied with plastic catheter.
- The dogs receive 20 ml/kg of water by gavage followed by hourly doses of 4 ml/kg of drinking water. Bladder is catheterized twice in an interval of 1 hr and urine is collected for analysis of initial values.
- The test drug and standard is applied either orally or i.v. hourly catheterization is repeated for 6hr without further water dosing, animals placed in metabolic cages over night. After 24 hr of test compound dogs catheterized once again. Urine collected through catheter measured together

Evaluation: Urine samples are analyzed for sodium, potassium and chloride.

- Osmolarity is measured through osmometer
- Urine volume also measured

Conclusion: For assessment of activity of test compound urine volume, electrolyte concentration and osmolarity of each animal recorded and averages for each group are calculated. Values plotted against time to allow comparison with pretreatment values as well as with water controls and standard drugs.

(iii) Stop flow technique: This is very useful in localization of transport processes along length of nephron. After clamping of ureter glomerular filtration rate GRF is decreased.

Aim: To determine diuretic activity of test drug by using clamp which is inserted to ureter.

Requirements:

Animals required	:	Male Wistar rats (150-200 gm)
Equipments required	:	Metabolic cages – wire mesh at bottom and funnel for collection of urine
Chemicals required	:	Insulin

Procedure:

- The ureter of animal undergoes intense osmatic diueresis, it is damped for several minutes allowing a relatively static column of urine to remain in contact with various tabular segments for longer than useful period of time. This way the operation of each segment on tubular fluid is exaggerated.
- Then the clamp is released and urine sample sequentially. Small serial samples collected rapidly.
- Earliest samples represent fluid which had been in contact with most distal nephron segment.
- Substances to be examined are administered along with insulin before the application of ureteral occlusion.
- The tubular segments downstream from proximal segments may modify the tubular fluid composition during its degrees. For assessment in each sample the concentration of a glomerular marker such as insulin and concentration of substance under study are measured.

Evaluation: Fractional exertion of substance and glomerular market are plotted against the cumulative urinary volume. This method has been found useful in the evaluation of uricosuric compounds.

5.7.2 Anti Urolithiatic Activity

Introduction

An urolithiasis or kidney stone is formation of urinary calculi at any level of urinary tract. Urolithiasis is complex process that occurs in kidneys. The main factors affecting stone formation are urine output (hence the concentration), the concentration of specific constituent, urine pH, infection or damage within the urinary tract. In this disease increased urinary excretion of stone forming constituent eliminates like calcium, phosphorus, uric acid, oxalate and cysteine will occur.

And also low urine output (1 liter/day) in this condition. Various drugs that increase the risk of stone formation are:

Decongestants	:	Ephedrine, guaifenesin
Diuretics	:	Triamterene
Protease inhibitors	:	Indinavir
Anticonvulsants	:	Felbamate, topiramate etc.

There are several types of renal stones that differ in composition and pathogenesis.

Example: Calcium stones, uric acid stones, struvite or triple phosphate stones, cysteine stones, protease related stones.

Screening methods:

(i) Antiurolithiatic activity of ethylene glycol and ammonium chloride induced urolithiasis

Aim: Ethylene glycol and ammonium chloride induced urolithiasis.

Requirements:

Animals required	:	Male Wistar albino rats (150-200 gm)
Chemicals required	:	Ethylene glycol

Procedure:

- Animals are divided into 2 groups (6 in each).
- 1st group is treated with ethylene glycol (0.75%) and drinking water. (It produces renal calculi within 34 days).
- 2nd group is treated with ethylene glycol (0.75%), drinking water and test drug.
- All animals are kept in individual metabolic cages urine samples for 24 hr periods were collected up to 34th day. Urine was analyzed for calcium, oxalate and total proteins.
- 2nd group of animals simultaneously treated with test drugs at the time of inducer administered. After 35 days two groups of animals sacrificed and blood samples were taken ad analyzed for sodium, calcium and creatinine and phosphorous.

Conclusion:

- Two groups of animal's samples are compared to determination of potency of test drugs. (By estimating of sodium, calcium, creatinine, and phosphorus levels in blood).
- Test drug potency is determined by reduced and prevented growth of urinary stones on ethylene glycol induced lithiasis.

5.8 SCREENING METHODS OF DRUGS ACTING ON GASTRO INTESTINAL SYSTEM

5.8.1 Screening Methods for Antiulcer Agents

Peptic Ulcer refers to Gastric ulcers
Duodenal ulcers
Post operative ulcers

- These ulcers normally at or near to the site of surgical gastro intestinal anastomosis.
- Pathogenesis of peptic ulcers involve disturbance in acid pepsin status of gastric contents.
- Due to high morbidity associated with this disease, there is continuous need for newer anti ulcer drugs. Peptic ulcers mean excess secretion of HCl.
- Main reasons for peptic ulcers are:
  Aggressive factors - which increases gastric acid secretion.
  Defensive factors - which decreases gastric acid secretion.

When the levels of aggressive factors equal to defensive factors levels, then there is not problematic. If the increased levels of aggressive factors or decreased levels of defensive factors lead to ulcer formation.

Aggressive factors are - Acetylcholine
Histamine
Gastrin
H. Pylori

Defensive factors are - Prostaglandins
Mucus
HCO_3^-

CCK_2 - Cholecystokinin receptor.

HCO_3^- - Used to neutralize H^+ ions.

Mucus - used to protect of gastric mucosa.

Drug which decreases gastric acid secretions:

- Anti histamine, proton pumps inhibitors, Anti cholinergics
- PG analogue, gastrin antagonists
- Anti *H. Pylori* drugs

- Antacids (to neutralize gastric acid)
- Ulcer protective, ulcer healing drugs are used to treat ulcers.

***In vitro* methods**

(i) Gastrin binding assay

(ii) H^+/K^+ ATPase inhibition Assay

(iii) Tiotidine binding assay for histamine H_2 receptors

***In vivo* methods**

(i) Stress ulcer models

(ii) Pylorus ligation in Rats

(iii) Histamine induced gastric ulcers

(iv) Ethanol induced mucosal Damage

(v) Acetic acid induced gastric ulcers

(vi) Reserpine induced chronic ulcers

(vii) Cysteamine induced duodenal ulcers

(viii) Dimaprin_induced duodenal ulcers

(ix) Mepirizole induced deodenal ulcers

(x) Gastric mucosal injury by local Ischemia – Reperfusion in Rats

***In vitro* methods**

(i) Gastrin binding assay

Gastrin is one of major stimuli for gastric acid secretion. Gastric acid by binding to its receptor on parietal cells as well as by releasing histamine from enterochromaffin like cells.

Aim: Compounds with Gastrin receptor antagonistic activity can prove to be useful antiulcer drugs.

Animals required	:	Guinea pig
Chemicals required	:	Centrifuge tubes, fundic gland suspension. Gastrin, ice cold buffer.

Procedure:

- The assay is done fundic gland suspension obtained from guinea pig stomach for binding and competition assays, the gland suspension is incubated with 50 μl gastrin.

- In presence of either buffer (for total binding) or in presence unlabeled gastrin (for non specific or in presence of test compound binding) for 90 min at 37 °C.
- Subsequently, ice cold buffer, in micro centrifuge tubes, is layered with incubated mixture and centrifuged for 5 min at 10,000 rpm.
- Radioactivity is quantified in pellet after discerning the supernatural.

Conclusion: Total binding, non – specific Binding are calculated.

Specific binding are determined by % of specifically bound {^{125}I} gastrin displaced by a given concentration of test compound is calculated and it IC_{50} and dissociation constant (Ki) values are calculated.

(ii) H^+/K^+ ATPase inhibition assay

H^+/K^+ ATPase Pump are also called as proton pump.

It is final step in synthesis of acid by parietal cells. Its exchanges intracellular H^+ with extracellular K^+ in canaliculi of parietal cells in response to stimulation by all gastric acid secretagogues those are histamine, acetylcholine and gastrin.

Proton pump inhibitors like Omeprazole, lansoprazole etc. are now established anti ulcer drugs.

Aim: Test drugs proton pump inhibitory activity is compared with standard drug activity.

Animals required	:	Pigs (gastric mucosa)
Chemicals required	:	Malachite green colorimetric reagent
		Citrate buffer
Equipment required	:	Microtiter plate
		Colorimeter (570 nm)
		15% sodium citrate

Procedure:

- Assay is carried out using homogenates of microsomal gastric H^+/K^+ ATPase obtained from pig gastric mucosa for inhibition assay.
- 80 ng Microsomal H^+/K^+ ATPase incubated with 100 ml buffer (pH 7.4) 1mM ATP and test compounds in microstate plate for 30 min at 37 °C.
- After 30 min of incubation, the reaction is stopped by adding of Malachite green colorimetric reagent and then after 10 sec 15% sod. citrate is added for 45 min.

- Release of orthophosphate from ATP is quantified by colorimeter at 570 nm.
- For study of Omeprazole (used as standard) which produce active metabolic at acidic pH, the microsomal homogenate is initially suspended in buffer at pH 6.1 along with drug and incubated for 30 min.
- The homogenate is then transferred to buffer at 7.4 and the procedure is followed.

Conclusion: % inhibition of H^+/K^+ ATPase is calculated.

***In vivo* methods**

(i) **Stress ulcer models:** Stress plays significant role in pathogenesis of gastric ulcers in human being. Several methods used involvement of production of gastric ulcers using these models.

- Restraint induced ulcers
- Cold water immersion induced ulcer
- Stress and NSAID's immersion induced ulcer
- Swimming stress ulcers

(a) Restraint induced ulcers

Animals required	:	Albino rats (150-200 gm)
Chemicals required	:	NaOH
Equipments required	:	Cork plate
		Galvanized steel window
		Binocular microscope

Procedure:

- Rats are taken, after 36 hr fasting, and test drug is administered. 30 min later animals are subjected to restraint by molding a special galvanized steel window screen around the animal and typing the limbs of animals in pair so that the animal cannot move.
- The animals are kept under restrained for 24 hr, the animals are then sacrificed their stomachs dissected out.
- The stomachs are opened along greater curvature and fixed to cork plate.
- The contents of stomach are drained into acidity determined by titration with 0.1N NaOH.
- Inner surface of stomach examined for ulceration with binocular microscope.

- Ulcer index is calculated and ulcer severity graded as mentioned:

0 – No ulcer	1 – Superficial ulcer
2 – Deep Ulcer	3 – Perforation

Ulcer index

$U_I = U_N + U_S + U_P \times 10^{-1}$

U_N = Average of no. of ulcers or animal

U_S = Average of severity scores

U_p = % of animals with ulcers

Conclusion: Ulcer index and acidity of gastric content of treated animals compared with control.

(b) Cold water immersion induced ulcers

It shortens the immobilization time.

Animals required	:	Wistar rats
Chemicals required	:	Evan's blue
		Water at 22 °C
		Saline
Equipment required	:	Restraint cages

Procedure:

- Wistar rats (150-200 gm) are taken and after 16 hr fasting the test compound is administered orally.
- Animals placed individually in restraint cages vertically and immersed in water at 22 °C for 1 hr.
- Azovan blue (Evans blue) in a dose of 30 mg/kg is injected i.v. *via* tail vein after removing rat from cage.
- They are sacrificed 10 min later.
- Stomach is removed and ligated at both ends filled with formal saline and kept overnight.
- On the next day stomach is opened along the greater curvature, washed with warm water and examined for ulcerative lesions.
- Evans blue helps in evaluation of lesion score, which is calculated by adding the lengths of longest diameter of the lesions.

(c) Stress and NSAIDs induced ulcers

Animals required	:	Wistar rats
Chemicals required	:	NSAIDs
		1% CMC

Procedure:

- Wistar rats fasted before 24-36 hr given the test agent (in 1% carboxymethyl cellulose) *via* gastric incubation and NSAIDs such as aspirin, indomethacin or diclofenac.
- After placing the rats in stress cages they are immersed in water up to the level of xiphoid process at 23 °C for 7 hr. The animals are then sacrificed their stomach removed and evaluated for ulcer index.
- The dose of NSADs required to increase gastric erosion by 100% relative to immobilization is compared with that of NSAIDs required to produce 100% increase in gastric erosion under the protective effect of test drug.

(d) Swimming stress ulcers

- Albino rats fasted for 24 hr with free access to water.
- The rats are forced to swim in a deep concrete tube filled with water at 23 °C for 5 hr.
- The animals are removed from tube after 5 hr, sacrificed and their stomach removed.
- The stomachs are opened along the greater curvature and severity grading is done and ulcer in dose calculated. Severity of ulceration lesions is graded as follow.

  0 – No lesion
  1 – Lesion with diameter less than 1 mm
  2 – Lesion with diameter less than 1-2 mm
  3 – Lesion with diameter less than 2-4 mm
  5 – Lesion with diameter more than 4 mm

Conclusion: Ulcer index is calculated by summation of scores for individual erosions and ulcers.

5.9 SCREENING METHODS FOR DRUGS ACTING ON LIVER

Main adverse effect of most using drugs is liver injury. Some drugs are withdrawn from market because of causing severe liver injury.

Drug induced hepatotoxicity because of different mechanisms like - Disruption of hepatocytes, Disruption of transport proteins, Cytolytic T Cell activation, Apoptosis of hepatocytes, Mitochondrial disruption or bile duct injury.

- Drugs get metabolized in liver only in phase 1, phase 2 reactions, these processes tend to increase solubility of the drug and can generate metabolites that are more chemically activate and potentially toxic.
- Liver diseases are so many types

Cirrhosis: A chronic disease of liver, characterized replacement of liver tissue by fibrosis (scar tissue) symptoms include jaundice, fatigue, weakness, loss of appetite, itching and easy bruising.

Hepatitis: Characterized by inflammation of liver caused by hepatitis A, B and C and also caused by alcohol and other toxins.

Fatty liver: It is reversible condition coherence in large volumes of triglyceride fat accumulate in liver

(i) Screening methods for CCl_4 induced hepatic toxicity

Aim: Screening for drugs which treat CCl_4 induced hepatic toxicity. These drugs are called as hepatoprotectives.

Requirements:

Animals	: Albino Rats (150- 200 gm)
Chemical	: CCL_4
Equipments	: SGOT, SGPT, ALP, Bilirubin kits etc.

Procedure:

- Liver damage is induced by CCL_4 (0.5 ml/kg i.p.) once daily for 7 days.
- After 7 days animals are subjected by liver damage.
- Then animals are divided into 2 groups, one group is remains like that only, second group is treated with test drug at the dose of 200 mg/kg, p.o.
- Then the 2nd group animals are examined for estimation of levels of marker enzymes like ALP, and ACP and also for total proteins (TP), albumin (Alb) in serum.
- After that lipid peroxidation is estimated by measuring of thiobarbituric acid reactive substances (TBARs) and glutathione levels (GSH).

Result: Serum GOT, GPT, ACP, ALP levels increases, when animals treated with CCL_4, if the test drug is potent these levels comes nearer to normal level while treating with test drug, to normal level while treating with test drug, and albumin. Serum total proteins, levels and albumin are decreases when animals treated with CCl_4 these levels comes nearer to normal when treated with potent test drug.

ALP	:	Alkaline Phosphatase
ACP	:	Acid Phosphatase
SGOT	:	Serum Glutamate Oxaloacetate Transaminase
SGPT	:	Serum Glutamic Pyruvate Transaminase

Some drugs list which causes hepatotoxicity

- Statins (Atorvastatin, flurvastatin)
- Oral hypoglycemics (Acarbose, pioglitazone)
- Anti epileptics (carbamazepine, valproic acid)
- Anti fungal (ketoconazole)
- Anti tuberculosis (Isoniazid & Rifampcin)
- Diclofenac, halothane, methyldopa etc.

5.10 SCREENING METHODS FOR DIABETIC DRUGS

The pancreas is an organ composed of 98% exocrine and 2% endocrine cells. Islets of Langerhans which form the endocrine parts of pancreas consists of 4 types of cells, they are

- α cells
- β cells
- δ cells
- PP cells

These cells secrete glucagon, insulin, somatostatin and pancreatic polypeptide. Glucose stimulates the β cells to release insulin which then promotes glucose uptake and storage in various tissues. Diabetes mellitus is a disease characterized by derangement which is caused by the complete or relative insufficiency of insulin secretions and or insulin action.

Two major types of diabetes

Type I (or) Insulin Dependent Diabetes Mellitus (IDDM)

Type II (or) Non Insulin Dependent Diabetes Mellitus (NIDDM)

Type I is associated with a specific and complete loss of pancreatic β cells.

Type II is the most common type and is associated with obesity, hyperinsulinemia and Insulin resistance.

The β cell mass is overall balance of β cell growth and cell loss depending on the mechanism as

- Replication of existing differential β cells
- Neogenesis of β cells from precursors located in the pancreatic ductal epithelium
- β cell size
- β cell death

Screening methods

(i) Chemically induced diabetes
    - Alloxan induced diabetes
    - Streptozotocin induced diabetes

(ii) Hormone induced diabetes

(iii) Insulin antibodies induced diabetes

(iv) Diabetes induced by viral agents

(v) Surgically induced diabetes

(vi) Genetic models
    - The NOD mouse
    - The BB rat

(vii) Models for NIDDM
    - Neonatal STZ model of NIDDM (chemically induced diabetes)

(viii) Genetic models of NIDDM
    - Monogenic models of obesity and NIDDM
    - Yellow mouse (The agouti mouse)
    - Obese and diabetic mouse

***In vitro* methods**

These are done on isolated organs, cells and membranes

- Isolated rat pancreatic islet
- Isolated pancreas of rat
- Isolated rat liver
- Isolated Hepatocytes
- Fructose 2,6- diphosphate production in rat Hepatocytes
- Isolated target tissue muscle
- Muscle cell lines

- Glucose uptake by isolated diaphragm from mice and rats
- Insulin receptor binding assays

(i) Alloxan induced diabetes

Aim: A cyclic urea analog was the first agent in this category which was reported to produce permanent diabetes in animals.

Mechanism of action: Alloxan is a highly reactive molecule that is readily reduced to dialuric acid which is then auto oxidized back to alloxan resulting in the product in of free radicals. These free radicals damage the DNA of β cells and cause cell death. Second mechanism proposed for alloxan is its ability to react with protein SH groups especially the membrane proteins like glucokinase on the β cells, finally resulting in cell necrosis. However there are major species differences in response to alloxan.

Animals required	:	Rabbits (2-3 kg)
		(or)
		Wistar or Sprague Dawley rat (150-200 gm)
		(or)
		Male Beagle dogs (15-20 kg)
Chemicals required	:	Alloxan, insulin

Procedure

- Rabbits weighing 2-3 kg are used Alloxan is infused *via* ear marginal vein at a dose of 150 mg/kg for 10 mints. About 70% of animals become hyperglycemic and uricosuric. The remaining animals either die or are temporarily hyperglycemic.
- Rats are injected with alloxan in s.c. in the dose of 100-175 mg/kg.
- For dogs-i.v. at a dose of 60 mg/kg.
- Alloxan has been given to non human primates like monkeys and baboons in the dose of 65-200 mg/kg i.v. induce diabetes.

  All the animals which are given alloxan receive glucose and regular insulin for one week and food ad libitum.

  There after single daily dose of 28 IU insulin is administered s.c. The blood glucose level shows triphasic change first a rise at 2 hr, followed by hypoglycemic phase at 8 hr ad finally an increase at 24 hr probably due to depletion of β cells of insulin.

(ii) Neonatal STZ model of NIDDM (chemically induced diabetes)

Aim: Estimation of treating capacity of test drug on chemically induced diabetes

Animals required : Wistar or Sprague Dawley rats
Chemicals required : STZ (80-100 mg/kg)

Procedure: Animals are treated with STZ at birth or within 5 days following birth. There is severe pancreatic β cells destruction, accompanied by a decrease pancreatic insulin stores and rise in plasma glucose levels. However in contrast to adult rats treated with STZ, the cells of the treated neonates particularly regenerate.

Following an initial spike in plasma glucose the STZ treated neonatal rats becomes normoglycemic by 3 weeks of age. In the next few weeks, the β cell number increases mainly from the proliferation of cells derived from ducts, the extent depending upon both the age at which the animal is treated with STZ and the species of the treated rats.

In vitro Methods

(i) Isolated rat pancreatic islet

Aim: This method is used for studying chronic modulation of α cells function has been performed

Animals required : Male Wistar rats (weighing 200-250 gm)
Chemicals required : Bovine albumin
Theophylline
Kreb's solution
Equipment required : Stereomicroscope
Microfuge tubes
Tuohy Borst adaptor
Perfusion chamber
Catheters
Water bath

Procedure: Two male Wistar rats act as donors of pancreas, which is removed under Phenobarbital anesthesia.

The islets are obtained by the collagenase method and collected under stereomicroscope.

In every test, up to 10 chambers each with 15 islets are perfused. Cut off Microfuge tubes sealed with Tuohy Borst adaptors, serve as perfusion chambers.

- Two thick-walled, small diameter teflon catheters are passed through the adapter into the chamber.
- One of the catheters extends to the bottom of chamber and acts as the perifusate inlet, the other extends to the lower edge of the adaptor cone and acts as outlet.

- The latter is connected to multichannel peristaltic pump, which delivers the perifusate to a fraction collector. The chamber volume is 0.15 ml
- The perifusate flow rate is 0.1 ml/minute
- The perifusate consists of Kreb's-ringer bicarbonate buffer with 1.0 mmol/l glucose, 0.25% bovine albumin and 5 mmol/l theophylline.
- The storage vessels for the perifusate, the chambers and the inlet catheters are immersed in a water bath of 37 °C.
- After a Pre-perifusion phase of one hour, the perifusate is collected every minute for 46 minutes.
- From the 2nd until the 18th min, the test compound is added at concentrations between 0.1 and 2.5 μmol/l and from the 34th to 46th minute, the glucose concentration is raised to 20.0 mol/l.
- Insulin is determined by Radio immunological methods.
- The determination is done immediately after the end of an experiment.

5.11 SCREENING METHODS FOR ANTIFERTILITY DRUGS

Antifertility agents are the agents which prevents the fertility by interfering with various normal reproductive mechanisms in males and females. If an ideal contraceptive were available that contraceptive could be 100% effective safe and easy to use its effect would be reversible. It would be aesthetically and personally acceptable in variety of social, political and religious settings. It would be suitable culturally in term of local attitudes concerning sexuality reproduction, menstruation roles and responsibilities of men and women.

Screening methods for females

The Antifertility drugs Acting through these following mechanisms

(i) Inhibition of ovulation

(ii) Prevention of fertilization

(iii) Interference transport of ova from oviduct to endometrium of uterus

(iv) Interference with implantation of fertilized ovum

(v) Distraction of early implanted embryo

Anti ovulatory activity

(i) HCG induced ovulation in rats

(ii) Cupric acetate induced ovulation in rabbits

Estrogenic activity

In vivo

(i) Vaginal opening

(ii) Assay for water uptake

(iii) Four day uterine cut assay

(iv) Vaginal cornification

(v) Chick oviduct method

In vitro

(i) Estrogenic receptor – binding assay

(ii) Dextran Coated Charcoal (DCC) –absorption technical and potency assay

Anti estrogenic activity

In vivo

Antagonism of physiological effects of estrogen

In vitro

Aromatize inhibition

Progestational activity

In vivo

(i) Pregnancy maintenance test

(ii) Proliferation of uterine endometrium in estrogen- primed rabbits

(iii) Carbonic anhydrase activity in rabbit's endometrium

(iv) Deciduoma reaction in rats

(v) Prevention of abortion in oxytocin treated pregnant rabbits

In vitro

(i) Progesterone receptor binding assay

(ii) Anti progestational activity in immature rabbits

(iii) Anti implantation activity

(iv) Abortifacient activity

Screening methods for males

(a) Emergent spermatozoa made non functional

(b) Fertility test

(c) Subsidiary test

In vitro

(i) Spermicidal activity

(ii) Immobilization assay

(iii) Non specific aggregation estimation

(iv) Sperm revival test

(v) Assessment of plasma membrane integrity

(vi) Evaluation of acrosomal status

Androgenic activity

In vivo

(i) Chicken comb method

(ii) Wight of ventral prostate, seminal vesicles and musculus deviator

(iii) Nitrogen retention

Anti androgenic activity

In vivo

(i) Chicken comb method anti androgenic activity in female rats

Screening Methods for Females

(i) HCG induced ovulation in rats

Aim: Evaluation of efficacy of anti ovulatory agents.

Animals required	:	Female albino rats (24-26 days)
Chemicals required	:	Test drugs
		HCG
		Buffered formalin

Procedure:

- Immature female albino rats 24-26 days are used for experiment.
- The animals are treated with various test drugs in different dose levels.
- After administration of test drug, HCG is given exogenously for ovulation.
- After 2 days animals sacrificed ovaries are dissected out, preserved in 10% buffered formalin and subjected to Histopathological parameter evaluation.

Evaluation: Test drug results compared with control group.

(ii) Estrogenic activity

The primary therapeutic use of estrogen is contraception. The rationale for these preparations is that excess exogenous estrogen inhibits FSH and LH thus prevents ovulation.

Vaginal opening: In this vaginal opening occur in immature female albino mice and rats by treating estrogenic compounds. Sign of complete vaginal opening is observed as sign of estrogen activity.

Procedure: Immature female animals are used for study the test and standard drugs are administered to animals in cotton seed oil. The time of complete vaginal opening can be observed as a sign of estrogenic activity.

(iii) Anti estrogenic activity

Antagonism of physiological effect of estrogen: Inhibits physiological effect of estrogen such as water uptake of uterus uterotrophy and vaginal certification.

Procedure: The assay techniques used for anti estrogens are modifications of estrogenic activity.

- The dose of estrogen used is that which is required to produce 50% of maximum possible response.
- The test compound can be injected simultaneous or at varying times before or after estrogen.
- The procedure for assay of water uptake, uterotrophy and vaginal cornification are followed as described earlier except that the test comp are given along estrogen.

(iv) Progestational activity

Pregnancy maintenance test: Progesterone is responsible for maintenance of pregnancy. This principle is used for screening of progestational compound.

Procedure:

- Ovariectomy is done on day 5/10/15 of pregnancy in different groups of pregnant rats. The animals are treated as different test and standard drugs.
- Pregnant rats are killed 5/10/15 days later.
- An average of living fetuses as end of experiment is compared standard and control group (without Ovariectomy).
- The ED_{50} of progesterone is 5 mg/day in rat and less than 0.5 mg/day in mouse.

(v) Abortifacient activity

- Adult female albino rabbits are used for study. The pregnancy date is counted from the date of observed mating.
- The existence of pregnancy may be confirmed by palpation after 12th day of pregnancy.
- Intra amniotic and intraplacental info are performed on rabbits under ether anesthesia on day 20 of pregnancy.
- The uterus is exposed through the midline incision, a particular site is chosen for injection and its various parts are identified by transilluminations from a strong source of light.
- Then material is injected in 0.1 ml of solvent into the amniotic fluid or in 0.05 ml of solvent into placenta.
- Alternatively the drugs can be given through any route and duration from day 20 of pregnancy.
- The effect of drug is determined by looking for vaginal bleeding, changes in weight, abdominal population and by postmortem examinations.

Screening methods for males

Developing male anti-fertility agent involves interference spermatogenesis loss of libido and secondary sexual characteristics.

***In vivo* methods**

Emergent spermatozoa made non functional/oligospermia/aspermia.

(i) Fertility test: Evaluation of average litter anti-fertility agents negatively affects the average litter size.

Procedure:

- Groups of 5-10 male rats of proven fertility are treated with drug and are paired with fertile female in ratio of 1:3.
- Daily vaginal smears are examined for presence of sperms.
- All females passed through estrus cycle must have mated. The mated animals are kept separately till the completion of gestational period. The litters are counted.
- Average litter size: Total number of litters/number of females mated.
- If vaginal smear shows leukocytes for 10-14 days, pseudo pregnancy is confirmed. If insemination is not detected then inhibition of libido or aspermia copulation might be cause. Fertility pattern can be obtained from changes in average litter size.

(ii) Androgenic activity

Chicken comb method

This assay is based in principle of growth of capon comb by androgenic compounds. This method has been useful for isolation and structural elucidation of natural androgens.

Procedure:

- In the beginning of assay, the sum of length plus height of each individuals comb is determined by measurement with a millimeter rule placed directly on the comb.
- The capons are injected daily i.m. for 5 consecutive days with a solution or suspension of test compound or the standard in 1 ml olive oil.
- After 24 hr the last injection the comb is re-measured and growth of comb is expressed as the sum of length and height in millimeter.
- Group of 8 animals are used for at least 2 doses of test compound.
- The lot of control and test group is compared with suitable statistical analysis.

(iii) Anti androgenic activity

Chicken comb method

Inhibition of growth of capon comb by anti androgenic compounds.

Procedure:

- One or 3 days old male or female white leghorn chicks are housed at constant temperature in heated incubator.
- Testosterone is incorporated into the finally ground chick starting mash at concern of 80 mg/kg food.
- Chicks are placed on this diet on day1.
- The test compound is dissolved in sesame oil.
- Each day for 4 days 0.1 ml of the oil solution is injected s.c.
- Control chicks receive only the vehicle.
- 24 hr after the last injection the animals are sacrificed, the combs removed and after blotting of cut edge, weighed rapidly to the nearest 0.5 mg. The weight of control and test groups are compared using suitable statistical method. In a shaking bath maintained at 25 ^{0}C, 50 ml ^{3}H pyrilamine (2x10^{-9} m), 50 ml membrane suspension from guinea pig whole brain (10 mg/ml) per sample are incubated for 30 min.

5.12 SCREENING METHODS OF DRUGS FOR MALARIA

Introduction

Malaria is one of oldest recorded disease. It is a protozoal disease caused by parasites like plasmodium species. Clinical manifestations of malaria include fever, chills, prostration and anemia. Severe disease can include delirium, metabolic acidosis, cerebral malaria and multi organ system failure and coma, death may ensure. Blood stage infection also generates sexual stage parasites (gametocytes) that are infectious for mosquitos leading to fertilization and genetic recombination in mosquito midgut. This is followed by production of haploid sporozoite forms that invade the salivary gland and are subsequently transmitted back to humans.

The main goal of antimalarial drug discovery is to develop safe and affordable new drugs to counter the spread of malaria parasites that are resistant to existing agents. Drug efficacy, pharmacology and toxicity are important parameters for selection of compounds for development, yet little attempt has been made to review and standardize antimalarial drug efficacy screening. Different *in vitro* and *in vivo* screening methods for antimalarial drug discovery are useful for evaluating new compounds. Cytosol, parasite membrane, food vacuole, mitochondrion apicoplasts are target compounds when preparing antimalarial drugs.

Screening methods: *In vitro* screening for activity constitutes a key component for antimalarial drug screening. It is based on ability of culture *plasmodium falciparum* in human erythrocytes *in vitro*. The development of techniques for continuous cultivation of *plasmodium falciparum* is a reliable source for continuous stock culture of parasite.

(i) [^{3}H]-Hypoxanthine uptake test

(ii) Giemsa stained slide method

(i) [^{3}H]-Hypoxanthine uptake test

***Aim*:** [^{3}H]-Hypoxanthine uptake is a standardized method to screening of antimalarial drugs. [^{3}H]-Hypoxanthine as a marker for inhibition of parasite growth. [^{3}H]-Hypoxanthine is taken up by parasite for purine salvage and DNA synthesis to determine the level of *plasmodium falciparum* growth inhibition.

Requirements: Radio labeled hypoxanthine

Parasite culture

Beta plate reader

Procedure:

- Radio labeled hypoxanthine uptake by parasite is an indicator of its growth and multiplication.
- Parasites are cultured in presence of different concentrations of test compounds in media containing reduced concentration of hypoxanthine.
- After that 3sub Hypoxanthine is added for an additional incubation period before cell harvesting and measurement of radioactivity by 1205betaplate reader.
- Mean count per minute (CPM) are generally in range of 20,000-60,000.
- % reduction in mean CPM is calculated for test samples.

Conclusion: % reduction is used to plot % inhibition of growth as a function of drug concentration.

- IC_{50} are determined by linear regression analyses on the linear segments of dose response curve.

This is the common method used for assessing antimalarial efficacy of a compound *in vitro*. Main disadvantage of this method are- it is very expensive, complicated and involve usage of radioactive substances (those are harmful).

(ii) Giemsa stained slide method

It is the method at low cost alternative for testing, used for small number of compound.

Aim: In this method parasites are incubated with test compound and then parasitemia of control and treated group are compared by counting Giemsa stained parasites by light microscopy.

Requirements	:	Parasites culture
		Erythrocytes suspension
Equipments	:	Light microscopy
		Incubating chamber

Procedure:

- In this model parasites are incubated in 5% suspension of erythrocytes with an initial parasite density of 1-2% at 37 ^{0}C.
- A sealed incubation chamber, continuously gassed with a mixture of 2% O_2, 8% CO_2, 90% N_2 is used.

- Increase in proportion of infected RBCs is assessed at the end of 72 hours incubation period in control samples and at various concentrations of each drug.

Conclusion:

- This method relies on a morphological criterion of response and reports a single concentration as the end point and concentration of drug in first sample showing complete inhibition of growth.
- This measurement is classically known as the minimum inhibitory concentration (MIC), method which is suitable for distinguishing susceptible and resistant isolates.

5.13 SCREENING METHODS OF DRUGS ACTING ON EYE

In ocular toxicity studies the number of drugs used to treat different conditions of eye was studied. To screen those drugs collection of treated and untreated eyes are required for that collection of surrounding ocular structures including both upper and lower eyelids, nictitating membrane, harderian glands, lacrimal glands, optic nerve and adjacent muscles. Those isolated parts usually be collected, fixed and evaluated microscopically.

Collection & dissection:

- Before dissection the right upper eye lid can be identified with a structure and circular, palpebral skin incision is made surrounding the eye, eyelids and medial and lateral canthus. The palpebral rim is reflected back to expose the orbit, the bulbar conjunctiva.
- The palpebral rim is reflected back to expose the orbit, the bulbar conjunctiva is grasped above the globe, the optic nerve and remaining muscle attachments are cut, the globe is removed in toto, and extraneous tissues are trimmed away except for 1 to 2 mm of optic nerve attached to the globe.
- The orbit is gently dissected from extraocular tissue at the reflection of the bulbar and palpebral conjuctiva in the back of the eye.

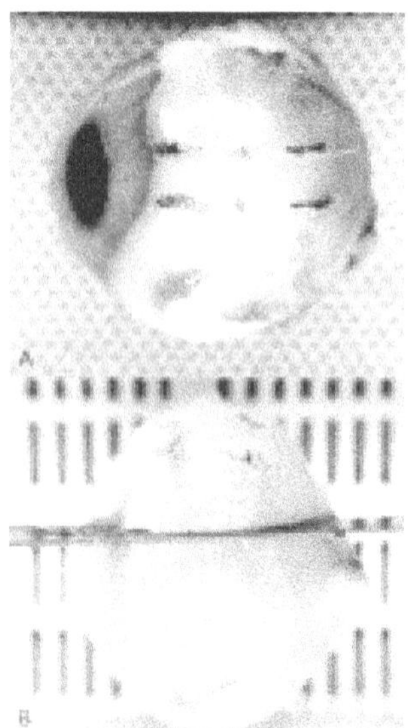

Fig. 5.5 Eye collection.

- For implant studies, implant sites are marked with indelible dye before fixation, so that they can be sectioned and examined. Scleral injection sites for intravitreal studies are usually too small to be identified macroscopically and are not sectioned unless visible and specifically requested.
- For microsphere studies by subconjunctival injection, the test article is usually identifiable macroscopically beneath the palpebral conjunctiva attached to the globe.
- The globes are placed in Davidson's fixative for 24 hours, 70% alcohol for 24 hours and processed or stored in formalin. A pluck of extraocular tissue containing remaining optic nerve, extraocular muscles, lacrimal glands, and Harderian glands is fixed in 10% normal buffered formalin.

View larger version

Ocular implant-site evaluation, rabbit eye with cornea on the left.

(a) Indelible marks are made on each side of two injection sites for ocular implantation in the vitreous before fixation.

(b) Plane of section for trimming eye for evaluation of injection sites.

(i) Trimming and sectioning

- For topical or intravitreal injection studies, the nasal and temporal edges of each eye are trimmed away perpendicular to the posterior ciliary arteries by cutting closer to the nasal side than the temporal side of the optic nerve and through the cornea. The injection site is not usually processed and examined for intravitreal injection studies. The trimmed eye is placed in a deep cassette

(ii) Morphometric species comparisons

- NZW rabbits and cynomolgus monkeys are two of the most common strains or species used in ocular toxicity studies for posterior-segment diseases, and anatomical difference must be factored in for correct interpretation of test-article effects.
- The rabbit eye is essentially a fisheye lens system with significantly greater corneal area to accommodate greater peripheral vision, with corresponding lens differences. An essential absence of ciliary muscle in the rabbit indicates that the focal length in this species is essentially fixed.
- In contrast, the monkey eye has a rather small lens coupled to a smaller cornea that occupies a smaller area of the globe, with a markedly greater vitreal volume compared to the rabbit.

- Although globe size was similar between the two species, the anterior chamber and lens of the rabbit eye were 2.3-fold and 3.9-fold larger, respectively, than similar areas of the monkey eye.
- Conversely, the rabbit vitreous is one-half the size of the monkey vitreous, and the ratio of the vitreous-to-globe area was 0.4 in the rabbit eye and 0.7 in the monkey eye. The monkey eye is more similar than the rabbit eye to humans, which is consistent with the ratio of vitreous-to-globe of 0.3 in rabbits and 0.6 in humans.
- The ciliary body and pars plana region is important in intravitreal implant studies, because it is the preferred site for surgical penetration of the posterior segment.
- The monkey eye is distinctive in two essential ways:
    1. The lens is positioned more forward and is volumetrically smaller than in the rabbit. Accordingly, the monkey lens is less likely to come in direct contact with the implant or be damaged by the method used for placement.
    2. Monkey ciliary muscle is significantly more developed than in the rabbit.

Glaucoma: Glaucoma is the important eye disorder. It is characterized by intraocular pressure associated optic neuropathy. Normal ocular pressure is 14-16 mm of Hg. It increases more than 20 mm of Hg in glaucoma. Draining capacity of ocular fluids are decreased. Increased fluid pressure in eye (aqueous humor). This can permanently damage vision in affected eyes and lead to blindness if left untreated. The term ocular hypertension is used for people with consistently raised intraocular pressure (IOP) without any associated optic nerve damage.

Screening methods

(i) Microbead-induced ocular hypertensive mouse model for screening and testing of aqueous production suppressants for glaucoma.

(ii) Establishment of a rabbit short-term dry eye model.

(i) Microbead-induced ocular hypertensive mouse model

Aim: This method is used to characterize the microbead induced ocular hypertension (OHT) mouse model. This method also useful to investigate its potential use for preclinical screening and evaluation of ocular hypotensive agents.

Requirements:

Animals required	:	Mice
Chemicals required	:	Microbeads Hypotensive agents Immuno fluorescence recognizer Spectral-domain optical coherence tomography (SD-OCT)

Procedure:

- In this method adult mice are taken to produce ocular hypotension. Intracameral injection of microbeads is induced to mice to produce OHT.
- After incubation of few mints, induction of commonly used ocular hypotensive drugs to be evaluated (e.g., timolol, brimonidine, brinzolamide, pilocarpine and latanoprost etc.) on IOP and glaucomatous neural damage of eye.
- Degeneration of retinal ganglion cells (RGCs) and optic nerve axons were quantitatively assessed using immunofluorescence labeling and histochemistry.
- Thickness of ganglion cells complex (GCC) was also assessed with SD-OCT.

Result:

- In this method, if the drug lowers the IOP through suppressing aqueous humor production & improved RGC and axon survival as compared to vehicle control.
- SD-OCT detected significantly less reduction of GCC thickness in mice treated with all their aqueous production suppressants as compared to vehicle control treated group.
- The drugs used to treat glaucoma are gives this positive result.

(ii) **Establishment of a rabbit short-term dry eye model:** The dry eye syndrome is chronic disease which can become a serious threat to useful vision. Established treatment is not there to cure this disease.

Aim: This method is used to prevent mechanical prevention of blinking and methylene blue staining.

Requirements	*:*	Methylene blue 3% chondroitin sulfate solution Microscope

Procedure:

- By using this method clinical signs of dry eye can be observed after a few hours on the form of acute desiccation.
- Corneal damage can easily be evaluated both qualitatively by chronic assay.
- After that visually observed corneal epithelial thinning was confirmed by scanning electron microscopy (SEM) to be due to loss of epithelial integrity.
- Using a 3% chondroitin sulfate solution, an already proven effective agent for dry eye, this already proven effectively demonstrated an 80% inhibition in development of methylene blue positive lesion after a period of only 2 hours
- This short term dry eye model is valuable in primarily screening the efficacy of potential therapeutic agents in prevention and treatment of dry eye.

5.14 SCREENING METHODS OF ANTI STRESSOR AND ANTI OXIDANT ACTIVITY

Introduction

Anti oxidants are the molecules which inhibit the oxidation of other molecules. Oxidation is a chemical reaction that transfers electrons or hydrogen from a substance to an oxidizing agent. Oxidation reactions can produce free radicals. Anti oxidants are chemicals that block the activity of other chemicals known as free radicals.

Vitamin C, E and beta carotene and the most commonly used dietary anti oxidant (Vitamin E is fat soluble). These free radicals are unstable products in body, they can cause DNA mutations, sometimes they may leads to serious conditions like heart disease, Parkinson's and cancers. Sometimes pollutants, cigarette smoke and sun over exposure may generate more free radicals. An antioxidant is a vitamin, mineral or other nutrient that may protect and repair cells in body against damage caused by free radicals.

Food rich with antioxidant source

B carotene	:	Spinach, Sweet potato, tomatoes, broccoli, carrots, corn, peaches, pink grape
Vitamin C	:	Peppers, strawberries, berries
Vitamin E	:	Broccoli, carrot, spinach, mustard & sunflower

Zinc : Red meat, beans and nuts, seafood, whole grains, fortified cereals, dairy products

Selenium : Brazil nuts, beef other grain

Anti oxidant property of test drugs are screened by

(i) Scavenging effect on DPPH radical

(ii) Scavenging effect on hydrogen peroxide

(i) Scavenging effect on DPPH radical

Aim: Test drug was screened for free radical scavenging activity using the "stable" free radical 2,2-diphenyl-1-picryl hydrazyl radical (DPPH). Radical scavenger activity was calculates as % inhibition of DPPH discoloration.

Requirements: DPPH, Methanol extract

Procedure:

- DPPH (3.94 mg) was dissolved in 100 ml methanol to give 100 μM solutions.
- Methanol solution DPPH (3.0 ml) was added to 0.5 ml of methanol extract taken from stock solution.
- The stock solution was prepared by dissolving 3.0 mg of crude methanol extract (test during) into 3 ml of methanol.
- This was shaken well and left to stand for 10 minutes.
- This preparation was done by test drug and also with standard drug.
- Some absorption was decreased by DPPH was measured at some frequency is measured and also some frequency is measured by standard drug.
- And also other concentrations of methanol extracts (0.5 mg/ml, 0.25 mg/ml, and 0.125 mg/ml) also prepared from stock solution and analyzed the same way and average was taken as result.

Result: The radical scavenging activity (RSA) was calculated as percentage inhibition of DPPH discoloration using the equation below.

$$\% \text{ RAS or } \% \text{ inhibition} = (A_{DPPH} - A_s) / A_{DPPH} \times 100$$

A_s: absorbance when test drug add at particular concentration to DPPH,

A_{DPPH}: absorbance of DPPH solution.

CHAPTER 6

TOXICOLOGY

Introduction

Toxicology is the science that deals with the adverse effects of drugs and study of poisons. Poisons are harmful substance which are dangerous or fatal to the living organism as such it is difficult to differentiate a drug and poisons since any drug may be poisonous if not used properly or used in toxic doses.

6.1 PRINCIPLES OF TOXICOLOGY

Drugs used to counteract the poisons effects are called antidotes. Drugs used in such measures, as to impart deleterious effects which may even prove fatal, incorporate toxicology. Toxic signs, symptoms, diagnosis and treatment are all included in the study of toxicology.

Such studies are done on experimental animals, to study the toxicity of drugs.

- When drug is used in therapeutic dose it may manifest some unwanted actions simultaneously, these are called side effects. The unwanted or adverse effects produced at higher doses are called toxic effects.
- Toxic manifestation produces functional disturbances and organ damage for more greater and serious than those of side effects. Side effects are less serious as compared to toxic effects. They demanded stoppage of drug. Excess of morphine, producing Cheyne-stokes breathing result in toxicity of morphine but constipation and miosis (constriction of pupils) produced by morphine are side effects of this drugs.
- Belladonna group when used as spasmolytics may produce dryness of mouth which is side effect but it produces delirium by its central action and it is toxic effect.
- Organ damage often occurs when toxicity is produced prolonged use of

streptomycin. For example, it may produce vertigo and deafness due to damage of the auditory nerve branches, sometimes mercurial's used as diuretics produce nephritis and anti-tubercular drugs like PAS may damage the liver cells. Chloramphenicol on prolonged use is known to produce aplastic anemia which is serious consequence.

- Humans live in a chemical environment and inhale, ingest or absorb from the skin many of those chemical toxicology is concerned with the deleterious effects of these chemical agents on all living systems.

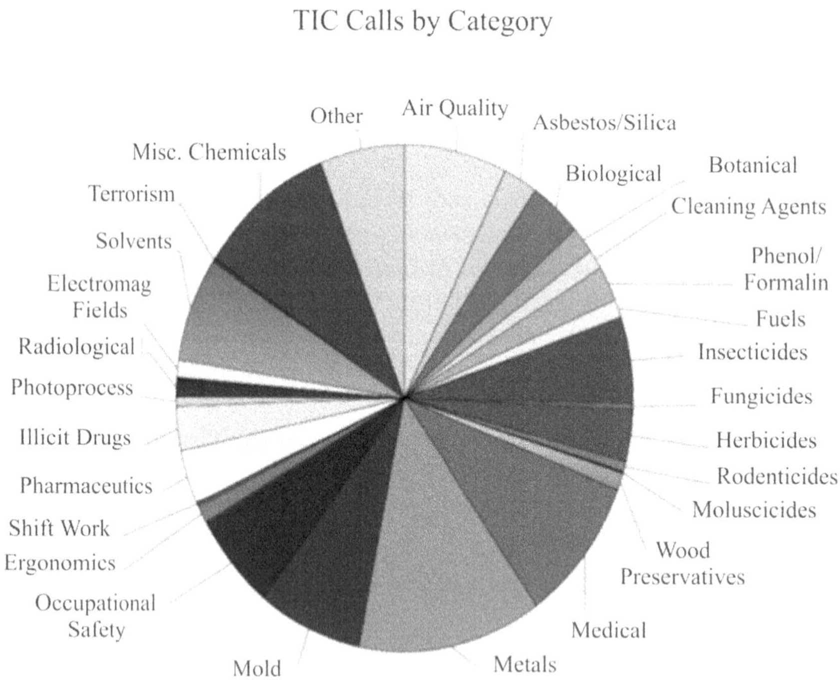

Fig. 6.1 Some types of toxic effects.

Some types of toxic effects

Occupational toxicology: Deals with chemical found in the work place occupational toxicologist may also define and carry out programs for surveillance of exposed workers and environment in which they work regulatory limits and voluntary guidelines how been elaborated to establish safe ambient our concentrations for many chemicals found in the work place.

Environment toxicology: Deals with the potentially deleterious impact of chemicals present as pollutants of the environment on living organisms.

The term environment includes all the surrounding of an individual organism but particularly the air, soil and water.

Ecotoxicology: Is concerned with the toxic effects of chemicals and physical agents on population and communities of living organism with in defined ecosystem it includes the transfer pathways of those agents on individual with the environment. Traditional toxicology is concerned with toxic effects on individual organisms ecotoxicology is concerned with the impact on popularity of living organisms or an ecosystem.

Toxicity testing: Although testing for toxicity, usually for the purposes of human health risk assessment, might be expected to be one of the more routine aspects of toxicology.

Toxicity Assessment is the determination of potential of any substance to act as a poison.

Summary of toxicity tests and related end points

(i) Chemical and physical properties.

(ii) Exposure and environment fate.

- Degradation studies, degradation in soil, water and air.
- Mobility and dissipation in soil and air.
- Accumulation in plants, aquatic animals, wild terrestrial animals, food plants.

(iii) *In vivo* tests:

(a) Acute

- LD_{50} and LC_{50} - Oral, Dermal, Haled.
- Eye irritation.
- Dermal irritation.
- Dermal sensitization.

(b) Sub Chronic

- 90 Day feeding.
- 20 to 90 day Dermal and Inhalation Exposure.

(c) Chronic/Reproduction

- Chronic feeding.
- Teratogenicity.
- Reproduction.

(d) Special Tests.

- Neurotoxicity.
- Potentiation.

- Metabolism.
- Pharmacodynamics, Behaviour

(iv) *In vitro* tests:

- Mutagenicity - Prokaryote.
- Mutagenicity - Eukaryote.
- Chromosome absorption.

(v) Effects on wild life

- Accumulation.

Modes of toxic action

This includes the consideration, at the fundamental level of organ, cell and molecular function, of all events leading to toxicity *in vivo*: Uptake, distribution, metabolism, mode of action and excretion.

- ***Biochemical and molecular toxicology:*** Including enzymes that metabolize xenobiotics, generation of reactive intermediate, interaction of xenobiotics or their metabolites with macromolecules, Gene expression in metabolism and mode of action and signaling pathways in toxic action.
- ***Nutritional toxicology:*** Deals with effects of diet on the expression of toxicity.
- ***Carcinogenesis:*** Chemical, bio chemical and molecular events that lead to large number of effects on cell growth collectively known as Cancer.
- ***Teratogenesis:*** Includes the chemical, biochemical and molecular events that lead to deleterious effect on development.
- ***Mutagenesis:*** It is converted with toxic effects on genetic material and the inheritance of these effects.
- ***Organ toxicity:*** Consider effect at the level of organ function. [Neurotoxicity, Hepatotoxicity, Nephrotoxicity etc.]

Applications of toxicology

Various aspects of toxicology

1. ***Academic applications:*** Academic concerns include all the public health areas in which progress in understanding sciences is necessary and include the elucidation of mechanistic, clinical and descriptive toxicological theories.
2. ***Industries applications:*** Toxicity testing in biotechnology and pharmaceutical industries performs for the screening of chemicals, preclinical testing's.

3. ***Regulatory toxicology:*** It is employed primarily in government administrative agencies. The guiding principles are promulgated through laws enacted by appropriate federal, state and local jurisdictions.

   Thus through these regulations, an agency determines who is accountable and responsible for manufacturing, procurement, distribution, marketing ultimately release and dispensing of chemical substance to public.

4. ***Forensic toxicology:*** This technique to identify compounds arising from mixtures of sometimes unrelated poisons as a result if incidental or deliberate exposure.

   - Used for identification of controlled substance of body fluids this is useful to perform antigen - antibody interaction for paternity testing. By using the principles of blood grouping and exclusion of possible outcomes of paternal contributions to off spring antigen - antibody interactions also became possible to eliminate a mole as a possible father of a child.
   - Antigen - Antibody interactions also became the bases for Enzyme Linked Immunosorbent Assay [ELISA] currently used for specific and sensitive identification of drugs in biological fluids.
   - RIA's [Radio Immuno Assay] utilize similar antigen - antibody reactions while incorporating radio labelled ligands as indicatory.
   - DNA separation and sequencing techniques have now almost totally replaced traditional paternity exclusion testing.
   - These methods are also the basis for inclusion or exclusion of evidence in criminal and civil cases.

5. ***Clinical toxicology:*** It is a branch of forensic counterparts. Clinical toxicologist is interested in identification, diagnosis and treatment of condition, pathology or disease resulting from environmental, therapeutic or illicit exposure to chemicals or drugs.

6. ***Nanotoxicity:*** It is a study of toxicity of nanomaterials. Because of quantum size effects and large surface area, nanomaterial has unique properties compared with their large counterparts.

6.2 MUTAGENESIS

Mutagenesis refers to the ability of a virus or chemical agent to induce changes in the genetic sequences of mammalian or bacterial cells, thus altering the phenotic expression of cell characteristics.

Genotoxicity: Genotoxic substances means sometimes indirectly altering the DNA sequence, some other times genotoxic substances induce by binding directly to DNA, it causes irreversible damage to cell. Genotoxicity refers to ability of an agent to induce heritable changes in genes that exercise homeostatic control in somatic cell while increasing the risk of influencing benign or malignant transformation. Those genotoxic substances are not necessarily carcinogenic. Sometimes genotypic and phenotypic consequences also produced because of addition of interaction of chemical, physical or viral agent with nucleic acids results in disruption of transfer or genetic information transfer interaction. This leads to mitogenesis; it is induction of cell division (mitosis) with in eukaryotic or prokaryotic cells by continuous exposure to through the cell cycle. Prolonged and continuous exposure to growth factor is required to commit cells to the cell cycle.

6.3 MULTISTAGE CARCINOGENESIS

Carcinogenesis is the process experimentally divided into 3 defined stages:

(a) Tumour initiation

(b) Tumour promotion

(c) Tumour progression

This multi stage development requires malignant conversion of benign hyper plastic cells to malignant state, involving of further genetic and epigenetic changes.

(a) **Tumor initiation:** Irreversible genetic alteration indicates that initial changes in chemical carcinogenesis are the early concept of tumor initiation. Activation of proto oncogene or inactivating of tumor suppressor gene by DNA adducts formation method is categorized as a tumor initiating event. According to recent data of molecular studies of pre neoplastic human lung and colon tissues, in early event in carcinogenesis, that is implicate epigenetic changes. Some tumor suppressor genes are also present, they are because of DNA methylation of promoter regions of genes can transcription all of tumor suppressor genes. Thus carcinogen DNA adduct formation is central to the theory of chemical carcinogenesis and may be necessary but not sufficient prerequisite for tumor initiation. One important step of this stage is its irreversibility. In this stage the cell is conferred in genotype or phenotype of imitated cell during the process. The initiating cells required more chemicals called as initiating agents. Subsequent promotion and progression rarely yields malignant transformation.

(b) **Tumor promotion:** Tumor promotion comprises through a mechanism of gene activation of initiated cells by selective clonal expansion in multi stage carcinogenesis process. Clonal expansions of initiated cells produce a large population of cells that are at risk of further genetic changes and malignant conversion. In this accumulation rate of mutations is proportional to rate of cell division.

Tumor promoters, they do not directly interact with DNA, generally non-mutagenic are not solely carcinogenic, often able to mediate their biologic effects without metabolic, activation. Examples of typical tumor promoters are

TPA (Tetradecanoyl Phorbol Acetate)

TCDD (2,3,7,8 – Tetra Chlorodibenzo Digoxin and Phenobarbital)

These are the reversible tumor promoters, although the continued presence of promoting agent maintains the state of promoted cell population (pre-neoplastic lesion). This is the stage appears to have a long duration, especially in humans and is preferred target for experimental manipulation.

At the time of tumor promotion, malignant conversion may occur in which pre neoplastic cell is transformed into malignant phenotype. Further genetic changes requires in this process. In this process tumor promoters are very important, these promoters are requires in repeated administration than the total dose. Malignant or benign lesions are regress if tumor promoter is discontinued before malignant conversion. Tumor promotions contribute to process of carcinogenesis by expansion of a population of initiated cells that are then at risk for malignant conversion. In part these genetic changes result from infidelity of DNA synthesis. Conversion of fraction of these cells to malignancy is accelerated in proportion to rate of cell division of the quantity of divided cells in the benign tumor or pre-neoplastic lesion.

(c) Tumor progression: In tumor progression process comprises the expression of malignant phenotype and tendency to malignant cells to acquire more aggressive characteristics over time. Metastasis is may involve the ability of tumor cells to secrete proteases that allow invasion beyond the immediate primary tumor location. This malignant phenotype is propensity for genomic instability and uncontrolled growth after that genetic and epigenetic change occur, this includes proto-oncogenes and functional loss if tumor suppress or genes.

In this process tumor suppressor genes functional loss may occur in a bimodal fashion, point mutations occurs frequently in one allele and loss of second allele by deletion, recombination event of chromosomal non disjunction. This process confers growth advantage to cells along with capacity for regional invasion and ultimately distant metastatic spread. In further stage of tumor genesis mutational events, and accumulation of these mutations can occur they appears as determine factor. In these three stages of chemical carcinogens, illustrates events can occurs and requirements necessary for completion of multistage process.

Carcinogenic and genotoxic agents: Environmental toxicity may occur because of collective and individual exposures. Various risk factors are determined by experimental investigation. For these investigation, supported epidemiological research. These profiles are perpetually in complete because humans incessantly modify the environment, thus increasing the risk of interactions with agents against which there may be no protective mechanisms. There are many causative agents are and physical carcinogenic agents does not render them easy to study. In humans cancer risk factors has highest causal relationship with various environmental hazardous compounds, cigarette smoke etc. Tobacco smoking plays a major role in the etiology of lung, oral cavity and esophageal cancers and a variety of other chronic degenerative diseases. Although cigarette smoke is mixture of about 4000 chemicals in those 60 known human carcinogens are present.

E.g., 4-(methylnitrosamino)-1-(-3-pyridyl)-1-butanone (nicotine-derived nitrosaminoketone, NNK) and NNN (N-Nitrosonoricotine)

These are known as human carcinogens.

NNK is metabolically activated by CYP450 enzymes in lungs and generates 06-methylguanine in DNA. The reaction generates G-C to A-T mutation with subsequent activation of K-ras proto-oncogene and development of tumor initiation. In human cancers most causative physical factors includes radiation, it plays significant role. Radiation promotes double strand breaks (DSBs) in DNA that lead to chromosome aberrations and cell death and also generators a variety of oxidative DNA damage. Because of Genotoxicity, radiation at high doses evidently results in appearances of various tumors in humans.

Carcinogenicity testing *in vivo*: Principles of *in vivo* carcinogenicity testing:

In human carcinogenicity risk assessment need improvement, the toxicity community generally agrees carcinogenicity testing and its application in human. In risk assessment process addition of more information is necessary about incorporation of mechanisms and modes of actions.

Number of proto-oncogenes and tumor suppressor genes are advances in molecular biology that are highly across species and are associated with an extensive variety of mammalian cancers.

In vivo transgenic rodent models incorporate these mechanisms are used to identify path ways involved in tumor formation. Transgenic methods are considered extensions of genetic manipulation of selective breeding-a technique that has long been employed in science and agriculture with carcinogenicity testing, the use of two rodent species is especially important for identifying trans-species carcinogens.

6.4 TERATOGENICITY

A single interactive exposure to a drug can affect the fetal structures undergoing rapid development at the time exposure.

Thalidomide is an example of a drug that may profoundly affect the development of limbs after only brief exposure. This exposure however must be at a critical time in the development of limbs.

6.4.1 Predictable Toxic Drug Actions in the Fetus

Chronic use of opioids by the mother may produce dependence in the fetus and new born. This dependence may be manifested after delivery as a neonatal withdrawal syndrome. A less well understood fetal drug toxicity is caused by the use of angiotensin converting enzyme inhibitors during pregnancy. These drugs can result in significant and irreversible renal damage in the fetus and are therefore contraindicated in pregnant women; adverse effects may also be delayed, as in the case of female fetuses exposed to diethylstilbestrol, which may be at increase risk for adenocarcinoma of the vagina after puberty.

6.4.2 Teratogenic Drug Actions

A single intrauterine exposure to a drug can affect the fetal structures rapid development at the time of exposure. Thalidomide is a drug used for morning sickness in pregnant women. Thalidomide is an example of a drug that may profoundly affect the development of the limbs after only brief exposure. This exposure however must be at a critical time in the development of the limbs. The thalidomide phocomelia risk occurs during the fourth through the seventh weeks of gestation because it is during this time that the arms and legs develop.

6.4.3 Defining a Teratogen

To be considered teratogenic, a candidate substance or process should result in a characteristic set of malformations, indicating selectivity for certain target organs. Exerts its effects at a particular stage of fetal development e.g., during the limited time period of organogenesis of the target organs and show a dose dependent incidence. Some drugs with known teratogenic or other adverse are not limited only to major malformations, but also include intrauterine growth restriction, miscarriage, still birth and neurocognitive delay (Example: Alcohol).

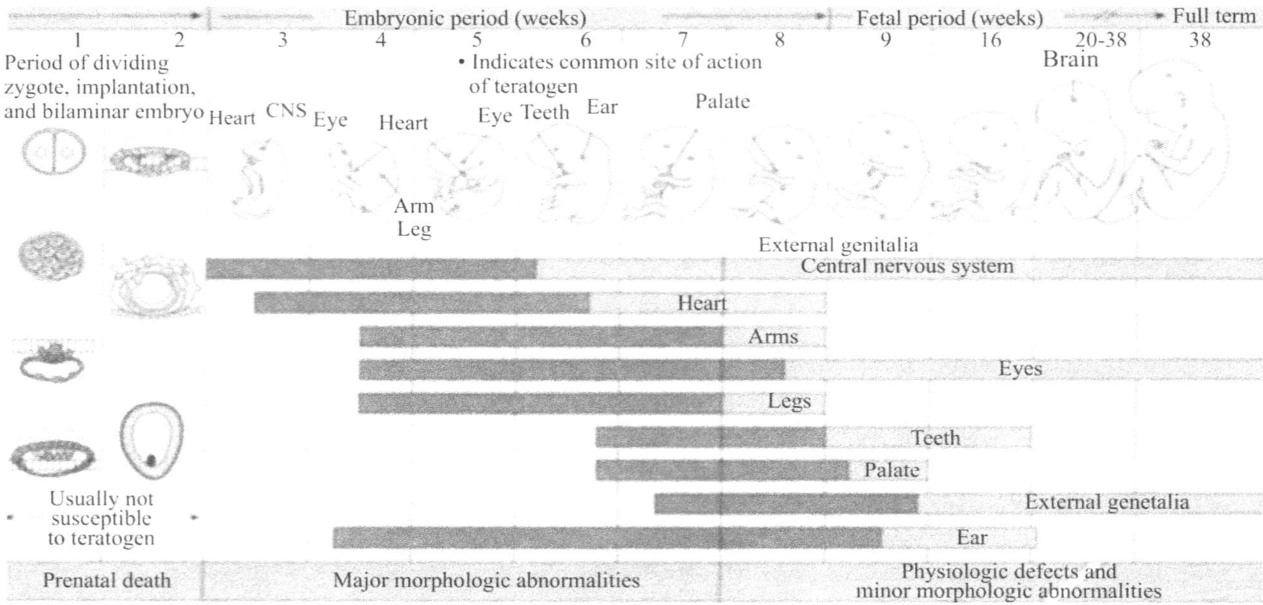

Source: Lange

Fig. 6.2 Various stages of pregnancy

The widely cited Food and Drug Administration (FDA) system for teratogenic potential is an attempt to quantify teratogenic risk from A (safe) to X (definite human teratogenic risk). This system has been criticized as inaccurate and impractical. For example, several drugs have been labeled "X" despite extensive opposite human safety data (e.g., Oral contraceptives). Diazepam and other benzodiazepines are labeled as "D" despite lack of positive evidence of human fetal risk. Presently the FDA is changing its system from the A, B, C grading system to narrative statements that will summarize evidence based knowledge about each drug in terms of fetal risk and safety.

6.4.4 Teratogenic Mechanisms

The mechanisms by which different drugs produce teratogenic effects are poorly understood and are probably multi factorial. For example, drugs may have a direct effect on maternal tissues with secondary or indirect effects on fetal tissues. Drugs may interfere with the passage of oxygen or nutrients through the placenta and therefore have effects on the most rapidly metabolizing tissues of the fetus. Finally, drugs may have important direct actions on the process of differentiation in developing tissues. For example, Vitamin A (retinol) has been shown to have important differentiation – directing actions in normal tissues. Several Vitamin A analogs (isotretinoin, etretinate) are powerful teratogens, suggesting that they alter the normal process of differentiation. Finally, deficiency of a critical substance appears to play a role in some types of abnormalities. For examples, folic acid supplementation during pregnancy appears to reduce the incidence of neural tube defects.

Continued exposure to a teratogen may produce cumulative effects or may affect several organs going through varying stages development. Chronic consumption of high doses of ethanol during pregnancy, particularly during the first and second trimesters may result in the fetal alcohol syndrome. In this syndrome, the central nervous system, growth and facial development may be affected.

6.4.5 Counseling of Women about Teratogenic Risk

Since the thalidomide disaster, medicine has been practiced as if every drug were a potential human teratogen when, in fact fewer than 30 such drugs have been identified, with hundreds of agents proved safe for the unborn. Owing to high levels of anxiety among pregnant women and because half of the pregnancies in North America are unplanned every year many thousands of women need counseling about fetal exposure to drugs, chemical and radiation.

Table 6.1 Drugs with significant teratogenic or other adverse effects on the fetus.

Drug	Trimester	Effect
ACE inhibitors	All, especially second and third	Renal damage
Aminopterin	First	Multiple gross anomalies
Amphetamines	All	Suspected abnormal development patterns, decreased school performance
Androgens	Second, third	Masculinization of female fetus
Antidepressants, Trycyclics	Third	Neonatal withdrawal symptoms have been reported in a few cases with clomipramine, desipramine, and imipramine
Barbiturates	All	Chronic use can lead to neonatal dependence
Busulfan	All	Various congenital malformations; low birth weight
Carbamazepine	First	Neural tube defects
Chlorpropamide	All	Prolonged symptomatic neonatal hypoglycemia
Clomipramine	Third	Neonatal lethargy, hypotonia, cyanosis, hypothermia
Cocaine	All	Increased risk of spontaneous absorption, abruptio placentae, and premature labor; neonatal cerebral infarction, abnormal development, and decreased school performance
Cyclophosphamide	First	Various congenital malformations
Cytarabine	First, second	Various congenital malformations
Diazepam	All	Chronic use may lead to neonatal dependence
Diethylstilbestrol	All	Vaginal adenosis, clear cell vaginal adenocarcinoma
Ethanol	All	Risk of fetal alcohol syndrome and alcohol-related neurodevelopmental defects
Etretinate	All	High risk of multiple congenital malformations
Heroin	All	Chronic use leads to neonatal dependence
Iodide	All	Congenital goiter, hypothyroidism
Isotretinoin	All	Extremely high risk of CNS, face, ear, and other malformations
Lithium	First, third	Ebstein's anomaly, neonatal toxicity after third trimester
Methadone	All	Chronic use may lead to neonatal absrinence

Source: Lange

In the mother risk program in Toronto, thousands of women are counseled every month, and the ability of appropriate counseling to prevent unnecessary abortions has been documented. Clinicians who wish to provide such counsel to pregnant women must ensure that their information is up to date and evidence based and that the woman understands that the baseline teratogenic risk in pregnancy (i.e., the risk of a neonatal abnormal in the absence of any known teratogenic exposure) is about 3%. It is also critical to address the maternal – fetal risks of the untreated condition if a medication is avoided. Recent studies show serious morbidity in women who discontinued selective serotonin reuptake inhibitor for depression in pregnancy.

Table 6.2 Teratogenic risk categories according to FDA.

FDA Teratogenic risk categories	
Category	**Description**
A	Controlled studies in women fail to demonstrate a risk to the fetus in the first trimester (and there is no evidence of a risk in late trimesters), and the possibility of fetal harm appears remote.
B	Either animal-reproduction studies have not demonstrated a fetal risk, but there are no controlled studies in pregnant women, or animal-reproduction studies have shown an adverse effect (other than a decrease in fertility) that was not confirmed in controlled studies in women in the first trimester (and there is no evidence of risk in later trimesters).
C	Either studies in animals have revealed adverse effects on the fetus (teratogenic or embryocidal or other) and there are no controlled studies in women or studies in women and animals are not available. Drugs should be given only if the potential benefit justifies the potential risk to fetus.
D	There is possible evidence of human fetal risk, but the benefits from use in pregnant women may be acceptable despite the risk (e.g., if the drug is needed in a life-threatening situation or for a serious disease for which safer drugs cannot be used or are ineffective).
X	Studies in animals or human beings have demonstrated fetal abnormalities or there is evidence of fetal risk based on human experience or both, and the risk of the use of the drug in pregnant women clearly outweighs any possible benefit. The drug is contraindicated in women who are or may become pregnant.

6.5 ACUTE, SUB ACUTE, CHRONIC TOXICITY STUDIES

6.5.1 Acute Toxicology Testing

Objective of acute toxicity testing

Chemicals sometimes produce toxicity to human and other life forms acute animal studies gives some information, which is essential for determining the potential toxicity of chemical. These chemicals are normally whether commercially available or some available by development. The potential toxicology of chemicals identified by objective of acute studies. The system also implies the short-term tests in animals parallel acute exposure in human population. In general selection animal species, time of chemical exposures, dose of chemical and biological parameters are flexible in acute studies. These tests are preferable to comparison of human situations. The toxic effects correlate with increasing doses. The doses are given by any routes like orally, locally, parenterally or *via* inhalation etc. The potency of toxicants was determined by toxicology studies, the potency of toxicant as correlative dose response relationship.

Acute toxicity test methods measure the adverse effects that occur within a short time after administration of a single dose of a test substrate. This testing is performed principally in rodents and is usually done early in the development of a new chemical or product to provide information of its potential toxicity. Acute toxicity data can help identify the mode of toxic action of a substance and may provide information of doses associated with target-organ toxicity and lethality that can be used in setting dose levels for repeated-dose studies.

This information may also be extrapolated for use in the diagnosis and treatment of toxic reactions in humans.

The results from acute toxicity tests can provide information for comparison of toxicity and dose-response among members of chemical classes and help in the selection of candidate materials for further work. They are further used to standardize certain biological products such as vaccines.

Acute oral testing

Traditionally acute oral toxicity testing has focused on determining the dose that kills half of the animals (i.e., the median lethal dose or LD_{50} values are presented as estimated doses (mg/kg) with confidence limits.

The simplest method for the determination of the LD_{50} is a graphic one and is based on the assumption that the effect is a quantal one (all or none), that the percentage responding in the experimental group is dose related, and the cumulative effect follows a normal distribution.

Organization of studies

The study depends on practical consideration than biological imperatives by considering of all these laboratory animal (may be rats or mice etc.).

Rodents technically easier to handle, and rodent species are more economic to use than other animals, have fewer interspecies variations and also they are readily available and also for rodents housing and caring are more easily and practical than they are for other species. All though this suggests species differences in absorption, distribution, biotransformation or elimination of a toxicant, this information is obtained from mechanistic studies rather than through the performance of additional LD_{50} tests.

Protocols for acquiring and acclimating animals are important to ensure study success. Animals should be purchased form dependable breeders and placed in quarantine area of an animal care facility for 7 to 14 days prior to initiation of an experiment. They are examined at appropriate stages for gross pathology and general health a protocol includes the enthonsia of organs. At the time of purchase animals there is necessary to purchase extra animals, because in screening process necessitates elimination of some animals.

Acute studies should be conducted for 24 hr in rodents and non-rodents. It can be extended to 78 hr. In this acute studies conducted for 96 hr. After the study 7-14 days observation should be needed for survived animals.

Parameters to be mentioned:

Behavioural aspects: Sedation, dropping head, sitting position with head up, depression, restlessness, irritability, aggressiveness, defensive hospitality and confusion.

Sensory aspects: Writhing reflex, sensation to pain corneal reflex sensitivity to sound and touch.

Neuromuscular changes: Tremors, weakness, increase or decrease in activities of muscle tone and convulsions.

Cardiovascular changes: Heart rate, vasoconstriction, dilation, arrhythmias.

Respiration changes: Gaspe, dyspnea, apnea.

Ocular changes: Lacrimation, mydriasis, miosis, alopecia, pilocarpine reflex.

GIT: Diarrhea, constipation, emesis, defecation.

Cutaneous changes: Piloerection, alopecia, arrhythmia, edema swelling necrosis.

Determination of acute lethality

The path by which a dose elicits a particular response is known as the dose-response (or concentration-effect) relationship. The observed response is a calculated observation, assuming that the response is a result of exposure to a chemical and is measured and quantified. The response also depends on the quantity of chemical exposure and administration within given period. Two types of dose-response relationships exist, depending on number of subjects and does tested.

The graded dose-response describes the relationship of test subjects to logarithmic increases in the dose or concentration of the chemical is proportional to the number of surviving subjects in the experimental systems or any other parameter of morbidity.

Quantal dose-response is determined by the distribution of responses to increasing dose in a population of test subjects. This relationship is generally classified as an all-or-none effect and the animals are quantified as either responders or non-responders. A typical graph shows about comparing ED_{50} (median effective dose 50%) to LD_{50}. Because the LD_{50} statistically calculated dose of a chemical that causes death in 50% of the animals tested, it is an example of a typical quantal dose-response curve. The doses administered are continuous or at different levels and the response is generally mortality (although gross injury, or formation, or other measurable criterion is used to determine a standard deviation or out-off value).

Support of the LD_{50} Test.

Continued use of the test has been advocated, however, on the grounds that it is of use in the following ways:

Properly conducted, acute toxicity tests yield not only the LD_{50} but also information on other acute effects such as cause of death, time of death, symptomatology, non-lethal acute effects, organs affected, and reversibility of non lethal effect.

- Information concerning mode of action and metabolism detoxification can be inferred from the slop of mortality curve.
- The results in form the basis for the design of subsequent sub-chronic studies.
- The test is useful as a first approximation of hazards to workers.
- The test is rapidly complete.
- Possible target organ toxicity can be known.
- Duration and intensity of toxic effects can be known.
- Help full for conducting sub-acute and sub-chronic studies.

This data can be applied by health physicians for therapeutic formulations

And staff of emergency treatment units.

6.5.2 Sub-Acute/Sub-Chronic Studies

1. To examine the biological nature of toxic effects from low doses. At cellular level measuring parameters which cannot be usually obtained in acute study, because of the high dose administration and the rapidity of onset of toxicity of signs and symptoms.

2. Variation in species response to repeated exposure to the agent looking for commonality response and distinct species difference.
3. Accesses possible cumulative effects of the repeated exposure to the agents or the biotransformation products of the agents (cell necrosis path also estimated).
4. To determine microscopic and macroscopic organ, tissue damage as it develops depending up on the dose of effects.
5. To identify the approximate dose which causes morphological changes.
6. To predict the long term adverse effects.

Parameters to be monitored

In-life Data. Interim tests are carried out at intervals before the study to establish baselines, at intervals during the study, and at the end of the study.

1. ***Appearance:*** Mortality and morbidity as well as the condition of the skin, mucous membranes, and orifices should be checked at least daily. Presence of palpable masses or external lesions should be noted.
2. ***Eyes:*** Ophthalmologic examination of both cornea and retina should be carried out at the beginning and at the end of the study.
3. ***Food consumption:*** Weekly.
4. ***Body weight:*** Weekly.
5. Behavioural abnormalities.
6. Respiration rate.
7. ECG Particularly with the larger animals.
8. ***Hematology:*** Assessment should be made prior to chemical administration (pretest) and at least prior to termination. Hemoglobin, hematocrit, RBC, WBC, differential counts, platelets, reticulocytes, and plotting parameters should be assessed.
9. ***Blood chemistry:*** Pretest, and at least prior to termination, electrolytes and electrolyte balance, acid-base balance, glucose, urea nitrogen, serum lipids, serum proteins (albumin-globulin ratio). Enzymes indicative of organ damage such as transminases and phosphatases should be measured. Toxicant and metabolite levels should be assessed as needed.
10. Urine analysis, pretest and at least prior to termination, microscopic appearance (sediment, cells, stones, etc.) pH specific gravity, chemical analysis for reducing sugars, proteins, ketones, and bilirubin should be measured. Toxicant and metabolite levels should be assessed as needed.

11. ***Fecal analysis:*** Occult blood, fluid content, and toxicant and metabolite levels should be assessed if needed.

Termination test: Because the number of tissues that may be sampled is large and the number of microscopic methods also large, it is necessary to consider all previous results before carrying out the pathological examination. For example, clinical tests or blood chemistry analyses may implicate a particular target organ that can then be examined in greater detail. These lesions and this method continue until a no effect group is reached. Because pathology is largely a descriptive at the beginning of the study and the same pathologist examine the slides form both treated and control animals. Pathologist is not an agreement on the necessity or the wisdom of coding slides so that the assessor is not aware of hazard in a procedure that depends on subjective evaluation. Other items of most importance are quality control, slide must be prepared. Because each of these may yield many slides to be stained, comparable quality of staining and the accurate correlation of a particular slide with its parent block, tissue, and animal is critical.

Table 6.3 Tissues and organs to be examined histological in chronic and sub-chronic toxicity tests.

Adrenals	Larynx	Salivary gland
Bone and bone marrow	Liver	Sciatic nerve
Brain	Lungs and bronchi	Seminal vessels
Cartilage	Lymph nodes	Skin
Cecum	Mammary glands	Spinal card
Colon	Mandibular lymph node	Spleen
Duodenum	Mesenteric lymph node	Stomach
Esophagus	Nasal cavity	Testis
Gall bladder	Parathyroid	Thymus
Illeium	Pituitary	Uterus
Jejunum	Prostate	
Kidneys	Rectum	

1. ***Necropsy:*** This must be conducted with care to avoid post-mortem damage to the specimens. Tissues are removed weighed, and examined closely for gross lesions, masses, and so on. Tissues are then fixed in buffered formalin for subsequent histological examination.

2. ***Histology:*** The tissues listed in table plus any lesions, masses, or abnormal tissues are embedded, sectioned, and strained for light microscopy. Paraffin embedding and staining with haematoxylin and erosin are the preferred routine methods, but special stains may be used for particular tissues or for more specific examination of certain lesions or cellular changes after their initial localization by more routine methods.

Evaluation of sub-acute and sub-chronic toxicities:

- For evaluation of biological effects.
- Establish dose effect relationship between biochemical, physiological and morphological effects.
- To explore the possible mechanisms for toxic effects of toxicants.
- To know the general impairment of the health.
- Cachexia – loss of body weight.
- Anorexia – loss of appetite.
- Debility – indicate the alteration of normal features of organ.

6.5.3 Chronic Toxicity Tests

Objectives and definition

Chronic exposure is any relative time period for which continuous or repeated exposure beyond the acute phase is required for the same chemical to induce a toxic response.

Objectives of chronic studies are to:

The goals of conducting chronic toxicity studies are similar to those of acute studies, with a few important differences. The objectives that overlap with acute studies include.

1. Determination of the lethal and toxic concentrations of a chemical and its effect on organs and tissues.
2. Identifications of the usual relationship between the administered dose and the altered physiological, biochemical, and morphological changes.
3. Monitoring of animal species variations in response to an agent.

Major differences between chronic studies and acute experiments, however, rarely on frequency, accumulation, and length of exposure to a toxic agent. For instance chronic studies are generally conducted to:

1. Measure or assess the toxic effects of lower, more frequently administered doses of a chemical, thus analyzing for repeated cumulative exposure.
2. Determine cumulative effects of repeated exposure.
3. Examine the toxicological effects of increasing does of chemicals over extended periods.
4. Identify recovery of subjects after removals of the source of exposure.
5. Predict long-term adverse health effects in the species arising from intermittent, repeated, or continuous exposure.

Finally, chronic studies generally complement acute studies assuming that the conditions are structured to enhance the results obtained in acute experiments.

Experimental design

As noted above, chronic often relative terms, especially in relation to the species historically, 2 yr is a typical period for conducting chronic studies in rodents. However , 2 yr does not represent a significant portion of the total life spans of other species such as dogs average life expected 9 to 10 yr or rabbits (5 to 6 yr) Even in rodents sustaining calorie-restricted diets, the 2 year exposure period of significantly less representative of their healthier, longer life spans. In general as the life expectancy of the mammalian species increases the exposure period must be adjusted to mimic a chronic exposure.

Thus it becomes more difficult to assign and extrapolate the chronic time period in a particular species to adequately correlate the results of such a study to human risk assessment. Consequently, the lengths of chronic studies (6 months to 3 yr) are variable and flexible and are determined according to the appropriateness of the objectives of a project.

Selection of dosage levels

Dosage levels for chronic toxicology studies are selected based on existing information available about a chemical from acute studies, known toxicological effects, animal and human epidemiological data knowledge of the species reaction to chemicals of similar classes, and known toxic concentrations of chemicals from similar classes. In addition, *in vitro* data is also recommended and as a method for screening chemicals for *in vivo* studies. Thus familiarity and awareness of dose measured response from a control in an *in vitro* system, values for the chemical aid and investigator in identifying proper does for a chronic *in vivo* study.

Understanding the details of the target end point is also essential for determining dosage levels. As the dosages established in studies whose objectives involve the evaluation of histological or pathological monitoring for toxicity may be different from carcinogenic projects. As with acute studies, an investigator has some flexibility in the selection of dosage levels, usually numbering up to five groups plus a vehicle and/or blank onto. In addition, preliminary experiments with small numbers of animals with repeated dosages are necessary to establish lowest and highest life statistically calculated dose of a chemical that causes death in 50% of the animals tested, it is an example of a typical quantal dose-response effect groups.

Those are then selected based on preliminary range-finding pilot projects. Finally, recognition of the pharmacokinetics of the chemical, if available, contributes to the perditions of its behavior of physiological compartments during the course of a study. Consequently, a pilot study on limited numbers of animals for several weeks supplies the necessary information to commence a full study. It also reduces the chances of altering the parameters during the course of the project such as adjustment of doses, significant changes in the number of animals, or modification of the study parameters to accommolate for excessive mortality or lack of effects.

Duration of studies

During the course of chronic and studies it is important to understand that selection of a termination time period should prevent interpretation of age related changes and pathologies as changes due to chemical induction. Sub-chronic studies are generally 21 to 90 days in duration, depending upon the route of administration and toxicological and points of interest. Time periods for the duration of chronic studies, however, have not been clearly defined.

Traditionally, based on the approximate life spans of rodents, chronic experiments have been designated to continue for the FDA recently suggested that these studies should be reduced to 6 to 18 months, depending on the animal species. This is similar to that seen during the first year. In fact, since age-related mortality and morbidity are uncommon in the early months of chronic experiments, most toxicity observed during this time is causal and dose-dependent.

This approach however may not adequately mimic the level of life time exposure for a rodent. In addition, the susceptibility of an animal to chemical in result increases with age, thus obviating pathological consequences of chemical administration in older animal populations. Consequently, it may be necessary to design separate projects whose objectives focus on detecting age-dependent, toxicant induced pathology. These studies may need to highlight different starting ages for the animals, continuing with exposure for 6 to 12 months. A primary concern, therefore, is that chronic studies are designed according to the expected life spans of the species involved.

CHAPTER 7

POISONS

A poison is defined as any substance which when administered, inhaled or swallowed or applied locally causes deleterious effects on the body. Thus a medicine in a toxic dosc is a poison and a poison in small dose may be a medicine.

Hence, if any substance is administered with the intention to save the life, it is called medicine and if it is given to cause the harm to the body (in large quantity), it is poison.

Laws governing the possession and sale of poison: under following acts the poison can be purchased, stored and sold.

- Poisons Act 1919.
- Drug Act 1940.
- Pharmacy Act 1948.
- Drugs and magic remedies Act 1954.
- Narcotic Drugs and Psychotropic substance Act 1985.

7.1 CLASSIFICATION OF POISONOUS SUBSTANCES

The purpose of poisoning in case of human being may be suicidal, homicidal, stupefying or accidental.

Depending on mechanism of action of poisonous substance these are classified as:

(a) Irritant substances

1. Inorganic
   - Non metallic – Phosphorus, Chlorine, Bromine, Iodine.
   - Metallic – Lead, Mercury, Copper, Zinc, Arsenic, Manganese.

2. Organic
    - Animal origin – Snake, Scorpion, Insects, Cantharides.
    - Vegetable origin – Ergot, Aloe, Capsicum and Caster oil seeds etc.
3. Mechanical - Powdered glass.

(b) Corrosive substances

Strong acids and alkaline, Such as:

- Hydrochloric acid
- Sulphuric acid
- Carbolic acid
- Oxalic acid
- Caustic soda
- Sodium carbonate
- Ammonium carbonate etc.

(c) Neurotic (substance act on CNS)

- **Cerebral poisons:** Opium, Sedative and Hypnotics, Insecticides, Cocaine, Hyoscyamus.
- **Special poisons:** Nuxvomica.
- **Peripheral poisons:** Curare alkaloids, Conium.

(d) Cardiac substances

- Digitals
- Strophanthus
- Aconite
- Tobacco

(e) Pulmonary depressants (lungs)

Gases such as

- Carbon monoxide
- Coal gas

(f) Miscellaneous

- Analgesics
- Anti pyretics
- Stimulants
- Antidepressants
- Antihistamine
- Hallucinogens etc.

Poisoning in human beings is 2 types

(a) Acute poisoning

(b) Chronic poisoning

(a) Acute poisoning: Symptoms appear immediately after the ingestion of poison they increase in severity and may flow death. The poison can be detected in the ingested substances or vomit, stool and urine of victim. The main symptoms are vomiting and diarrhea or convulsions and coma.

(b) Chronic poisoning: The symptoms of chronic poisoning appear gradually, the symptoms may disappear after removal of victim from his surroundings. Poison can be detected in the ingested substance or stool, vomit and urine of victim. The main symptoms are chronic ill health, malaise, repeated attacks of GI irritation and increased cachexia.

Specific chemicals

Air pollutants: Five major substances account for about 98% of air pollution. They are

- Carbon monoxide - 52%
- Sulfur oxides - 14%
- Hydrocarbons - 14%
- Nitrogen oxides - 14%
- Particulate matter - 14%

The sources of these chemicals include transportation, industry, generation of electric power, space heating and refuse disposal.

(i) ***Carbon monoxide(CO):*** It is a colorless, tasteless, odorless and non irritating gas, a byproduct of incomplete combustion. The average concentration of CO in the atmosphere is about 0.1 ppm, in heavy traffic, the concentration may exceed 100 ppm.

Principals' signs of CO intoxication are hypoxia:

- Psychomotor impairment.
- Headache and tightness in temporal area.
- Confusion and loss of visual activity.
- Tachycardia, tachypnea, syncope and coma.

(ii) ***Sulphur dioxide:*** It is colorless, inherent gas generated primarily by the combustion of sulfur-containing fossil fuels.

Clinical effects of SO_2 intoxification:

- Eyes, nose and throat and reflex bronchi construction.

- Asthmatics exposure to SO_2 - results acute asthmatic episode.
- Pulmonary edema observed.

(iii) ***Nitrogen oxides:*** It is brownish irritant gas sometimes associated with fires and also from fresh silage. Exposure of farmers to nitrogen dioxide in confines of silo can lead to silo - fillers disease. Signs and symptoms are nitrogen oxides produces irritation to eyes and nose, cough, mucous or frothy sputum production, dyspnea and chest pain.

(iv) ***Ozone (O_3)***

- It is a bluish irritant gas that occurs normally in the earth's atmosphere, where it is an important absorbent of ultraviolet light.
- In the work place, it can occur around high - voltage electrical equipment and around ozone producing devices used for air and water purification.
- It is also an important oxidant found in polluted urban air.
- Signs and symptoms of O_3 is an irritant of mucous membranes. Mild exposure can cause deep lung irritation, with pulmonary edema when inhaled at sufficient concentration.

7.2 COMMON POISONING AGENTS

(a) Solvent

(i) Halogenated aliphatic hydrocarbons.

(ii) Aromatic hydrocarbons.

(i) Halogenated aliphatic hydrocarbons: It is used as industrial solvents, degreasing agents and cleaning agents.

Example

- Carbon tetra chloride
- Chloroform
- Trichloroethylene
- Tetrachloroethylene
- Trichloroethane

These are carcinogenic to human. They found in ground water and drinking water.

Signs and symptoms: These symptoms are depressants of CNS. Chronic exposure produce

- Impaired memory
- Peripheral neuropathy

- Hepatotoxicity
- Nephrotoxicity

(ii) Aromatic hydro carbons

- Benzene
- Toluene
- Xylene

Benzene

- It is used for solvent properties and intermediate in synthesis of other chemicals.
- Acute toxic effect of benzene is depression of CNS.
- Exposure to 7500 ppm for 30 minutes can be fatal.
- Exposure to concentrations larger than 3000 ppm may cause euphorbia, nausea, locomotors problems and coma.
- Vertigo, drowsiness, headache and nausea may occur at concentration ranging from 250 – 500 ppm.
- Chronic Exposure to benzene – Results very serious toxic effects.
- Aplastic anemia, leukemia, pancytopenia and thrombocytopenia and several leukemias.

Toluene

- It is CNS depressant.
- Symptoms are eye, skin irritant, phototoxic. Exposure to 800 ppm can lead to severe fatigue and toxia, at 1000 ppm can produce loss of consciousness.

Xylene (Dimethylbenzene)

It is also CNS depressants, skin irritant.

(b) Pesticides

(i) Organochlorine pesticides
(ii) Organophosphorus pesticides
(iii) Carbomate pesticides
(iv) Botanical pesticides

(i) Organochlorine pesticides: These agents are usually four groups.

- Chlorophenothane DDT
- Benzene Hexachloride

- Cyclodienes
- Toxophenes

They are aryl, carboxylic or heterocyclic compounds contain substituent. They absorb from skin, inhalation or oral ingestion chronic administration results oncogenesis like brain cancer, testicular cancer, breast cancer etc.

(ii) Organophosphorus pesticides

Azinphos methyl	Fenitrothion
Chlorfenvinphos	Malathion
Diazinon	Parathion
Dimethioate	Trichlorfon etc.

These agents are based on compounds such as soman, sarim and tabum which are developed for use as war gases.

Signs are burning and tingling sensation

- Particularly in feet.
- Sensory and motor difficulty in legs and hands.
- A toxic may be present.
- CNS and ANS change may develop.

(iii) Carbonate pesticides: These compounds inhibit acetylcholine esterase by Carbamoylation of the Esteratic site. They are

Aldicarb	Carbaryl
Aminocarb	Dimension
Carbofuran	Methomyl etc.

The clinical effects due to carbonates are of shorter duration than those observed with organophosphorus compounds.

(iv) Botanical pesticides: These are pesticides derived from natural sources include

- Nicotine – obtained from *Nicotiana tabacum*
- Rotenone – obtained from *Lonchocarpus nicou*
- Pyrethrum – Synthetic.

These are rapidly absorbed from skin.

Nicotine: Absorbed from mucosal surface. Reacts with acetylcholine receptors of post sympathetic membrane [sympathetic, parasympathetic ganglia, neuromuscular junction] results in depolarization of membrane.

Toxic doses cause stimulation rapidly followed by blockade of transmission.

Rotenone: Produce GIT irrigation, conjunctivites, dermatitis, pharyngitis and rhinitis can also occur.

Pyrethrum: Consists of six known insecticidal esters:

Pyrethrin-I	Cinerin-II
Pyrethin-II	Jasmolin-I
Cinerin-I	Jasmolin-II

Pyrethrum pesticides are not highly toxic. But it causes CNS excitation, convulsions and tetanic paralysis.

(c) Herbicides

(i) Chlorophenoxy herbicides.
(ii) Glyphosate.
(iii) Bipyridyl herbicides.

(i) ***Chlorophenoxy herbicides:*** 2,4-dichlorophenoxy acetic acid (2,4-D).

2,4,5-trichlorophenoxy acetic acid (2,4,5-T) and their salts and esters.

2,4-D in large doses cause coma and generalized muscle hypotonic, rarely causes muscle weakness, and also chances to cause Non-Hodgkin's lymphoma.

2,4,5-T is a carcinogen.

(ii) ***Glyphosate (N-phosphonomethyl glycine):*** It is most widely used herbicide. It functions as a contact herbicide and absorbed through the important crops. Glyphosate is significant eye and skin irritant.

(iii) ***Bipyridyl herbicides:*** Best example is paraquat. It accumulates slowly in lungs by an active process and causes lung edema, alveolitis and progressive fibrosis. It probably inhibits superoxide dismutase, resulting in intracellular free radical oxygen toxicity.

(d) Environmental pollutants

(i) Polychlorinated biphenyls
(ii) Endocrine disruptors
(iii) Asbestos

(i) ***Polychlorinated biphenyls (PCBs):*** These compounds have been used in a large variety of applications as transfer fluids, lubricating oils, plasticizers, wax extenders and flame retardants. Unfortunately PCBs persists in environment, chronic exposure may cause Non-Hodgkin's lymphoma and also number of cancers such as soft tissue sarcomas lung cancer.

(ii) ***Endocrine disruption:*** The potential hazardous effects of some chemicals in the environment are receiving considerable attention because of their estrogen like or antiandrogenic properties. Compounds that effect thyroid function are also of concern. These chemicals mimic, enhance or inhibit hormonal action. The appearance of bioaccumulation of these compounds causes toxic effects. These substances cause reproductive cancers.

(iii) ***Asbestos:*** In many of its forms has been widely used in industry for over 100 years. They are causing lung diseases that are characterized by fibrotic process. Cigarette smoking and exposure to random daughters increase the incidence of asbestos caused lung cancer in synergistic fashion.

(e) Metals

(i) Beryllium

(ii) Cadmium

(iii) Arsenic

(iv) Lead

(v) Mercury

- Occupational and environmental poisoning with metals, metalloids and metal compounds is a major health problem.
- Exposure in work place. Classical metal poisons are arsenic, lead and mercury. Occupational exposure and poisoning due to beryllium, cadmium, manganese, uranium.

(i) ***Beryllium (Be):*** Beryllium is a light alkaline metal. One attractive property of beryllium is its non sparkling quality, which makers it useful in such diver is highly toxic by inhalation and produce carcinogenic effect. Inhalation of beryllium cause progressive pulmonary fibrosis and may lead to cancer and also cause skin diseases and chronic granulomatous pulmonary fibrosis.

(ii) ***Cadmium (Cd):*** Cd is a transition metal widely used in industry. Cd is toxic by inhalation or ingestion may cause cadmium fume fever (shaking chills, cough, fever and malaise) and also pneumonia. Chronic exposure of Cd cause progressive pulmonary fibrosis and sever kidney damage.

Table 7.1 Toxicology of selected arsenic, lead, and mercury compounds

Metals	Form entering body	Major route of absorption	Distribution	Major clinical effects	Key aspects of Mechanism	Metabolism and Elimination
Arsenic	Inorganic arsenic salts	Gastrointestinal, respiratory (all mucosal surfaces)	Predominantly soft tissues (highest in liver, kidney). Avidly bound in skin, hair, nails	Cardiovascular, shock, arrhythmias. CNS encephalopathy, peripheral neuropathy. Gastroenteritis, pancytopenia; cancer (many sites)	Inhibits enzymes; interferes with oxidative phosphorylation; alters cell signaling, gene expression	Methylation, Renal (major); sweat and faces (minor)
Lead	Inorganic lead oxides and salts	Gastrointestinal, respiratory	Soft tissues; redistributed to skeleton (> 90% of adult body burden)	CNS deflects; peripheral neuropathy; anemia; nephropathy; hypertension; reproductive toxicity	Inhibits enzymes; interferes with essential cations; alters membrane structure	Renal (major); feces and breast milk (minor)
	Organic (tetraethyl lead)	Skin, gastrointestinal, respiratory	Soft tissues, especially liver, CNS	Encephalopathy	Hepatic dealkylation (fast) → trialkyl metabolites (slow) → dissociation to lead	Urine and feces (major); sweat (minor)
Mercury	Elemental mercury	Respiratory tract	Soft issues, especially kidney, CNS	CNS; tremor, behavioral (erethism); gingivostomatitis; peripheral neuropathy; acrodynia; pneumonitis (high-dose)	Inhibits enzymes, alters membranes	Elemental Hg converted to Hg^{2+}, urine (major); feces (minor)
	Inorganic Hg^{+} (less toxic); Hg^{2+} (more toxic)	Gastrointestinal, skin (minor)	Soft tissue especially kidney	Acute tubular necrosis; gastroenteritis; CNS effects (rare)	Inhibits enzymes; alters membranes	Urine
	Organic alkyl, aryl	Gastrointestinal, skin, respiratory (minor)	Soft tissues	CNS effects, birth detects	Inhibits enzymes; alters microtubules, neuronal structure	Deacylation, Fecal (alkyl, major); urine (Hg^{2+} after deacylation, minor)

7.3 PRINCIPLES OF MANAGEMENT OF ACUTE POISONING, TREATMENT OF POISONING

An understanding of common mechanisms of death due to poisoning can help to prepare the care giver to treat patients effectively. Many toxins depress the CNS, resulting in obtundations or coma. Comatose patients frequently lose their air way protective reflexes and their respiratory drive. They may die as a result of airway obstruction by the may die as a result if airway obstruction by the flaccid tongue, aspiration of gastric contents in to the trachea bronchial tree or respiratory arrest. These are the most common causes of death due to overdose of narcotics and sedative hypnotic drugs (Examples: Barbiturate and Alcohol).

Initial management

Initial management of patient with coma, seizures or any other symptoms is supported by ABCD's of poisoning treatment.

- 1st airway should be cleared of vitamins or any other obstruction oral air way or end tracheal tube inserted, if need.
- Breathing should be assessed by observation and pulse oximetry.
- The circulation should be assessed by continuous monitoring of pulse rate, blood pressure, urinary output and evolution of peripheral perfusions.
- An i.v. line should be placed and blood drawn for serum glucose and other routine determinations. At this point, every patient with alerted mental status should receive a challenge with concentrated dextrose.

The five basic principles of general treatment of poisoning.

(a) To remove unabsorbed poison from the body.

(b) For to use antidote.

(c) To excrete absorbed poison.

(d) To treat the general symptoms of the victim.

(e) To maintain the victims general condition.

History and physical examination: It is also needed history oral statements about the amount and even the type of drug ingested in toxic emergencies may be unreliable.

There is a need to search for any syringes, empty bottles, household products or ever the computer dedicatory in immediate vicinity of possible poisoned patient's premises.

Physical examination: Should be performed, emphasizing those areas most likely to give clues to the toxicology diagnosis. This includes vital signs, eyes and mouth, skin, abdomen and nervous system.

Vital signs

- Blood pressure, pulse, respiration, temperature evolution of vital signs is essential in all toxicological emergencies. Occurrence of hypertension and tachycardia with amphetamines, cocaine, anti muscarinic drug.
- Hypotension and bradycardia are characteristic features of over dose with calcium channel blocker, beta blockers, clonidine, and sedatives, hypnotics.
- Hypotension and tachycardia is common with tricyclic antidepressants, trazodone, quetiapine, vasodilators and beta agonists.
- Hyperthermia may associated with sympathomimetics, salicylates, anti cholinergics.
- Rapid respirations are typical of salicylates, carbon monoxide.
- Hypothermia can be caused by CNS depressants.

Eyes

- Eyes are the valuable toxicological information. Constriction of pupils (miosis) is typical of opioids, clonidine, phenothiazines, choline esterase (example: organophosphate insecticides). Deep coma due to sedative drug.
- Mydriasis is common with amphetamines, cocaine, LSD and atropine and other anticholinergic drugs.
- Horizontal nystagmus is characteristic of intoxication with phenytoin, alcohol, barbiturates.
- The presence of both vertical and horizontal nystagmus is strongly suggestive of phencyclidine poisoning.

Mouth

- The mouth may show signs of burns due to corrosive substances or soot from smoke inhalation.
- Typical odours of alcohol, hydrocarbon solvents or ammonia may be noted.
- Poisoning due to cyanide can be recognized by some examiners as an odor like bitter almonds.

Skin

- The skin often appears flushed, hot and dry in poisoning with atropine and other anti muscarinics.

- Excessive sweating occurs with organophosphates, nicotine and sympathomimetics.
- Cyanosis may be caused by hypoxemia or by methemoglobinemia.

Abdomen

Abdominal examination may reveal, which is typical of poisoning with anti muscarinic, opioid and sedative drugs.

Hyperactive bowel sounds, abdominal cramping and diarrhea are common in poising with organophosphates, iron, arsenic, and theophylline.

Nervous system

A careful neurological examination is essential.

- Focal seizures or motor deficits suggest a structural lesion [intracranial hemorrhage due to trauma] rather than or metabolic encephalopathy.
- Nystagmus, dysarthria, a toxic is typical of phenytoin, carbamazepine, alcohol and sedative intoxication.
- Twitching and muscular hyperactivity are common with atropine and the anti cholinergic agents, cocaine and other sympathomimetic drugs.
- Muscular rigidity can be caused by haloperidol and other antipsychotic agents.
- Generalized hypertonicity of muscles and lower extremity clonus are typical of serotonin syndrome.
- Seizures are often caused by overdose with antidepressants.

Laboratory and imaging procedures

A. Arterial blood gases

- Poor tissue oxygenation due to hypoxia, hypotension or cyanide poisoning will result in metabolic acidosis.
- The PaO_2 measures only oxygen dissolved in the plasma and not total blood oxygen dissolved in the plasma and not total blood oxygen content or hemoglobin saturation and may appear normal in patients with severe carbon monoxide poisoning.
- Pulse oximetry may also give falsely normal results in carbon monoxide intoxication.

B. Electrolytes

- Sodium, potassium, chloride and bicarbonate should be measured; the anion is then calculated by subtracting the measured anions from cations.

- Normally the sum of cations exceeds the sum of the anions by not more than 12 - 16 mEq/lit. A larger than expected anion is calculated by the presence of unmeasured anions (lactate, acetates etc.). Accompanying metabolic acidosis. This may occur with numerous conditions, such as diabetic ketoacidosis, renal failure or shock - induced lactic acidosis includes aspirin, metformin, methanol, ethylene glycol is ionized iron.
- Alteration in serum potassium level is hazardous because they can result in cardiac arrhythmia.
- Drugs that may cause hyperkalemia despite normal renal function include potassium itself, B-blockers, digitals glycosides, potassium sparing diuretics and fluoride.

C. Renal function tests

- Some toxins have direct nephrotoxic effects, renal failure due to shock or myoglobinuria.
- Blood urea nitrogen and creatinine levels should be measured and urinalysis performed.
- Elevated serum creatinine kinase (CK) and myoglobin in urine suggest muscle necrosis due to seizures or muscular rigidity.
- Oxalate crystals in large numbers in the urine, suggest crystals in large numbers in the urine, suggests ethylene glycol poisoning.

Serum osmolality

The calculated serum osmolality is dependent mainly on the serum and glucose and the blood urea nitrogen.

Electrocardiogram

- Widening of the QSR complex duration (to more than 100 mins) is typical of tricyclic antidepressant and quinidine over dose.
- A plain film like imaging finding film of abdomen may be useful because tablets, particularly iron and potassium may be radioopaque.
- Chest radio graphs may reveal aspiration pneumonia, hydrocarbon pneumonia or pulmonary edema.
- When head trauma is suspected a computed tomography (CT) scan is recommended.

Toxicology screening test

It is a common misconception that a broad toxicology "Screening" is the best way to diagnose and manage an acute poisoning. But it is expensive and time consuming. Although screening tests may be helpful in conforming a suspected intoxication or for ruling out intoxication as a cause of apparent brain death, they should not delay needed treatment.

Decontamination

Procedures should be undertaken simultaneously with initial stabilization. Diagnostic assessment and laboratory evaluation. Decontamination involves removing toxin from the skin or gastrointestinal tract.

7.4 GENERAL TREATMENT OF POISONING

When the poison is known, the specific treatment should be given but when poison is unknown, aim of the treatment is to save the life of the victim by maintaining the respiration and circulation or beating of the heart.

The five basic principles of general treatment of poisoning are.

- To remove unabsorbed poison from the body
- To use antidotes
- To excrete absorbed poison
- To treat the general symptoms of the victim
- To maintain the victims general condition

(a) **To remove unabsorbed poison from the body:** Following measures should be taken for the removal of unabsorbed poison entered by different routes.

- ***Poison entered through nose (Inhalation):*** When any toxic gas has been inhaled, the victim should be removed immediately to fresh air. Artificial respiration should be given immediately.
- ***Poison entered through contact with skin, eye or wound:*** Wash out the poison with plain warm water and if specific antidote is available, neutralize it.
- ***Poison entered through injection:*** The unabsorbed poison may be removed by inducing vomiting and washing the stomach (gastric lavage)

Vomiting: Emetics are the agents which produce vomiting. The emesis should not be done if the poisoning is by strychnine, corrosives or in coma condition. The common household emetics are mustard powder (15 gm), Common salt 2- tablespoon, Ipecac 1-2 gm, Ammonium Carbonate 1-2 gm, Zinc Sulphate 1-2 gm in 200 ml water are the emetics. The dose of 6 mg of Apomorphine by s.c. injection followed by 5 -10 mg Naloxone hydrochloride by i.m. or i.v. (to contract the narcotic effects of apomorphine) is widely used emetics. Apomorphine has following advantages:

- Quick onset of action i.e., within 5 min.
- It facilitates gastric lavage.
- It produces reflux of upper intestinal contents into the stomach.

The disadvantage of apomorphine is, it should not be used in depressed patients or in coma condition. Its effect after oral administration is slow.

Vomiting is contained in case of acid or alkali poisoning since it may cause rupture of the stomach.

Gastric lavage (Stomach wash): It is the best method for the removal of unabsorbed poison from the stomach. It is used only up to 4 to 6 hr after ingestion of poison.

Method: The patient should be prone on his side with the head down. This will help in rcspiratory drainage and prevent the material entering the respiratory tract. The stomach tube is a flexible rubber tube about 1.5 meter in length, 12.7 m in diameter. A filter funnel is provided at upper end, the suction bulb to suck the contents and remove any obstruction in the tube. A mouth gage with a central hole at the level of 50 cm from lower end (to avoid biting of tube) of tube is provided. The lower end of the tube is perforated. The lower end is lubricated with liquid paraffin or glycerin and passed through the hole in mouth gape down the esophagus. At the level of mark the tip of tube lies in the stomach. Make sure of it and run about 0.5 lit of plain warm water through funnel which is held above the level of patient's mouth. Then lower the funnel down the level of mouth to allow the gastric contents to be removed out. The process is repeated with warm water or fluid containing specific antidote until the returned fluid is of same colour as the lavage fluid. After lavage, some of antidote may remain in the stomach. To remove it and other poison from intestine sodium sulphate or magnesium sulphate solution should be administrated to cause purgation. Activated charcoal should be given to absorb alkaloidal poison.

(b) **Antidotes:** These are the substances which neutralize the effects of poison. Whenever the poison has been absorbed in the systematic circulation use of only emesis or lavage is not sufficiently. The specific antidote must be administered to counteract the effects of poison. The antibodies are of four types.

(i) ***Physical antidote:*** These are the substances which inhibit the absorption of poison.

Examples: Demulcents such as fats, oils and egg albumin. The demulcents form the coat on the mucous membrane if GIT and thus inhibit the absorption of poison. Fats and oils should not be used as antidote in phosphorus poisoning since phosphorus is soluble in it. Banana is the best antidote for glass poisoning. Charcoal is used to absorb alkaloid poison.

(ii) ***Chemical antidote:*** It is a substance which interacts chemically with poison to form an insoluble precipitate which is non toxic or it oxidizes the poison to its non – toxic form.

(iii) ***Physiological antidote:*** It is a substance which produces the effect opposite to that of the poison without interacting chemically with it.

These are antagonists of poison. Sometimes the antagonism may be incomplete and the antagonists itself may produce the adverse effects. Chelating agents are the substance which produces a form non ionized cyclic complex, called as chelate with cations. The important chelating agents are BAL, EDTA, penicillamine and desferioxamine - B.

1. *BAL (British anti – lewisite) (Dimercaprol):* It is a chelating agent used in the treatment of heavy metal poisoning. The heavy metals have the affinity for thiol (-SH) groups and combine with them in body tissues, displacing the hydrogen and depriving the body from these enzymes whose activities depends on thiol group. If BAL is administered sufficiently in excess amount, the heavy metals react with it and thus protect the enzyme system of the body. The resultant complex formed is stable and excreted without any damage to liver or kidney. BAL is administered in a dose of 3-5 mg/kg. i.m. at the internal of 4 hours for first 2 days, interval of 4-6 hr for additional 2 days and internal of 6 -12 hr for additional 7 days.
2. *EDTA (Ethylene Diamine Tetra Acetate):* It is a chelating agent which has great affinity for the lead. The chelated lead is excreted in the urine. Short courses of treatment are advised to avoid the depletion of metallic ions essential for metabolites.

   Dose: 75 mg/kg 24 hours i.m. or slow i.v. infusion given in 3 to 60 divided doses for 5 days may be repeated for a second course after a minimum of 2 days, each course should not exceed a total of 500 mg/kg.
3. *Penicillamine:* It has a stable SH group which confers the chelating action. It is less toxic than EDTA and can be given orally. It is used in copper, lead and mercury poisoning. It is also can be given orally. It is used in copper, lead and mercury poisoning. It is also used for treatment of Hepatolenticular degeneration (Wilson's disease).

Dose: 100 mg/kg/day (max 1 gm) in divided doses for up to 5days. For long term therapy it should not exceed 40 mg/kg/day.

4. *Desferioxamine:* It is a chelating agent which chelates iron in the stomach and binds the iron in the blood. Thus it is useful both orally and intravenously for avoiding systemic absorption and removing the absorbed iron.

   Dose: Oral 8-12 gm in 40 to 60 ml distilled water i.v. 2 gm in 5% laevous solution.

   [140mg of Desferioxamine can bind about 1 gm of ferrous sulphate 200 mg of iron].

(iv) *Universal antidote:* When the nature of ingested poison is unknown, the universal antidote is used:

- To neutralize the acids
- To absorb the alkaloidal poisons
- To precipitate or chelate the metals, certain glycosides and alkaloids.

Composition of universal antidote:

1. Magnesium oxide - 1 part.
2. Activated charcoal - 2 parts.
3. Tannic acid - 1 part.

The mixture should be given in a dose of 1 table spoon in 200 ml of water once or twice.

(c) To excrete absorbed poison

After 6 hours of ingestion of poison, are emesis and gastric lavage useless, the poison has entered the intestine and hence the following measures should be taken to excrete the poison through urine and seat and faeces.

- Forced Diuresis: Use i.v. chlorothiazide and or mannitol.
- Use of cathartics.
- Use of hot packs: For increase sweating.
- Peritoneal dialysis: For salicylate poisoning in children.
- Haemodialysis: For excretion of Barbiturates, Salicylates, Thiocyanates, Bromides.
- Exchange transfusion is only feasible with small children.

All types of poisons are removed by this technique.

(d) To treat the general symptoms of the victim

When the poison is unknown, the symptoms provide the best clue for treatment.

Symptom	Treatment
Pain	Morphine
Circulation Failure	Cardiac Stimulants
Respiratory Failure	Artificial Respiration
Dehydration	Saline infusion

Addition of glucose and sodium bicarbonate in saline infusion is beneficial for maintaining pH and glucose level in blood.

(e) **To maintain the victims general condition**

In case of unconscious victim, there is maximum danger of upper respiratory infection. To avoid this risk of infection, the prophylactic antibiotics therapy must be given. Also the management of hypothermia is necessary. Intensive supportive treatment and good nursing care is required to maintain the general condition of victim.

7.5 SPECIAL TREATMENT OF POISONING

Insecticide poisoning

Organophosphorus compounds: The compounds of this class include:

(a) ***Alkyl phosphates:*** Hexaethyl Tetraphosphate (HETP), Tetra Ethyl Pyrophosphate (TEPP), Octamethyl Pyrophosphoramide (OMPA) and malathion.

(b) ***Aryl phosphates:*** Parathion and Diazinon

A. Organophosphorus compounds

Symptoms	Fatal Dose	Treatment
Poison first affects the smooth muscles and glands and then vital brain centers.	**HETP:** i.v. , i.m. : 160 mg, oral -350 mg	Decontamination.
Initially headache, malaise, construction of chest with pin point pupils.	**OMPA:** i.v. , i.m. : 80 mg, oral -175 mg	Artificial respiration, positive pressure respiration. Tracheostomy if required
After few hours nausea, vomiting, diarrhea, abdominal cramps, sweating, salivation and muscular twitching.	**TEPP:** i.v. , i.m. : 45 mg oral -100 mg	Antidote therapy: Atropine - 2 mg i.m. or i.v. every 15-30 min to counteract muscarinic effects of Acetyl choline.

Table *Contd...*

Symptoms	Fatal Dose	Treatment
In severe poisoning, pulmonary edema, coma, convulsions and death may result.	**Malathion**: 1 gm **parathion**: HETP: i.v., i.m.: 80 mg oral - 150 mg **Diazinon**: 1 gm orally.	Cholinesterase reactivators therapy.- Pralidoxime chloride, Pralidoxime iodide and pyridine aldoxime methyl chloride (PAM) in a dose of 1-2 gm i.v. for adults. Repeated after 12 hours.

B. Dichloro Diphenyl Trichloroethane (D.D.T)

Symptoms	Fatal Dose	Treatment
Oral route: Salivation, nausea, vomiting and abdominal pain **Contact:** Irritation of eyes, nose, throat, blurred vision, pulmonary edema, dermatitis. Nervous symptoms include hyper irritability, muscle spasms and tremors, convulsions, paralysis of limb muscles, collapse and death due to respiratory failure.	150 to 1000 mg per kg of body weight.	If ingested then material must be removed from G.I.T by lavage and cathartics, fats and oils should be avoided. Adrenaline should not be used. Artificial respiration. If muscular twitching then give barbiturates i.v. diazepam.

C. Endrine

Symptoms	Fatal Dose	Treatment
Vomiting, abdominal pain, convulsions, oozing of white froth form mouth and nostrils, dyspnea, coma respiratory failure and death.	6 gm	Decontamination. Artificial respiration. Barbiturate to control convulsions. 10 ml 10% solution of calcium i,v., for every 6 hours .

D. Naphthalene

Symptoms	Fatal Dose	Treatment
Acute nephritis, hemolytic anemia, jaundice and optic neuritis. After ingestion it causes gastric irritation with nausea, vomiting and abdominal pain. Pains in urethra bladder and kidney. Urine may be brown or black.	Approximately 2 gm	Keep the patient warm. Stomach washes with warm water or saline. Use of magnesium sulphate to clear the bowels. Administer sodium bicarbonate to maintain the urine alkaline which prevents formation of acid hematin crystals.

Table *Contd...*

Symptoms	Fatal Dose	Treatment
Severe poisoning causes liver and kidney damage resulting in convulsions, cyanosis. Coma and death. After inhalation it causes headache it causes headache nausea vomiting, malaise, conjunctivitis, mental confusion and visual disturbance		Blood transfusion may be necessary. Hydrocortisone for haemolysis.

Heavy Metal Poisoning

Symptoms	Fatal Dose	Treatment
1. Arsenic acute poisoning: Wide spreading damage to the capillaries severe gastro enteritis, dysphasia, epigastric and abdominal pain, vomiting, watery or bloody diarrhea, jaundice, muscle cramps. Pale anxious face, sunken eyes, dilated pupils, rapid pulse sighing respiration followed by convulsions, coma and death.	100-200 mg.	Stomach washes with warm water. Freshly precipitated hydrated ferric oxide as antidote which forms harmless ferric arsenate. i.v. sodium thiosulphate 1 gm in 10 ml sterile water every 4 - 6 hours for first day. i.m. Dimercaprol as specific antidote. **Dose:** 3 mg/kg body weight every 3 hours. On third day and then same dose every 12 hours till symptoms disappear. Morphine for controlling pain.
Arsenic chronic poisoning: Peripheral or optic neurotics, diarrhea, conjunctivitis, pigmentation of skin, liver, cirrhosis and dependent of skin, liver, cirrhosis and dependent edema. It also causes palmer and plantar keratosis and carcinomas. A characteristics state of ill health appears. Four stages appear successively.	100 - 200 mg.	Removal of patient from exposure. i.v. Sodium thiosulphate, 1 gm, in 10 ml sterile W.F.I 2-3 times/week for many weeks.
Stage I : Related with nutritional type - anorexia, occasional vomiting diarrhea, easy fatigability.		Dimercaprol. Dose schedules same as cute poisoning.
Stage II: Catarrhal - conjunctivitis, running of eyes, running of nose, sense of fullness of head.		

Table *Contd...*

Symptoms	Fatal Dose	Treatment
Stage III: Skin rash, Hyper keratosis of foot, brittle nails falling of hair		
Stage IV: Related with CNS Convulsions, coma.		
2. Lead acute poisoning: Metallic taste, vomiting, colic pains in abdomen, constipation, black faces, urine suppressed, lead encephalopathy, Head ache loss of vision, hallucination, delirium and convulsion. Acute haemolytic crisis may occur.	500 mg	Stomach wash with 10 % solution of magnesium sulphate followed with plain water. Bowel should be washed at regular intervals. Calcium versenate (EDTA) or penicillamine should be used as antidote.
Chronic poisoning: (plumbism) Facial pallor, lead line 9 bluish- black line on the gums. Anemia with punctate basophilia (presence of dark blue spots in cytoplasm of R.B.C.) constipation paralysis of muscles of wrist: encephalopathy. hypertension, nephritis, menstrual disorders, Abortion General Symptoms: Metallic tase, norexia, dyspepsia, headache, weakness, vertigo drowsiness.		Excretion of lead I.e., deleading by acidosis. Deleading by acidosis - combination of EDTA and BAL is effective. EDTA 3 is mixed with saline and given i.v. drip. BAL - 4 mg Kg body weight ever 4 hours.
3. Mercury acute poisoning:		
The main feature is metallic taste in mouth. The tongue, mouth become, grayish white, nausea, vomit contains white mucus with blood. Cold skin, pale face dilated pupils, shock, renal failure and liver damage.	400 mg	
Chronic poisoning: Multiple neurological disorders such as shyness, irritability, tumors, loss of sleep, hallucinations and insanity. This disorder is also called as "Erythrism". Excessive salivation with metallic taste is peculiar symptoms. Loosening of teeth with painful gums.		Charcoal powder, 3 - 4 tablespoons with water. BAL in usual dose.

Table *Contd…*

Symptoms	Fatal Dose	Treatment
Colitis, anemia, hypertension, renal failure Mercuria lentis - Discolouration of lens of eye due to deposition of mercury.		Removal of patient from exposure. Promoting elimination of mercury by kidneys and bowels. Dimercaprol therapy for chelation For excessive salivation - Dry extract of belladonna 30 mg/3 times a day.
4. Copper acute poisoning: It is not poisonous in metallic state but some salts (e.g., copper sulphate) are poisonous. **Acute poisoning:** Metallic taste with excessive salivation and thirst abdominal pain diarrhea. Vomit: Green or blue. Stools: Brown without blood. Urine: Like ink containing albumin. **Chronic poisoning:** Symptoms are similar to lead poisoning	30 gm of copper sulphate	Same as mercury poisoning stomach wash with I potassium ferrocyanide. Same as for chronic mercury Poisoning.

Barbiturate Poisoning

Symptoms	Fatal Dose	Treatment
Nausea, mental confusion, respiratory depression, drowsiness, deep sleep, hypotension, skin rash, muscle spasm, cyanotic face. Barbitate automatism in few cases (Patient takes more drug automatically forgetting that he has already taken a dose) Alternate contraction and relaxation of the pupil, hypotension. Decreased urine fermentation Death occurs due to respiratory failure.	3-5 gm	1. Gastric lavage with potassium permanganate. 2. Artificial respiration. 3. To elevate B.P. 2.5 mg Metaraminol, i.v., 5% glucose saline i.v. drip. Coramine i.v. 5 ml 25% followed by 10 ml in 15 minutes and then 20 ml every 30 minutes till reflexes return. 4. Forced Diuresis 5. Haemodialysis 6. Enema

Narcotic drugs poisoning

Symptoms

1. **Opium:** The symptoms appear in three different stages.
   - (a) ***Excitement:*** Pleasurable mental excitement with increase in heart – rate.
   - (b) ***Sopor:*** Headache, giddiness, a sense of weight in limbs itching, cyanosis of face and lips and miosis strong tendency for sleep.
   - (c) ***Narcosis:*** Patient enters in deep coma, relaxation of muscles, loss of reflex pinpoint pupils, hypotension, hypothermia frothing from mouth and finally death.
2. **Cocaine:** Euphoria, dysphasia, mydriasis, dry mouth, numbness, heart rate increases, cyanosis, sweating, hallucinations, black tongue, homosexuality, nasal perforations.
3. **Belladonna alkaloids:** (Atropine) Datura, hyoscyamus.

   Dry mouth, bitter taste, dysphagia, abdominal pain, hot dry skin, mydriasis. Diplopia, vomiting, giddiness delirium, fever, vision blurred, heart rate increased with increase in respiration.
4. **Cannabis:** Excitement followed by hallucinates, increased muscular movements, mental confusion. Drowsiness, mydriasis, deep sleep.
5. **Pethidine:** Dry mouth, mydriasis, flush face, tachycardia, hyperthermia, drowsiness coma.

Fatal dose

1. Morphine - 2 gm
2. Hyoscine - 125 mg
3. Charas – 2 gm
4. Ganja – 8 gm
5. Bhang – 0.10 gm per kg body weight
6. Pethidine - 2 gm

Treatment

1. In early stage, stomach wash with tepid water first and then with solution of potassium permanganate.
2. Continue stomach wash till returned water is of pink colour.
3. Clear the intestine by enema.
4. Antagonist therapy 5 – 10 mg Nalorphine, i.v. every 15 minutes till dilation of pupil.
5. Naloxone 0.4 – 0.8 mg i.v. every 15 minutes.
6. For shock 1 litter 5% glucose saline solution.

Gastric lavage is done with $KMnO_4$ or tannic acid. In local application, wash the skin with water.

Artificial respiration or by cardiac stimulant therapy is given.

Medicinal charcoal can also be employed.

1. Stomach washes with 5% tannic acid.
2. Neostigmine – 2.5 mg i.v. every 3 hours. or
3. Physostigmine 1-4 mg every 1 – 2 hr.
4. Sponging for raised body temperature.
5. For excitement – Diazepam 10 mg i.v.
   - Gastric lavage, saline purgatives, i.v. fluid, hypodermic injection of strychnine. Artificial respiration.
   - Gastric lavage, Coramine i.v. symptomatic treatment.

INDEX

1-(3-chlorphenyl) piperazine, 159

19-25 G needle, 56

1K1C hypertension, 198

2,2-diphenyl-1-picryl hydrazyl radical (DPPH), 263

20G needle, 46

21 to 25G needle, 57

22G needle, 54

23G needle, 48

23G/27G needle, 47

25 ml Hamilton syringe, 193

25G needle, 51, 52

26G needle, 54, 56

26-gauge needle, 131

2-dimensional protein electrophoresis, 30

2K2C hypertension, 198

3D structures, 76

[^{3}H] GABA – receptor binding assay, 151

^{3}H pyrilamine, 219, 220

^{3}H-Dihydromorphine, 228

[^{3}H]- Hypoxanthine, 256

3r's, 73

3sub hypoxanthine, 257

4-(methylnitrosamino)-1-(-3-pyridyl)-1-butanone, 272

5-fold serial dilutions, 130

5HT (Serotonin), 164

5-HT, 225

5-HT_2 serotonergic, 160

96 well micro plate, 221

A

Abacavir, 26

Absence seizures, 149

Absorbance-based assay, 19

ACE inhibitors, 208

Acetylcholine, 203, 239

Acetylcholinestrase, 188

Aconitine antagonism, 206

Aconitine, 206

Activated charcoal, 301

Acute lethality, 95, 279

Acute poisoning, 289
Acute toxicity test, 93, 95, 277, 280
Acute, 277
Adenylyl cyclase, 168
Adrenal cortex, 198
Adrenaline, 120
Adrenergic receptor, 120, 160
Adult male wistar rats, 182
Aerosols, 222, 224
Affinity chromatography, 30
AIDS, 70
Air lift fermented culture, 82
Albino guinea pigs (300 gm), 131
Albino mice, 144, 165, 195, 227
Albino rats, 124, 144, 238, 242, 252
Albumin phosphate buffer, 137
Aldosterone, 197, 200
Alexander fleming, 5
Alkyl phosphates, 304
Allergen, 218
Allograft, 70
Allosteric site, 6
Alloxan, 248
Alternatives technique, 74
Alzheimer's disease, 64
Amitriptyline, 164
Ammonium carbonate, 288
Amphetamine, 162, 176, 177, 276, 297
Amphoterician-B, 88
Anaesthesia, 42, 187, 188
Anaesthetic, 42, 52, 93, 108, 119
Anaesthetized cat method, 121
Anaesthetized spleen strips, 184
Analgesics, 225, 288
Analgesiometer, 193
Anaphylactic shock, 141
Anastomosis, 239
Anesthesia, 35, 45, 136, 147, 163, 182, 190, 249
Anesthetic agent, 45, 51, 121
Anesthetics, 189, 209
Angiogram catheter, 211
Angiotensin, 273
Animal care, 16, 33, 35, 36
Animal facilities, 11, 16, 37, 61
Animal husbandry, 36, 39
Animal rooms, 37, 40, 42
Animal welfare act, 33, 58, 93
Anorexia, 283, 306
Anova, 148, 158
Anti androgenic compounds, 255
Anti angina, 141
Anti arrhythmic activity, 201, 206
Anti cholinesterase activity, 186
Anti depressants, 164
Anti diuretic activity, 106, 108
Anti epileptic activity, 148
Anti hypertensive agents, 196
Anti muscarinic agents, 218
Anti nociception, 193
Anti parkinsonism activity, 168

Anti stressor, 262
Anti-aggressive activity, 156
Anti-anxiety test, 156
Antibiotics, 6, 304
Antidote, 265, 296
Antihistamics, 168
Antihypertensive agent's, 7
Antihypertensive, 141, 197
Antileukemic, 141
Antimalarial drugs, 256
Antimicrobial activities, 142
Antipyretics, 225
Antispasmodics, 168
Antitumor agents, 6
Anxiolytic activity, 156
Anxiolytics, 159
Aorta, 197
Aortic cannula, 209
Apocynaceae, 171
Arachidonic Acid (A.A), 231, 233
Aromatize inhibition, 251
Array technology, 20
Arsenic acute poisoning, 306
Arsenic chronic poisoning, 306
Arsenic, 287, 294, 295, 298
Arthritic pain, 225
Artificial media, 78, 79
Artificial respiration, 120, 206, 211, 215, 300, 310
Aryl phosphates, 304
Asbestos, 293, 294
Aspermia, 254
Asthma, 27, 218
Ataxia, 177
Atherosclerosis, 64, 213, 215
Atorvastatin, 246
ATP, 89, 225
Atropine sulphate, 116, 121
Atropine, 176
Attention, 20, 172, 293
Autopsy reports, 158
AV nodal calcium channel
blockers, 203
Azovan blue, 243

B

B cells, 70
Baclofen, 152, 153
Bacterial lip polysaccharide, 230
BAL (British anti – lewisite), 302
BAL fluid examination, 222
Balb/c mice, 222
Barbiturates, 276
Bead-based assay, 19
Beagle dogs, 236
Behavioural aspects, 279
Beige mice, 140
Belladonna alkaloids, 168, 309
Belladonna group, 265
Benzene, 291
Benzodiazepines, 143
Beryllium (Be), 294

Beta – adrenergic receptors, 203
Beta plate reader, 256
Bilirubin, 281
Bimodal fashion, 271
Binocular microscope, 242
Bio availability, 5, 7
Bio technology department, 75
Bioassay of digitalis, 135
Bioassay of vasopressin, 106
Bioassay, 101
Bioavailability, 1
Bioinformatics, 8
Bioisosteres, 8
Biological activity, 5
Biological assay, 101
Bioreactors, 139
Biotransformation, 278, 281
Bipolar disorders, 27
Bipolar sub cortical electrodes, 148
Blood chemistry, 281
Blood collection, 45
Blood pressure recorder, 108
Blood pressure, 120, 182, 206, 212
Blood sample, 14, 44
Blood vessel cannulation, 45
Blotting of cut edge, 255
Bond angles, 76
Bordetella pertussis, 126
Botanical pesticides, 291
Bracket method, 103, 104
Bradycardia, 187, 297
Bradykinesia, 168
Breeding problems, 62
Breeding techniques, 57
Brimonidine, 261
Broccoli, 262
Bronchi, 181
Bronchial alveoli, 222
Budesonide, 218
Buffer solution, 97
Buffer, 152, 175
Bulbar conjunctiva, 258
Butyrophenones, 160

C

Cachexia, 283, 289
Cadmium (Cd), 294
Cages, 37, 40, 144, 194
Camouflage, 142
Cancer metastasis, 70
Cancer pain etc, 225
Candida albicans, 231
Canis familiaris, 141
Cannabis, 309
Cannula, 45, 52, 111, 136, 182, 183, 204, 215
Capillary tube, 51
Carbachol, 122, 123, 189
Carbamazepine, 246
Carbon monoxide, 288, 289
Carbon tetra chloride, 290
Carbonate pesticides, 292

Carcinogen, 293
Carcinogenesis, 71, 268, 270, 271
Carcinogenicity, 10, 94, 272
Cardiac glycosides, 102, 208
Cardiac hyper trophy, 64
Cardiac puncture, 46, 202
Cardiac stimulants, 207
Cardiomyocytes, 86
Cardiomyopathy, 212, 213
Cardiovascular changes, 279
Carotid artery, 52, 120, 187
Carotid sinus denervation, 200
Carrageen, 231
Casein hydrolysate, 126
Catalepsy, 161, 162, 167
Catheterization, 236
CD4+, 69, 70
CD8+ Tells, 70
C_dcl_2, 201
Cell line techniques, 74, 77
Cell patch, 87
Central nervous system, 176, 275
Centrifuge tubes, 151, 184
Centrifuge, 78, 151, 161, 183, 219
Chemical and radiation, 275
Chemical antidote, 302
Chemical method, 102
Chemical stimuli, 225
Chemically defined media, 79
Chemically induced diabetes, 247, 248
Chick embryo fibroblast, 80, 85
Chimney test, 144, 195
Chloramphenicol, 266
Chloride silver curve, 86
Chlorine, 287
Chloroform, 183, 205, 290
Cholesterol-lowering efficacy, 26
Choline, 169
Cholinesterase inhibition, 172
Chromogenic assays, 18
Chromosome absorption, 268
Chronic discases, 22
Chronic pain, 225
Chronic poisoning, 289
Chronic renal failure, 234
Chronic studies, 283, 284
Chronometer, 204, 209, 214
Citric acid, 106
Clamping electrodes, 228
Clinical protocol, 13
Clinical trial, 9, 14, 16
Clinomics, 27
Clonal expansion, 270
Cloning genes, 97
Clorgilene, 164
Clostridium tetani, 132
CNS depressants, 291
CNS stimulants, 176
Coagulation factors, 23
Coal gas, 288
Cocaine, 177, 276, 309

Codeine solution, 224
Cogenic strains, 59
Cognition, 164, 172
Coisogenic strains, 59
Combinatorial chemistry, 5
Comparison, 28, 77, 178
Computed tomography, 299
Concentration, 169
Consomic strains, 60
Continuous cell line, 75, 85
Continuous flow culture, 82
Contractile force, 204, 209
Committee for the purpose of control and Supervision for Experiments on Animals (CPCSEA), 11, 33
Convulsions, 149, 155, 222, 279, 289
Coprophagy, 141
Corneal anesthesia, 190, 192
Corneal electroshock, 154
Coronary Artery Disease (CAD), 213
Coronary outflow, 214
Corticotrophin, 124
Cotton swab, 191, 192
Count per minute, 257
CPCSEA guidelines, 33
Cre – loxp recombination system, 68
Cre – loxp, 69
Cre gene, 68
Criminal procedure code, 58
CROs, 4
Cross over design, 92, 108
Culture plate, 170
Cumulative effects, 275
Curare alkaloids, 288
Cylinder cages, 176
Cysteine, 238
Cytochrome P450, 22
Cytotoxicity, 75, 93

D

DA (Dopamine), 164
d-amphetamine, 162
Dawley rats, 169
Day-night cycle, 167
DDT, 291
De Jalon's solution composition, 122
Decongestants, 238
Decontamination, 300
Delirium, 256, 265, 307
Dental drill, 228
Deoxy Nucleotide Triphosphates, (d ntps), 97
Deoxycorticosterone acetate (DOCA), 200
Deoxyephedrine, 178
Depolarization, 202
Depression in pregnancy, 277
Dermal irritation, 267
Desferioxamine, 303
Desipramine, 164
Dextran coated charcoal, 251
Dextran sulphate, 231
Dextrose saline, 124

Diarrhea, 279, 308
Diazepam, 147, 275, 276
Dibenzazepines, 160
Dichloro Diphenyl Trichloroethane (D.D.T), 305
Diclofenac, 244, 246
Dietary hypertension, 200
Digital counter, 178
Digitalis, 6, 135, 208
Dihydrogen tartrate, 232
Diphtheria vaccine, 133
Disruption of transport proteins, 244
DNA arrays, 29
DNA coding, 96
DNA copy, 97
DNA micro injection, 64
DNA polymerase, 97
DNA sequence, 62, 97, 269
Dodecyl phosphate, 98
Dopamine, 3, 163, 164, 168
Dorsal pedal vein, 45
Dosage levels, 284
Dose response curve, 21, 87, 104, 123, 192, 257
Double knock out (DKO), 67
Drug Act, 287
Drug codeine phosphate, 224
Drug Hypersensitivity Reactions (DHRs), 26
Drug metabolism and pharmacokinetics (DMPK), 27
Drug safety issues, 25
Drugs and magic remedies Act, 287
Dry eye model, 261
D-Tubocurarine, 115
Dulbecco's culture, 170
Dunnett's test, 160
Duodenal ulcers, 239
Duration of studies, 285

E

Eagle's medium, 79, 170
Easy bruising, 245
Ecotoxicology, 267
ED_{50}, 126, 127, 144, 146, 157, 193, 223, 228, 253
Edema, 231, 233, 279, 290
EDTA (Ethylene Diamine Tetra Acetate), 302
EEG, 147
Ejaculation plugs, 157
Electrical amplifier, 216
Electrical function, 208
Electrical stimulation, 121, 183
Electrical stimulator, 121, 153, 183, 185, 209, 215
Electro flow meter, 209
Electrode, 88, 87, 148
Electrolytes, 281, 298
Electromagnetic blood flow meter, 217
Electromagnetic flow meter, 217
Electromagnetic, 214
Electronic cell counter, 221
Electronic device, 143

Electronic properties, 5
Electrophoresis, 28, 30
Elimination, 279
ELISA (Enzyme linked immunosorbent assays), 18, 91
Embryo toxicity, 94
Embryo transfer, 63
Embryonic stem cell, 63
Emergent spermatozoa, 251
Endogenous factors, 230
Endogenous sources, 6
Endogenous, 5
Endothelial growth factor, 79
Endrine, 305
Enzymatic activities, 24
Enzyme activity, 175
Eosinophilia, 222
Eosinophils, 222
Ephedrine, 176, 238
Epicardial ECG electrode, 204
Epigenetic changes, 270
Erythema, 230, 233
Erythrocytes suspension, 257
ES cells, 63
Establish a transgenic strain, 63
Establish safe ambient, 266
Estrogenic receptor, 251
Ethanol, 276
Ethics, 34
Euthanasia, 14, 42, 92
Evan's blue, 243
Exaggerated, 237
Exogenous factors, 230
Exogenous, 5, 62
Experimental animals, 20, 36, 45, 265
Experimental area, 38
Expressional proteomics, 29
Exsanguinated rat, 232
Exsanguinations, 185, 189

F

Facial clonus, 155
FDA, 275, 285
Fecal analysis, 282
Federal and local laws, 33
Felbamate, 238
Female albino rats, 109, 252
Femoral veins, 52
Fertilized eggs, 64
Fetal calf serum, 170
Fetal risk, 277
Fetal structures, 273
FEV_1, 218
Fibrillation, 202, 203, 205
Fibroblast growth factor, 79
Fibroblasts, 94
Filter funnel, 225
Finite cell line, 75, 85
Fluorescence Anisotropy (FA), 19
Fluorescence Intensity Assay (FIA), 19
Fluorescence-based assay, 19

Fluorescent labels, 19
Fluorometer, 78
Food and bedding, 37
Food and Drug Administration (FDA), 275
Forced expiratory volume, 218
Forceps, 144, 190, 195
Forelimbs, 196
Fortified cereals, 263
Four point bioassay, 106
Foxni gene, 69
Fraternal twins, 160
Freezing point, 76
Fresh culture flask, 85
Frog rectus abdominous muscle, 104, 105
Frontal cortex, 162
Frontal writing lever, 118
Functional proteomics, 29
Furosemide, 236

G

GABA ($\tilde{\gamma}$ amino butyric acid), 164
GABA, 6
GABA-mimetic agents, 156
Gallbladder, 140
Galvanized steel window, 242
Ganglionic cholinergic nerves, 186
Gastric incubation, 244
Gastric lavage, 300, 301, 308
Gel electrophoresis, 99
Gene knockout embryonic stem cell lines, 98
Gene therapy, 64, 75
Genetic factors, 197
Genetic models, 160, 163, 212, 247
Genetic polymorphisms, 21
Genetic variations, 22
Genetic, 21
Genetically modified organism (GMO), 28
Genetically semi-defined strains, 59
Genetics of mammals, 57
Genome, 7, 27, 28, 29, 62
Genomics and proteomics, 5, 7
Genomics, 3, 7, 12, 20
Genotoxic agents, 272
Genotoxicity, 10, 272
Genotype, 20
Gestation, 142
GI irritation, 289
Glaucoma, 234, 260
Ganglion cells complex, 261
GLP (Good Laboratory Practices, 10, 11, 61
Glucocorticoids, 200
Glycerin, 132
Goldblatt method, 197, 198
Graft rejection, 70
Graphical method, 109
Grip strength, 144, 193, 195
Grollman hypertension, 199

Growth factors, 79
Growth rate, 85
Guaifenesin, 238
Guide for the care and use of laboratory animals (GUIDE), 58
Guinea pig method, 136
Guinea pig whole brain, 255
Guinea pig, 190, 203, 214, 240
Guinea pig's ileum, 119

H

H. Pylori, 239
H_1 receptor, 123
Haemolymph, 93
Hallocinogenation, 5
Hallucinations, 160
Hallucinogens, 288
Halogenated aliphatic hydrocarbons, 290
Hamilton syringe, 193
Hanging wire, 166
Haplotypes, 99
Harderian glands, 259
Hazardous agents, 36
HCG, 137
Head nodding, 155
Healthy volunteers, 25
Heart problems, 66
Heating pads, 182
Hebb's william, 172
Helper T cells, 69
Hematology, 65, 281
Hemicholinium, 169
Hemocytometer, 78
Hemodynamic data, 217
Hemorrhagic disease, 65
Heparin, 108, 109, 182, 183, 188, 209
Hepatotoxicity, 244, 268, 291
Herbicides, 293
Hereditary disorder, 163
Heroin, 276
Heterogeneity, 152
Heterogeneous assays, 18
Heterozygous mice, 63
HETP, 304
Hexobarbitone, 147
High salt diet, 210
High through put screening, 7, 18
Hind limb rigidity, 171
Hippocampal slices, 149
Histamine hydrochloride, 223
Histamine receptor assay, 219
Histamine, 6
Histology, 283
Histopathological, 252
HMG-CoA reductase, 25
HNO_3 0.1N, 206
Hole board, 143
Hologus recombination, 68
Homogeneous assays, 18
Homogenization, 152
Homogenize, 151
Homogenizer, 161

Homologous recombination (HR), 28
Homozygosis, 59
Horizontal thin metallic wire, 196
Hormones, 79
Horse red cells, 131
Hot plate, 226, 227
Housing and husbandry, 14
Human albumin, 106, 137
Human diploid cells, 86
Human neuroblastoma cells, 170
Humidity control, 38
Humidity, 142
Hyaluronidase, 130
Hybridization, 32
Hydrocarbons, 289
Hydrogen peroxide, 170
Hydrogen sulphite, 224
Hydrolysate, 126
Hygienic operation, 38
Hyoscyamus, 288
Hyperinsulinemia, 201
Hypersensitivity responses, 70
Hypertension, 171, 199
Hyperthermia, 167
Hypertrophic, 213
Hypertrophy, 212
Hypnotics, 146
Hypoglycemic, 113
Hypophagia study, 159
Hypophysectomise, 125
Hypophysectomy, 125
Hypothermia, 167, 297
Hypothesized, 1
Hypovolemia, 45

I

IAEC, 37
IC_{50} value, 176, 221
ICAT – Isotope coded affinity tagging, 31
Ice – cold tris buffer, 219
Ice cold kreb's solution, 169
Identical twins, 160
Identification, 17
IgA, 70
IgG, 70
IgM, 70
IHC assay validation, 4
Imipramine, 164, 165
Immature female albino mice, 253
Immobilization, 244
Immobilized cell system, 80
Immune deficiency, 70
Immuno fluorescence recognizer, 261
In vitro studies, 9
In vivo studies, 9
Inbreed strains, 59
Inbreeding, 201
Incubator, 169
Indian penal code, 58
Indomethacin or diclofenac, 244
Inflammation, 225
Inflammatory drugs, 229

Informatics, 18
Inhalation anaesthesia, 51
Inhalation cages, 222
Inhaled corticosteroids, 218
Inherent gas, 289
Inhibition, 115, 176
Inorganic, 287
Inotropic agents, 208
Insecticide poisoning, 304
Insecticides, 288
Inside out patch, 87
Insomnia, 147
Institutional Animal Ethical Committee (IAEC), 11
Institutional bio safety committee, 37
Insulin, 79
Intelligence, 172
Intensive area, 37
International Organization for Standardization (ISO), 62
Interpolation bioassay, 103, 105
Interpretation, 32
Intoxification, 289
Intraocular pressure, 260
Invasive model, 183
Invasiveness, 92
Investigational new drug application, 13
Involuntary tremors, 168
Iodide, 276, 305
Ion channels, 88
IPG (immobilized pH gradients), 30
IR region, 20
Irritant substances, 287
Ischemia – reperfusion, 240
Ischemia, 214
Islets of langerhans, 246
Isoflurane, 45
Isogenic, 59
Isogenicity, 59
Isolated hepatocytes, 247
Isometric strain gauge, 185
Isoniazid, 155
Isopropanol, 170
Isotonic frontal lever, 119
Isotonic frontal writing lever, 120
Isotonic, 123

J

Jugular Vein, 45, 51, 183, 216, 218

K

Keratinocytes, 94
Keratoacanthoma, 70
Ketamine, 45
Kidney cells, 88
Kidney damage, 294
Knocked out, 28
Knockout animals, 67
Knock-out mice, 57
Kreb's bicarbonate solution, 185
Kreb's solution, 184, 189
Krebs-ringer bicarbonate buffer, 216
Kymograph, 205

L

L- adrenaline dihydrogen tartrate, 232
L type channels, 203
Laboratory animal care, 33
Laboratory animal research, 58
Laboratory animals, 33, 34, 42, 91, 92, 142, 278
Laboratory technique, 86
L-Adrenergic receptor blockers, 108
Lagomorphs, 44
LAL test [Limulus Amebocyte Lysate Test], 93
Langendorff heart preparation, 9, 213, 214
Langendorff ringer solution, 209
Langendorff technique, 203, 204
Lansoprazole, 241
L-ascorbic acid, 125
LD_{50} tests, 279
LD_{50} values, 196, 278
LD_{50}, 127, 146
Lead compounds, 6
Lead II ECG, 206
Lead, 295
Leaky, 70
Left ventricular end diastolic pressure (LVEDP), 212
Leprosy, 70
Lethal complications, 196
Leukocytosis, 48
Levallorphan tartrate, 229
Libido, 254
Libitum, 235
Life span, 142
Li-Fraumeni syndrome, 68
Light-dark model, 158
Limbic areas, 163
Linked Immunosorbent Assay [ELISA], 269
Liposomes, 139
Lipoxygenase inhibitory, 233
Lipschitz test, 234, 235
Lipschitz value, 235
Liquid nitrogen, 126
Liquid scintillation photometry, 151
Liquiscint, 151
Lithiasis, 238
Lithium, 276
Local anaesthetic activity, 189
Local anaesthetic cream, 52
Local anaesthetic, 6, 42, 46
Local jurisdictions, 269
Local Lymph Node Assay (LLNA), 93
Locomotion, 179
Locomotor activity, 158
Log- probity analysis method, 144
Lox P, 68
Luminescence-based assay, 19

M

Macaca mulatta, 141
Malachite, 241

Male albino rats, 108
Male beagle dogs, 248
Male ivanovo rats, 206
Male sprague dawley rats, 159, 169, 193
Male swiss albino mice, 144
Male swiss mice, 146
Male wistar rats, 151, 161, 175, 229, 235, 249
Malignant transformation, 270
Mammalian cancers, 272
Mammalian organ bath, 123
Manganese, 287
Marginal ear vein/artery, 46, 54
Marine species, 91
Mass analyzer, 31
Mass spectrometry, 32
MAT test [Monocyte Activation Test], 93
Matching method, 103
Materia medica, 139
Maternal aggression, 157
Maximal electroshock seizures, 153
Maximum collection volume, 53
mCPP, 159
Mean responses, 106
Medicine, 287
Memory, 172
Mepirizole, 240
Mepyramine, 220
Mercury acute poisoning, 307
Mercury monometer, 121
Mercury swivel, 148
Mercury, 287, 295
Mesentery of ileum, 123
Metabolic acidosis, 299
Metabolic cages, 106
Metal rod, 171
Metallic taste, 308
Methanol, 263
Methohexital sodium, 215
Methyl phenidate, 176
Methyl xanthenes drugs, 218
Methylene blue, 261
Mice, 261
Micro meter, 86
Micro organisms, 91, 101
Micro plate assays, 7
Micro plate reader, 170
Micro-array technology, 7, 32
Microbead-induced, 260
Microbeads, 261
Microbiology laboratory, 78
Micropipette, 88, 150
Microscopy, 283
Microsomal enzyme inhibitors, 147
Microsphere, 211
Microtiter plate, 241
Mineralocorticoid, 200
Minimum inhibitory concentration (MIC), 258
Mobility, 267

Moclobemide, 164
Molecular modelling, 8, 76
Molecular-scale, 95
Monkey kidney cells, 86
Monoclonal antibodies, 85
Monogenic models, 247
Monolayer culture, 80
Morbidity, 196, 280
Morphine, 6, 265
Morphological criterion, 258
Morris method, 173
Morris water maze test, 172
Motility, 181
Motivation, 172
Motor coordination, 146
MP – Multiplexed proteomics, 31
Multi surface culture, 81
Mus musculus, 140
Muscarinic receptor, 186
Muscimol, 152
Muscle attachments, 258
Muscle relaxants, 193, 196
Mutagenesis, 98, 269
Mutagenicity test, 94
Mutant strains, 57
Mutations, 22
Mydriasis, 297, 309
Myocardial infarction, 202
Myocardium, 210
Myoclonic seizures, 149
Myofibrillar organization, 213
Myopathy, 25
Myosin heavy chain isoform, 210

N

N^1 Tetramethyl-P-phenylenediamine dichloride, 232
NaCl solution, 210
Naloxone, 309
Nanoparticles, 139
Nanosensors, 139
Nanotoxicity, 269
Naphthalene, 305
Narcotic drugs and psychotropic substance, 287
Narcotic drugs poisoning, 309
Narcotics, 296
National Institutes of Health (NIH), 45
Natural androgens, 255
Natural media, 78
NE (Nor epinephrine), 164
Nebulizer, 223
Necropsy, 282
Needle size, 53
Needle, 193
Neogenesis, 247
Neonatal STZ, 247
Neostigmine, 310
Nephrectomy, 200
Nephritic syndrome, 234
Nephritis, 266
Nephrotic syndrome, 234

Nephrotoxicity, 291
Neural tube defects, 275
Neurocognitive delay, 273
Neuroleptic drugs, 160
Neuroleptics, 160
Neurophysiology, 58
Neuroprotective agent, 170
Neuroprotective efficacy, 168, 170
Neurosteroids, 152
Neurotoxicity, 168
Neutrophils, 222
New drug discovery, 16
New zealand albino rabbits, 192
New zealand white rabbits, 205
Newman-keuls test, 160
Nicotine, 292
Nicotinic receptor, 117, 186
Nitrocellulose ligands, 88
Nitrogen oxides, 289
NK cells, 70
NMRI strain, 180
Noise control, 38
Nomifensine, 169
Non homologous and joining (NHJ), 28
Non-isogenic, 59
Nonrodents, 44, 140
Nootropics, 172
Noradrenalin, 186
Normal saline, 188
Northern blotting, 98
Nose-poking, 180
Nostrils, 192
Nucleic acids, 98
Nucleoside analogue reverse-transcriptase inhibitor, 26
Nude mice, 69, 140
Nude mouse, 71
Nutritional stabilization, 36
Nuxvomica, 288
NZW, 259

O

Ocular hypertensive mouse model, 260
Office of Laboratory Animal Welfare (OLAW), 59
Oligospermia, 254
Omeprazole, 241
Ophthalmic anaesthetic agent, 50
Opium, 309
Orbital sinus, 45, 46
Organ bath, 118, 122, 184, 189, 209
Organ bath, frontal writing, 118
Organ toxicity, 268, 278
Organic, 288
Organization for Economic Co-operation and Development (OECD), 62
Organization of Economic Cooperation & Development (OECD), 11
Organochlorine pesticides, 291
Organophosphates, 298

Organophosphorus pesticides, 292
Oryctolagus cuniculus, 141
Osmatic diueresis, 237
Osmolality, 80
Ouabain, 209
Out side out patch, 87
Ovalbumin, 222
Oxalic acid, 288
Oxotremorine, 201
Oxygen, 80
Oxygenated ringers solution, 204
Oxytocin, 109

P

P^{53} Knockout mice, 68
Palpation, 254
Palpebral rim, 258
Papillary muscle, 210
Paraffin, 184
Parallelism, 132
Parasitemia, 257
Parasympatholytic activity, 189
Parasympathomimetic activity, 189
Parasympathomimetics, 186
Pargyline chloride, 169
Parkinson's and cancers, 262
Partial seizures, 149
Particulate matter, 289
Partition coefficient, 5
Patch clamp technique, 74, 75
Pathogenesis, 242
Pathology, 103
PDGF – Platelet Derived Growth Factor, 79
PDGF, 79
Pelvic girdle, 193
Penicillamine, 302
Penicillin, 6, 141, 155
Penicillin, isoniazid, 155
Pentobarbitone sodium, 121, 216, 217
Pentylenetetrazole, 155, 176
Peripheral vein, 207
Peristalsis in G.I.T., 181
Peritoneal mast cells, 232
Personal hygiene, 36
Personalized medicine, 20
Perspex chamber, 150
Pertussis vaccine, 126
Pesticides, 291
Pethidine, 309
Petridish, 119, 123
P-glycoprotein, 24
Pharmacodynamic, 142, 268
Pharmacogenomics, 8, 25, 27
Pharmacokinetic, 142
Pharmacological profile, 11
Pharmacy act, 287
Phencyclidine poisoning, 297
Phencyclidine, 161
Phenobarbital anesthesia, 249
Phenol, 137
Phenoxybenzamine, 109
Phentolamine, 162, 184

Phosphate buffer, 188
Phosphoric acid, 125
Photocell equipped zone, 158
Photocell, 179, 180
PHS policy, 15
Physical examination, 297
Physicochemical properties of culture media, 80
Physicochemical, 5
Physiological antidote, 302
Pigs (gastric mucosa), 241
Pigeon method, 136
Pin prick, 191
Pipette, 119, 123
Plague vaccine, 127
Plaque, 213
Plasma exudation, 233
Plasma Renin Activity (PRA), 198
Plasmodium falciparum, 256
Plastic catheter, 236
Plexiglas perfusion apparatus, 204
Plexiglass cage, 180
Plexiglass shaft, 165, 166
Plexiglass water tank, 165
Ploidy, 85
Pluripotent embryonic stem cells, 63
Poison, 287
Poisons act, 287
Poly graph, 204
Polychlorinated biphenyls (PCBs), 293
Polyethylene catheter, 182, 183
Polymerase Chain Reaction (PCR), 97
Polymorphisms, 22
Polythene catheters, 188
Post marketing studies, 15
Posterior vena cava, 46, 57
Postganglionic, 186
Potassium channel, 89
Potency, 101
Potter-Elvehjem homogenizer, 175
Pravastatin, 25
Prazosin, 162
Preclinical studies, 9
Preclinical testing’s, 268
Preclinical tests, 11
Preganglionic, 186
Prevention of cruelty to animals act, 58
Primary culture, 77
Primary tumor location, 271
Progesterone receptor, 251
Pronuclear method, 63
Prostaglandins (PG), 79, 225
Protein free media, 79
Protein-protein interactions, 29
Proteins C, 23
Proteomics, 3, 7, 12, 20, 29
Protocol design, 13
Protocol, 12, 34, 279
Proximal tubule, 89
Psychosis, 171

Ptosis test, 176
Ptosis, 167
Public Health Service (PHS) Policy, 33
Purification, 17
Purine salvage, 256
Pyrex glass cylinder, 144, 195
Pyridoxine, 233

Q

QRS complex, 202
Quadra pole knockouts (QKO), 67
Qualitative bioassay, 103
Quantities bioassay, 103
Quarantine, 36

R

Rabbit head – drop method, 116
Rabbit, 185, 228
Rabies vaccine, 128
Radio activity, 184, 221
Radio Immune Assay (RIA), 18
Radio ligand, 162
Rat Ileum, 119
Rat tail cuff, 10
Rational drugs design, 2
Rattus norvegicus, 140
Rauwolfia serpentina, 160
Rauwolfia serpentine, 171
Reactors, 63
Recombinant DNA, 65
Recombinant-Cogenic strains, 60
Recombinant-Cogenic, 60
Record keeping, 41
Rectal body temperature, 167
Rectus abdomen's muscle, 117
Referred pain, 225
Refinement, 73
Remobilization, 212
Renal arteries, 198
Renal function tests, 299
Renal parenchyma, 199
Renin Angiotensin-Aldosterone System (RAAS), 197
Renovascular hypertension, 198
Repolarization, 202
Reserpine, 167, 171, 177
Respiration changes, 279
Retinal regeneration, 66
Retrovirus mediated gene transfer, 63
Reverse-transcriptase inhibitor, 26
RIA's Radio Immuno Assay, 269
Rifampcin, 246
Rigidity, 168
Ringer solution composition, 122
Ringer solution, 115, 204, 205, 209
Rodents, 44, 140, 284
Roller bottle, 81
Rotarod apparatus, 194
Rotarod, 143, 146
Rotenone, 293

Roux bottle, 81
Runway test, 176

S

Sacrificed, 110
Saline, 193, 200
Saliva solution, 210
Salivation, 304
Salmonella, 128
Saluretic, 234, 236
Sandauswurf, 176
Sanitation and cleanliness, 40
Sanitizing equipment, 38
Saphenous vein, 45
Sarcoplasmic reticulum calcium pump, 210
Scanning electron microscopy, 262
Schizophrenia, 3, 163
Scintillation counter, 183
Scintillation vials, 229
Scintillation, 221
Scleral injection, 259
Screening techniques, 139
Second dimension separation (SDS), 30
Secretagogues, 241
Sedative and hypnotics, 288
Sedative drugs, 196
Sedative hypnotic drugs, 296
Sedatives, 143
Seizures, 296
Self-regulation, 35
Sensory aspects, 279
Separation, 36
Serendipity, 5
Serology, 57
Serotonergic pathway, 166
Serotonin, 3
Serum containing media, 79
Serum free media, 79
Serum Glutamate Oxaloacetate Transaminase, 246
Serum lipids, 281
Serum osmolality, 299
SH – SY5Y cells, 170
Simvastatin, 25
Single Nucleotide Polymorphism (SNP), 8, 23
Skeletal muscles, 187
Skin irritant, 291
Small forceps, 190
Small steel hook, 214
Social environment, 39
Sodium bicarbonate, 304
Sodium channels, 89, 202
Sodium chloride, 134, 200
Soft-Pac module, 175
Somatic pain, 225
SOPs (Standard Operating Procedures/guidelines), 41
Sound-attenuating box, 179
Southern blotting, 98
Special laboratories, 37

Species, 35
Spectrophotometer, 185
Speed, 179
Spinal anesthesia, 190
Spinal cord, 216
Spleen capsule, 181
Spontaneous hypertension, 141
Sprague Dawley rats, 188, 210
Squamous carcinoma, 70
Stage carcinogenesis process, 270
Staphylococci, 131
Statistical design, 92
Statistical methods, 12
Stereo chemical properties, 5
Stereotoxic instrument, 163
Stereotype activity, 163
Stereotypic sniffing, 155
Sterilization areas, 37
Stevens Johnson syndrome (SJS), 26
Stimulants, 288
Stirred suspension culture flow, 82
Stock solution, 263
Streptococci, 131
Streptomycin, 266
Striatal slices, 168
Structural proteomics, 29
Strychnine, 176
STZ, 249
Sub acute, 277
Sub culture, 77
Sub strain, 12
Substance P, 225
Substantia Nigra Compacta (SNC), 163
Sucrose, 151
Sulfur oxides, 289
Sulphuric acid, 288
Super fusion chamber, 169
Superior mesenteric veins, 184
Surgical blade, 52, 57
Suspension culture, 80
Swiss albino mice, 143, 147, 156, 167
Symmetrical Y shaped runway, 177
Sympathomimetics, 181
Synaptosomes, 168
Syrian Hamster Embryo (SHE), 94
Syrian hamster, 209

T

Tachycardia, 216, 297, 309
Tail cuffs, 182
Tail flick assay, 193
Tail snip, 45, 49
Tail suspension, 164
Tail vein, 45, 147
Target identification, 3
Target validation, 4
Tarsal vein, 46, 54
Teflon coated steel wires, 148
Temperature detector, 167
Temperature, 38, 80
Temporary cannula, 45

Teratogenesis, 268
Teratogenic risk, 277
Teratogenicity, 10
Termination test, 282
Test or standard, 194
Test-article effects, 259
Tetanus antitoxin, 132
Tetra Chlorodibenzo Digoxin and Phenobarbital, 271
Tetracycline, 6
Tgfβ – Tissue Growth Factor, 79
Thalidomide, 273
The minimum inhibitory concentration (MIC), 258
Theophylline, 218, 249
Therapeutic confirmation, 15
Therapeutic exploration, 15
Thiobarbituric acid, 245
Thiol ester, 188
Thiomersol, 137
Thiopental, 228
Thiopurine methyltransferase (TPMT), 24
Thioxanthenes, 160
Thoracic cage, 214
Thoracotomy, 56, 210, 212
Three – point method, 124
Three point bioassay, 105
Threshold models, 153
Tiotidine binding, 240
Tissue chopper, 169
Tissue culture, 74
Tissue extracts, 79
Tissue slices, 74
Tobacco, 288
Toluene, 291
Tonic – clonic, 149
Topical anesthetics, 190
Topiramate, 238
Torsion angles, 76
Toxicity studies, 9
Toxicogenomics, 27
Toxicologist, 266
Toxicology, 21, 265
Trachea, 181, 189
Tracheostomy tube, 188
Traditional approach, 22
Traditional drug discovery research, 16
Traditional therapy, 208
Traditional toxicology, 267
Tranquilizers, 42, 93
Transforming ES cells in culture, 63
Transgenic animals, 62
Transgenic cells, 90
Transgenic fish, 66
Transgenic mice line, 68
Transgenic microbes, 65
Transgenic pigs, 66
Transgenic techniques, 75
Transgenic, 57, 62, 208
Transilluminations, 254
Transplantation, 65

Trans-species carcinogens, 272
Tranylcypromine, 164
Traumatic antigen challenge, 230
Tremors, 279, 305
Trimming, 259
Triple Knockout (TKO), 67
Tris HCL buffer, 162, 220
Tris maleate buffer, 151
Tris–HCl buffer, 162
Triton x-100, 233
Trypsin, 221
Tuberculosis, 27, 141
Tumor promoters, 271
Tumorogenicity, 70
Tuohy borst adaptor, 249
Twin cross over test, 114
Typhimurium cultures, 91
Tyrode solution, 119, 120, 123

U

Ulcer protective, 240
Ulcerative lesions, 243
Ultra high throughput screening, 18
Ultrasound nebulizer, 222
Unilateral nephrectomy, 199
Universal antidote, 303
Ureter glomerular, 237
Urethane, 45, 206
Uricosuric compounds, 237
Urination, 187
Urine analysis, 281
Urolithiasis, 237, 238
U-shaped silver ribbon clip, 198
Uterus uterotrophy, 253
UV light, 99

V

Vaccine, 126, 134
Vagal nerves, 141
Vagotomy, 200
Vasoconstrictors, 192
Vasodilators, 56
Vegetable origin, 288
Venoms and toxins, 7
Venous cannula, 111, 112
Ventricle strip, 185
Vertebral column, 193
Veterinary care, 35, 36
Victim, 289, 300
Vinyl tubing, 182
Viral infection, 161
Virgin fcmalc, 122
Visceral pain, 225
Vital signs, 297
Vitamin A (retinol), 275
Vitamin K, 23
Vitreous-to-globe area, 260
Voltage clamp studies, 76, 90
Voltage gated ion channels, 87

W

Warfarin, 23
Warm copper plate, 111, 112

Warm paraffin, 183
Warming chamber, 52
Washing, 18, 37
Waste disposal, 41
Water container, 166
Water wheel, 164
Whatman GF/B filters, 229
Wheezing, 218
Whole board, 143
Whole cell patch, 87
Wild life protection act, 58
Wild terrestrial animals, 267
Wire cages, 162
Wire mesh at bottom, 235
Wistar or Sprague Dawley rat, 248
Wistar rats, 162, 177, 193, 244
Woolen box, 171
World health organization, 133

X

Xanthine, 176
Xenografts, 70
X-ray crystallography, 77
Xylazine, 45

Y

Y-maze, 174
Yohimbine, 156

www.ingramcontent.com/pod-product-compliance
Ingram Content Group UK Ltd.
Pitfield, Milton Keynes, MK11 3LW, UK
UKHW061534190726
13845UKWH00005B/94

9 789385 433818